Workbook to Accompany

CLINICAL MEDICAL ASSISTING:

A Professional, Field Smart Approach to the Workplace

Workbook to Accompany

CLINICAL MEDICAL ASSISTING:
A Professional, Field Smart
Approach to the Workplace

Prepared by:

Michelle E. Heller, CMA (AAMA), RMA

Melinda Parker

Lynette M. Veach, MLT (ASCP)

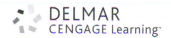
DELMAR
CENGAGE Learning™

Detroit • New York • San Francisco • New Haven, Conn • Waterville, Maine • London

DELMAR
CENGAGE Learning™

Workbook to Accompany Clinical Medical
Assisting: A Professional, Field Smart
Approach to the Workplace
Michelle E. Heller, Lynette M. Veach

Vice President, Career and Professional
  Editorial: Dave Garza

Director of Learning Solutions: Matthew Kane

Senior Acquisitions Editor: Rhonda Dearborn

Managing Editor: Marah Bellegarde

Senior Product Manager: Sarah Prime

Editorial Assistant: Chiara Astriab

Vice President, Career and Professional
  Marketing: Jennifer McAvey

Executive Marketing Manager:
  Wendy E. Mapstone

Marketing Manager: Nancy Bradshaw

Marketing Coordinator: Erica Ropitzky

Production Director: Carolyn Miller

Senior Content Project Manager:
  Stacey Lamodi

Senior Art Director: Jack Pendleton

Senior Technology Product Manager:
  Mary Colleen Liburdi

Technology Project Manager: Ben Knapp

For product information and technology assistance, contact us at
Cengage Learning Customer & Sales Support,
1-800-354-9706

For permission to use material from this text or product,
submit all requests online at **www.cengage.com/permissions**
Further permissions questions can be emailed to
permissionrequest@cengage.com

Library of Congress Control Number: 2007940733
ISBN-13: 978-1-4018-2720-5
ISBN-10: 1-4018-2720-9

Delmar
5 Maxwell Drive
Clifton Park, NY 12065-2919
USA

Cengage Learning is a leading provider of customized learning solutions
with office locations around the globe, including Singapore, the United
Kingdom, Australia, Mexico, Brazil, and Japan. Locate your local office at:
international.cengage.com/region.

Cengage Learning products are represented in Canada by
Nelson Education, Ltd.

To learn more about Delmar, visit **www.cengage.com/delmar**.
Purchase any of our products at your local college store or at our
preferred online store **www.ichapters.com**.

Notice to the Reader
Publisher does not warrant or guarantee any of the products described
herein or perform any independent analysis in connection with any of
the product information contained herein. Publisher does not assume,
and expressly disclaims, any obligation to obtain and include information
other than that provided to it by the manufacturer. The reader is expressly
warned to consider and adopt all safety precautions that might be indicated
by the activities described herein and to avoid all potential hazards. By
following the instructions contained herein, the reader willingly assumes
all risks in connection with such instructions. The publisher makes no
representations or warranties of any kind, including but not limited to, the
warranties of fitness for particular purpose or merchantability, nor are any
such representations implied with respect to the material set forth herein,
and the publisher takes no responsibility with respect to such material. The
publisher shall not be liable for any special, consequential, or exemplary
damages resulting, in whole or part, from the readers' use of, or reliance
upon, this material.

Printed in the United States
1 2 3 4 5 XX 10 09 08

CONTENTS

Chapter Assignment Sheets

C H A P T E R **1**

Journey to Professionalism

FIELD RELEVANCY AND BENEFITS

The health care industry represents some of the oldest and most respected medical professions in the world. And even though procedures have changed dramatically throughout the years, the ethical standards that shape its members remain constant. To be a successful member of the health care community, you must understand the mindset that is necessary to perform the types of duties that health care professionals perform.

You may have the best technical skills in your class, but if you lack professional skills you may never obtain an opportunity to use your technical skills.

This chapter will take you on a professional journey and provide you with a list of character qualities that are essential to succeed and flourish in the field of medical assisting.

NOTE SHEET

Professionalism and the Clinical Medical Assistant

_____

_____

_____

_____

Developing Your Professional Persona

_____

_____

_____

VOCABULARY REVIEW
Assignment 1-1: Matching
Match the term with its definition and place the corresponding letter in the blank.

____ 1. Empathy

____ 2. Initiative

____ 3. Compassion

____ 4. Attitude

____ 5. Tact

____ 6. Professionalism

____ 7. Dependability

____ 8. Appearance

____ 9. Service

____ 10. Integrity

A. To be reliable, dependable, or trustworthy

B. The conduct, aims, or qualities that characterize or mark a professional or a professional person

C. Having the ability to put yourself in another person's shoes

D. To possess character

E. To show concern and empathy

F. To extend help to others

G. A character trait; sensitive to what is appropriate and suitable when dealing with other individuals

H. To take the lead or to work independently

I. The way you feel about someone or something

J. The patient's initial impression about you as a professional

Assignment 1-2: Vocabulary Builder
Find the words below that are misspelled; circle them and then correctly spell them in the spaces provided. Then replace the highlighted words in the following sentences with the correct vocabulary terms from the list.

Appearance	Certification	Confidantiality
Attitude	Compassion	Credantialing
Dependebility	Integrity	Service
Education	Licencing	Tact
Impathy	Profesionalism	
Initiative	Registration	

_____   _____   _____

_____   _____   _____

In the development of professionalism, there are important traits or characteristics the medical assistant must evaluate in order to succeed in the profession. (1) Your _____ helps mold your personality and is the way you feel about someone or something. (2) _____ is one of the most important keys to possess as a professional; it means that you are reliable and dependable. (3) _____ is a character trait that you exhibit when you are sensitive to what is appropriate and suitable when dealing with other individuals. (4) _____ is what the patient bases his or her initial impression about you as a professional.

In the medical office, it is important to ensure patient (5) _____ at all times in order to protect the patient's private information. Truthfulness, honesty, and honor are all qualities of a person who possesses (6) _____.

As you become more seasoned in the field of medical assisting, you will be able to take more (7) _____, working independently and using observation and listening skills to expedite this process. The more you know, the better you can serve your employer and patients, so (8) _____ shouldn't stop at the time of graduation. You should continue this process through educational workshops and seminars and staying active in your professional organizations. Extending help to others is an example of providing (9) _____. (10) _____ demonstrates to your patients and supervisors that you are worthy to be working in the capacity in which you have been entrusted. Types of credentialing include: (11) _____, which is a *legal document* that permits or authorizes you to perform specific tasks. (12) _____ signifies that you have fulfilled the necessary requirements of a specific organization to perform specific tasks, usually through formal testing. (13) _____ means to enroll your name in a register, based on successful completion of a specific program and/or passing an examination designed specifically for that particular specialty.

CHAPTER REVIEW

Assignment 1-3: Acronym Review

Write what each of the following acronyms stands for.

1. ABHES: _____
2. AAMA: _____
3. AMT: _____
4. ARMA: _____
5. CMA (AAMA): _____
6. CAAHEP: _____
7. NCCT: _____
8. RMA: _____

Assignment 1-4: Short Answer

1. List five factors that may contribute to some patients holding clinical personnel to a higher degree of professionalism than those working in administrative settings.

   A. _____
   _____

   B. _____
   _____

   C. _____
   _____

   D. _____
   _____

   E. _____
   _____

2. List four organizations that credential medical assistants.

   A. _____
   B. _____
   C. _____
   D. _____

3. List six character qualities that are essential to possess as a professional medical assistant.

   A. _____

   B. _____

   C. _____

   D. _____

   E. _____

   F. _____

4. List two different types of communications.

   A. _____

   B. _____

5. List five external actions that must be taken in order to expand your technical knowledge, communicate more effectively, and demonstrate a caring attitude toward the patient.

   A. _____
   _____

   B. _____
   _____

   C. _____
   _____

   D. _____
   _____

   E. _____
   _____

6. How does empathy play a role in patient relations?

   _____
   _____
   _____

7. In order to share patient information with other individuals, you must first obtain _____ from the patient.

Assignment 1-5: True or False

Fill in the blank with a "T" for true statements and an "F" for false statements. Rewrite the false statements to make them true.

____ 1. In order to be eligible to sit for the CMA (AAMA) exam offered by the AAMA, the testing candidate must have graduated from either a CAAHEP or ABHES accredited institution.

   _____
   _____

____ 2. An NCMA is a nationally certified medical assistant through the AMT.

   _____
   _____

____ 3. A medical assistant is automatically certified to perform phlebotomy in programs that teach phlebotomy.

_____

_____

____ 4. Medical assisting students who graduate from a CAAHEP or ABHES accredited program are eligible to sit for the RMA exam offered by the AMT upon graduation.

_____

_____

____ 5. There is no formal testing required in order to obtain the RMA credential through the ARMA.

_____

_____

____ 6. The CMA (AAMA) is given throughout the year at Prometric testing centers throughout the country.

_____

_____

____ 7. Medical assistants are able to take x-rays once they become registered or certified as a medical assistant.

_____

_____

____ 8. The AMT offers the RPT or Registered Phlebotomy Technician credential.

_____

_____

____ 9. The CCMA credential is a specialized certification offered by the National Healthcareer Association and stands for Certified Clinical Medical Assistant.

_____

_____

Assignment 1-6: Certification Practice

Choose the best answer and place the corresponding letter in the blank.

____ 1. The CMA (AAMA) certification test is given:

    A. once a year.

    B. twice a year.

    C. three times a year.

    D. throughout the year.

____ 2. Medical assistants may take the AAMA examination to obtain which credential?

    A. AMT

    B. EMT

    C. RMA

    D. CPC

    E. CMA (AAMA)

____ 3. A person with integrity:

    A. is reliable.

    B. maintains high standards.

    C. is honest and dependable.

    D. all of the above.

____ 4. Persons who graduate from CAAHEP or ABHES accredited institutions may sit for:

    A. certification exam through the AAMA.

    B. registry exam through the AMT.

    C. both A and B.

    D. none of the above.

____ 5. Which of the following traits or characteristics would not be considered desirable in a medical assistant?

    A. Initiative

    B. A self-serving attitude

    C. Dependability

    D. Empathy

    E. Tactfulness

____ 6. Which of the following would convey a "professional appearance" to the patient?

    A. A clean uniform that is free of wrinkles

    B. Duty or athletic shoes that follow institutional guidelines

    C. A name tag worn on the uniform that identifies the medical assistant's name and credential.

    D. All of the above

____ 7. Which of the following would be considered unprofessional?

    A. Hair pulled back and away from the face

    B. Fingernails clean and trimmed

    C. Chewing gum while working

    D. Good hygiene

____ 8. This is the type of regulation for health care providers that is legislated by each state and mandated to perform duties.

    A. Registration

    B. Licensure

    C. Certification

    D. Both B and C

____ 9. Which of the following is a mandatory form of credential?

    A. Regulation

    B. Licensure

    C. Certification

    D. Registration

    E. Accreditation

____ 10. A term that signifies that one has fulfilled the necessary requirements of a specific organization to perform specific tasks; usually accomplished through some form of testing.

    A. Certification

    B. Licensure

    C. Registration

    D. Accreditation

____ 11. What type of consent is necessary in order to share information about a patient to another individual?

    A. Verbal consent

    B. Informed consent

    C. Written consent

    D. All of the above

____ 12. The term that means the ability to put yourself in another person's shoes.

    A. Compassion

    B. Integrity

    C. Empathy

    D. Initiative

____ 13. The term that means to be reliable or trustworthy is:
   A. initiative.
   B. dependability.
   C. tactful.
   D. all of the above.

SKILL APPLICATION CHALLENGES

Assignment 1-7: Projects

1. Research employment opportunities for medical assistants using the Internet, newspapers, and/or other sources. Find at least three openings for which a medical assistant would be qualified. Find at least one opening outside your state. Take note of the titles of the positions advertised. On each of the listings, highlight the information that identifies educational requirements, credentialing requirements, personal qualities, and other useful information.

2. Chapter 1 lists examples of professional and unprofessional appearance for a medical assistant. Using magazines, newspapers, the Internet, or any other sources available, find three pictures of medical assistants dressed in professional attire. Cut out each picture and secure it to a standard piece of 8½ × 11 paper. Describe in detail how each person looks professional. Is there anything in the photograph that looks substandard in regard to professional appearance?

FIELD APPLICATION CHALLENGES

Assignment 1-8

Read the following Field Application Challenges and respond to the questions following each scenario.

1. A medical assistant getting ready to perform an EKG notices that the disposable electrodes are missing from the stand that holds the EKG unit. The patient is in a hurry and needs to get back to work. The medical assistant remembers that there was a entire box of electrodes on the stand this morning when he ran an EKG on his first patient. The practice usually only goes through one pack of leads per month and the leads are only good for a certain amount of time after opening. He quickly searches areas in which the leads may be located but to no avail. Sarah is another medical assistant who just performed an EKG before him; she is now with a new patient and will not be out of the patient's room for several minutes. From the choices below, what would be the *best* solution for obtaining the leads?
   A. Confront the other medical assistant about the leads in front of the new patient.
   B. Open a new box of leads.
   C. Wait until the medical assistant comes out of the patient's room to inquire about the leads.
   D. Quietly knock on the door and ask the medical assistant to step out of the room for a moment before inquiring about the leads.

2. Your provider finishes up with patients early today. You notice that Megan, the medical assistant who works for Dr. Thompson is running severely behind schedule. The other medical assistants refuse to help her because they have other commitments and frankly they are not very fond of her. Megan mentioned to you that she was supposed to attend a birthday dinner for her mother tonight but that she is now going to be very late for the dinner. You have plans of your own and worked very hard to get done early so that you can leave early today as well. Are you committed to staying later to help Megan after you worked very hard to finish early so that you could leave on time?

_____

_____

_____

_____

_____

JOURNALING EXERCISE
Assignment 1-9

What content within this chapter was most meaningful to you? Why? List some examples of how you might apply information contained in this chapter, both during your training and after you enter the health care industry.

C H A P T E R **2**

Organization and Time Management in the Medical Office

FIELD RELEVANCY AND BENEFITS

Good professional and technical skills are essential to achieve success in the health care industry, but the addition of good organizational skills can make the difference between a medical assistant who is merely good and a medical assistant who is truly spectacular. This chapter will provide you with school and field organizational tips that will assist you with overall orderliness and good time management. The information in this chapter applies to all types of medical offices.

NOTE SHEET

Becoming Organized While You Are in School

_____

_____

_____

_____

Setting Up Your Work Station and the Clinical Area

_____

_____

_____

_____

Getting Acclimated to Your New Work Environment

_____

_____

_____

_____

Daily Procedures That Clinical Staff Members Perform

_____

_____

_____

_____

Clinical Assisting and Time Management Issues

_____

_____

_____

_____

Performing Routine Maintenance on Clinical Equipment

_____

_____

_____

_____

VOCABULARY REVIEW

Assignment 2-1: Spelling Review

Find the words below that are misspelled; circle them and then correctly spell them in the spaces provided.

Accolimate	Callbacks	Clinicean
Compotency	Critical Labs	Desktop Organizer
Drawer Organizer	Out Guide	Pending
Preventative Health Screenings	Protacol	Queri
Task Box	Task List	Time Management
To Do List	Workstation	

_____   _____   _____

_____   _____

Assignment 2-2: Fill in the Blank

Fill in the blanks below with Essential Terms from this chapter.

1. A(n) _____ refers to a checklist that is used by an evaluator to determine your knowledge of a specific skill.

2. _____ is a practice to improve efficiency and productivity.

3. A(n) _____ is a list of jobs that need to be completed, usually within a certain amount of time; it is meant to jog your memory so that you won't forget to perform the task.

4. Check to see if the patient is up to date on all _____, which are screenings that help to identify health concerns before they become problems, such as rectal exams, mammograms, cholesterol levels, and blood pressure screenings. Immunization status should also be checked.

5. A(n) _____ is a temporary file that replaces a chart that is removed from the file. This will assist other staff members who may need the chart for other purposes.

6. To _____ means to make a request for information.

7. _____ refers to a set of guidelines that should be instituted based on office policy and may include: urine testing for pregnant patients, setting up specific trays for various procedures, and disrobing instructions based on symptoms.

8. The term _____ means to become accustomed to a new environment or situation. Of course you will want to start by reading the office policy and procedure manuals. The information found in these manuals can save you many questions and a great deal of time if you will take the time to read them.

9. The term _____ usually refers to practitioners employed within the practice including the physician, the physician's assistant, and nurse. However, in this text, clinician is used to mean anyone working in a clinical setting.

Assignment 2-3: Matching

Match the term with its definition and place the corresponding letter in the blank.

____ 1. Critical labs

____ 2. Workstation

____ 3. Callbacks

____ 4. Pending

____ 5. To Do list or Task list

____ 6. Query

____ 7. Electronic task

____ 8. Time management

____ 9. Desktop organizers

A. A list of jobs that need to be completed, usually within a certain time frame

B. File folder holders, card holders, letter trays, and pen and pencil holders on top of the desk

C. A practice to increase efficiency and productivity

D. An area in the office supplied with equipment and furnishings for one person

E. Abnormal test results that require an immediate response from the provider

F. To await or something that is to occur

G. A group of tasks that usually requires a phone call such as: returning a patient's call, calling in a prescription, faxing reports to the hospital, etc.

H. A notation on a computer that alerts the user of a task that needs to be performed

I. To make a request for information

CHAPTER REVIEW

Assignment 2-4: Short Answer

1. List three ways that the medical assistant can become better acclimated to the medical office environment.

A. _____

B. _____

C. _____

2. List types of forms, equipment, and supplies that can help to create and maintain an organized workstation.

A. _____

_____

_____

B. _____

_____

_____

C. _____

_____

_____

_____

D. _____

_____

_____

_____

E. _____

_____

_____

_____

F. _____

_____

_____

_____

3. List common opening procedures for the clinical medical assistant.

A. _____

_____

B. _____

_____

C. _____

_____

D. _____

_____

E. _____

_____

F. _____

_____

G. _____

_____

H. _____

_____

4. List different ways that the medical assistant can organize his study area at home to make it more efficient.

_____

_____

_____

_____

_____

_____

_____

5. Why should basic examination rooms be set up and stocked exactly the same from one room to the next?

_____

_____

_____

_____

6. Explain how EMR reduces the amount of time in performing pending tasks.

_____

_____

_____

_____

7. List at least four different preventative health screenings that should be performed at regular intervals.

   A. _____

   B. _____

   C. _____

   D. _____

8. How does EMR assist with preventative health maintenance screenings?

_____

_____

_____

_____

Assignment 2-5: True or False

Fill in the blank with a "T" for true statements and an "F" for false statements. Rewrite the false statements to make them true.

____ 1. The out guide is used to replace the patient's chart that has been removed from the file.

_____

_____

____ 2. To keep up with your instructor, it is best to read the assigned information after the material has been covered in class.

_____

_____

___ 3. It is best to complete callbacks and any tasks from the pending file workstation at the end of the day.

_____

_____

___ 4. When calling in a prescription for a patient; the medical assistant will need to notify the patient once the task has been completed so that the patient can pick the prescription up.

_____

_____

___ 5. When discharging a patient with home care instructions, hand the information to the patient to read and document in the chart that the patient received the information.

_____

_____

___ 6. To become more efficient with your time and the amount of time you spend with each patient, you should prepare paper charts at least three days in advance before patients are scheduled.

_____

_____

___ 7. Most new equipment is purchased with a maintenance or service agreement.

_____

_____

Assignment 2-6: Certification Practice

Choose the best answer and place the corresponding letter in the blank.

___ 1. Which of the following procedures should not be instituted when organizing patient exam rooms?
   A. Reorganize the room to your specifications.
   B. Check with your supervisor regarding boundaries.
   C. Share your ideas with all staff members that share the room and ask for their input.
   D. Stock the room as needed.

___ 2. Which of the following procedures are not part of general closing procedures?
   A. Making certain examination rooms are ready to go for the next day
   B. Completing critical tasks
   C. Unlocking the drug room
   D. Setting the security code

___ 3. To await or something that is to occur is termed:
   A. Query
   B. Task list
   C. Pending
   D. Protocol

The following scenario applies to Questions 4–7: Dr. Yeager has three examination rooms and prefers that all exam rooms are filled at all times. He just finished with the patient in Room #2 and requested that you draw blood for a lab panel before allowing this patient to leave. You still have an EKG (part of an annual physical) to perform on the patient in Room #1 and Room #3 is empty. There are two patients waiting to come back from the reception area; one person is here for a BP check and refill on BP medication and the other person is here for her monthly allergy shot (which is listed as a medical assisting visit). List the order in which you will complete these tasks. There are no other patients scheduled for the next half hour.

____ 4. Which task will you perform first?

    A. EKG in Room #1

    B. Lab work in Room #2

    C. Patient who is here for weekly allergy shot

    D. Place patient waiting for the BP check and medication refill in Room #3

____ 5. Which task will you perform second?

    A. EKG in Room #1

    B. Lab work in Room #2

    C. Patient who is here for weekly allergy shot

    D. Place patient waiting for the BP check and medication refill in Room #3

____ 6. Which task will you perform third?

    A. EKG in Room #1

    B. Lab work in Room #2

    C. Patient who is here for weekly allergy shot

    D. Place patient waiting for the BP check and medication refill in Room #3

____ 7. Which task will you perform last?

    A. EKG in Room #1

    B. Lab work in Room #2

    C. Patient who is here for weekly allergy shot

    D. Place patient waiting for the BP check and medication refill in Room #3

The following scenario corresponds with Questions 8–11: You have 30 minutes until your next patient arrives for her appointment. You have time to catch up on a few charts in your pending file station and on your task list. Items include:

• Call back patient with lab results that are normal.

• Request maintenance on one of your two EKG machines.

• Call in a refill for a patient's BP medication.

• Call patient with a critical lab value to give instructions for a change in the way the patient is to take her medication.

____ 8. Which task would you perform first?

    A. Call back patient with lab results that are normal.

    B. Request maintenance on one of your two EKG machines.

    C. Call in a refill for a patient's BP medication.

    D. Call patient with a critical lab value to give instructions for changing the way she is currently taking her medication.

____ 9. Which task would you perform second?

    A. Call back patient with lab results that are normal.

    B. Request maintenance on one of your two EKG machines.

    C. Call in a refill for a patient's BP medication.

    D. Call patient with a critical lab value to give instructions for a change in the way she is currently taking her medication.

___ 10. Which task would you perform third?

    A. Call back patient with lab results that are normal.

    B. Request maintenance on one of your two EKG machines.

    C. Call in a refill for a patient's BP medication.

    D. Call patient with a critical lab value to give instructions for a change in the way she is currently taking her medication.

___ 11. Which task would you perform fourth?

    A. Call back patient with lab results that are normal.

    B. Request maintenance on one of your two EKG machines.

    C. Call in a refill for a patient's BP medication.

    D. Call patient with a critical lab value to give instructions for a change in the way she is currently taking her medication.

___ 12. The purpose of an OUT guide is:

    A. to act as a place holder for the chart that has been removed.

    B. to identify the current location of the chart.

    C. to assist with easy filing once the chart is re-filed.

    D. all of the above.

___ 13. The staff ran very late the night before and were unable to complete all of their daily tasks. The staff now has today's opening tasks and tasks that didn't get completed the day before. Which of the following tasks should have been performed the day before?

    A. Pulling off lab results that came in throughout the night and attaching them to patients' charts

    B. Running a set of lab controls on lab equipment

    C. Going through the charts of patients being seen today and making certain that each chart is updated with any outstanding lab results; inserting new forms for any forms that are full or getting full; and writing notations for any patients who are behind on preventative health screenings

    D. Turning on equipment in the lab and x-ray rooms

___ 14. All of the following equipment may contain a service maintenance contract and should be inspected following contract guidelines except the:

    A. microwave.

    B. pulmonary function unit.

    C. Holter monitor.

    D. AED.

___ 15. Surveyors for insurance companies and federal agencies will look for which of the following during inspections?

    A. Maintenance logs

    B. Equipment logs

    C. Fire extinguisher logs

    D. Service tags

    E. All of the above

___ 16. What is the best way to perfect the skills of time management?

    A. Procrastination

    B. Practice

    C. Ponder

    D. Take a time management course

SKILL APPLICATION CHALLENGE
Assignment 2-7: Project

Create an equipment maintenance log for the equipment in your school lab. Each piece of equipment should have a separate page. This can be written or typed. Place the log pages in a 1 inch notebook or folder and make a nice cover for the log.

FIELD APPLICATION CHALLENGE
Assignment 2-8

Read the following Field Application Challenge and respond to the question following the scenario.

You have just been hired for a new position and personal organization is not one of your strengths. You are determined to improve in this area and decide to purchase some organizers to assist you with organization. Your desk space consists of a small area of counterspace located within the medical assistant's workstation and you have only one drawer. What type of organizers would be best since you are very limited in space?

_____

_____

_____

_____

_____

JOURNALING EXERCISE
Assignment 2-9

What content within this chapter was most meaningful to you? Why? List some examples of how you might apply information contained in this chapter, both during your training, and after you enter the health care industry.

C H A P T E R **3**

The Complete Medical Record and Electronic Charting

FIELD RELEVANCY AND BENEFITS

The medical record is the most important record kept in the medical office. Whether you are working in an office that uses paper files or in a paperless office, understanding the components of the medical record and where information is stored in the record is essential. Electronic medical records (EMRs) are booming in today's health care culture, and having a basic understanding of how to use an EMR system should make you more marketable. Learning information in this chapter is applicable to all types of medical practices.

NOTE SHEET

The Medical Record

_____

_____

_____

_____

Contents of the Medical Record

_____

_____

_____

_____

Medical Record Formats

_____

_____

_____

_____

Creating and Maintaining the Medical Record

_____

_____

_____

_____

Laws That Affect the Medical Record

_____

_____

_____

_____

Ownership, Retention, and Disposal of Medical Records

_____

_____

_____

_____

VOCABULARY REVIEW

Assignment 3-1: Matching

Match the term with its definition and place the corresponding letter in the blank.

____ 1. Shingling

____ 2. Assessment

____ 3. Electronic health record

____ 4. Business associate agreement

____ 5. Notice of privacy practices

____ 6. Subjective impressions

____ 7. Problem list

____ 8. Reverse chronological order

____ 9. Progress note

____ 10. Objective impressions

____ 11. Flow sheets

____ 12. Plans

____ 13. Electronic medical record

____ 14. Personal health record

____ 15. Concierge medicine

A. A patient's medical record in digital format

B. Describes exactly how protected information is to be handled between business partners.

C. Provider's plans to perform diagnostic and lab testing to assist in confirming a diagnosis and plans for treating the patient

D. The heart of the patient record; a chronological listing of the patient's overall health status

E. The way information is stored within the patient's chart; the most recent notes, reports, and forms are always on top

F. The method for filing lab reports when reports are not the size of a standard piece of paper

G. An interpretation of the subjective and objective findings

H. Logs found in the patient's chart that assist the provider in monitoring specific repetitive information, at one glance

I. A record of specific problems that are identified from the patient history form; it should list new problems as they arise; each problem is numbered and should include the name of the problem or diagnosis

J. Patients should receive a notice for how their personal medical information may be used

K. "A generic term for all electronic patient care systems"

L. A type of medicine in which the patient pays an annual fee for special services

M. Patient's vital signs, height and weight, laboratory results, or other diagnostic data

N. A copy of the patient's own personal health information that can be shared with all providers

O. The patient's chief complaint or an explanation of why the patient is here

CHAPTER REVIEW

Assignment 3-2: Acronym Review

Write what each of the following acronyms stands for.

1. CCHIT: _____

2. HIT: _____

3. HIPAA: _____

4. IIPI: _____

5. PHI: _____

6. POMR: _____

7. SOAP: _____

8. SOMR: _____

Assignment 3-3: Short Answer

1. List the commission responsible for certifying electronic medical records.

   _____

2. Why are flow sheets used in the medical record?

   _____

   _____

   _____

   _____

3. List the two major types of formats which are used for documenting in the patient's record.

   A. _____

   B. _____

4. List what each of the letters stand for in the SOAP acronym and describe information that would be included in each section.

   _____

   _____

   _____

   _____

   _____

5. List four advantages of the POMR.

   A. _____

   B. _____

   C. _____

   D. _____

6. Describe how long medical records need to be retained and how to properly dispose of medical records.

   _____

   _____

   _____

7. EMR has many positives, but what may be some "pitfalls" associated with EMR?

   _____

   _____

   _____

8. Provide at least three examples of phone reports that may need to be documented either on a progress note or onto a special phone form.

   _____

   _____

9. List six functions of EMR.

   _____

   _____

   _____

   _____

   _____

   _____

   _____

   _____

   _____

   _____

   _____

   _____

   _____

   _____

10. Explain the shingling method for filing and list examples of some reports that may be shingled.

   _____

   _____

   _____

   _____

11. Why would an office manager conduct a comprehensive audit trail?

   _____

   _____

   _____

Assignment 3-4: Matching I

Information found in a SOAP note is listed below. Identify the part of the note in which the information would be found. Match the information with the answers listed. Record the answer in the blank provided. Each answer may be used more than once.

S—Subjective   A—Assessment

O—Objective   P—Plan

____ A. Temperature 99.9°F

____ B. Patient c/o sore throat

____ C. Lymph nodes enlarged upon palpation

____ D. Strep throat

____ E. Abdomen and groin area shows rash

____ F. Lungs are clear

____ G. Patient states slight headache above right eye

____ H. Will perform an EKG and run a metabolic panel

____ I. Results of rapid strep test

Assignment 3-5: Matching II

Match the section of the chart in which you would find the following information.

Sections of the chart:

____ 1. Patient's chief complaint   A. Demographic information

____ 2. CBC or complete blood count   B. Insurance section

____ 3. Referral form (This may vary from office to office)   C. Correspondence

____ 4. Registration form   D. Diagnostic/x-ray reports

____ 5. MRI report   E. Lab reports

____ 6. Letter from the cardiologist   F. Medication information

____ 7. Social history   G. Progress note

____ 8. Copy of the patient's insurance card   H. Medical history

____ 9. Notation that the patient no-showed for appointment.   I. Consultation report

____ 10. Prescription information

Assignment 3-6: Certification Practice

Choose the best answer and place the corresponding letter in the blank.

____ 1. This is an analysis of the patient's health status.

    A. Patient's record

    B. Medical record

    C. Flow sheets

    D. Objective impressions

____ 2. This is the person who developed the POMR system.

    A. Larry Word

    B. Larry Reed

    C. Lawrence Weed

    D. Robert Weed

____ 3. This is the section of the medical record that contains letters written about the patient from an assessment made by a specialist.

    A. Progress notes

    B. Discharge summary

    C. Correspondence

    D. Consultation reports

____ 4. This is the section of the chart in which you would find a biopsy study.

    A. Laboratory section (pathology report)

    B. Correspondence

    C. Insurance section

    D. Progress notes

____ 5. A Lipid Panel and Chem 21 would be filed in which of the following sections of the chart?

    A. Diagnostic section

    B. Laboratory section

    C. Progress notes

    D. Medication section

____ 6. Which of the following does not belong with the others?

    A. Assessment

    B. Impression

    C. Diagnosis

    D. Examination

____ 7. Which of the following is not a use of the medical record?

    A. Medical research and education

    B. Legal documentation

    C. Tracking patient's progress

    D. To check the patient's financial balance

____ 8. All of the following are found in the administrative section of the record *except:*

    A. demographics.

    B. patient insurance.

    C. correspondence.

    D. prescription info.

____ 9. The physical outer part of the medical record belongs to the practice; however, information stored within the chart is property of the:

    A. patient.

    B. practice.

    C. both A and B.

    D. none of the above.

____ 10. The information in a POMR includes:

    A. database.

    B. problem list.

    C. plans.

    D. progress notes.

    E. all of the above.

____ 11. When filing in *reverse* chronologic order, which of the following is the correct sequence?

    A. Radiology report from June 20, 2011, would be in front of a radiology report dated June 30, 2011

    B. A referral letter from June 15, 2011, would be behind a referral letter dated December 15, 2010

    C. Laboratory test result dated May 25, 2011, would be in front of a lab test dated March 23, 2011

    D. Progress note entry dated January 20, 2011, would be in front of a progress note dated July 16, 2011

___ 12. Which of the following would not be in a flow sheet?

    A. PT/INR results

    B. Drug allergies

    C. Blood pressure screenings

    D. Glucose results

___ 13. In an executive order from President Bush, by what year should the majority of Americans have access to EMR?

    A. 2010

    B. 2012

    C. 2014

    D. 2016

___ 14. An important rule for releasing medical records is:

    A. There is no need to gain written permission to release medical information as long as you have the patient's verbal consent to release information.

    B. Have the patient sign a release form before giving out any information and send a copy of the medical record, not the original.

    C. Always give the patient the original medical record and keep a copy of the record for the office.

    D. none of the above.

___ 15. Examples of internal security measures that should be implemented to protect the patient's health information include:

    A. Back up your computer at the end of each day and store the backup in a secure place outside the office, such as a bank deposit box.

    B. Use encrypted passwords.

    C. Create limited accessibility accounts for employees.

    D. Change pass codes on a regular basis.

    E. all of the above.

___ 16. Which of the following would *not* be an example of following HIPAA guidelines?

    A. Accessing the patient's chart only when it is absolutely necessary

    B. Leaving computer monitors in plain sight for other patients to see

    C. Using sign-in sheets that require a minimal amount of information

    D. Allowing the patient to review his medical record and make requests for changes

___ 17. In this system, there is no systematic cross-referencing of data from one section to the next.

    A. SOAP

    B. POMR

    C. POR

    D. SOMR

___ 18. A notice of how a patient's medical information will be used should be given to every patient and a form explaining that the patient received the information should be signed and filed in the chart. What is the name of the notice?

    A. Notice of Privacy Practices

    B. Notice of HIPAA

    C. Notice of Sharing Medical Information Practices

    D. None of the above

___ 19. Which of the following would *not* be included in the initial database of a POMR record?

    A. Patient profile

    B. Baseline readings for diagnostic and laboratory testing

    C. Treatment plans

    D. None of the above

___ 20. Important uses of the medical record include providing accurate, comprehensive medical information to assist the provider in:

    A. formulating an accurate diagnosis.

    B. planning an appropriate treatment.

    C. tracking the patient's progress.

    D. formulating disease prevention measures.

    E. all of the above.

___ 21. Penalties for violating HIPAA rules can be as high as:

    A. $50,000 and 1 year in prison.

    B. $100,000 and 5 years in prison.

    C. $250,000 and 10 years in prison.

    D. $500,000 and 20 years in prison.

SKILL APPLICATION CHALLENGE

Assignment 3-7: Documentation Exercise

From the following dictation put the information into a SOAP note format on the progress note provided on the next page.

"I have pain when I go to the bathroom. I go all the time, especially at night." +abdominal pain(6), -back pain, +fever ("99.6° to 101°F"), LMP 05-06-2010. OTC; Urostat (no relief). Rx: Accutane. Allergies: Latex and SULFA. Vital Signs: T 99.2°F. BP 110/76, R: 20 P 78. Abdominal tenderness and guarding in the mid hypogastric region of the abdomen. Urinalysis: Urine bright orange due to the urostat: Unable to read urine dipstick. Microscopic examination of urine revealed a large amount of white blood cells and bacteria. Few red blood cells. Diagnosis: Urinary tract infection. Will send urine out for a C & S and start the patient on Bactrim DS, sig 1 tab/day × 7 days. Pt. to return to office in 10 days for a recheck on urine.

S: _____

_____

_____

_____

O: _____

_____

_____

_____

A: _____

_____

_____

_____

P: _____

_____

_____

_____

FIELD APPLICATION CHALLENGE
Assignment 3-8
Read the following Field Application Challenge and respond to the questions following the scenario.

Mr. Snodgrass calls to request his wife's lab results. Mrs. Snodgrass is traveling today and will not have access to a phone until after the office is closed. Mr. Snodgrass states that his wife is most anxious about the results and does not want to wait until tomorrow for the results. Mr. Snodgrass is listed on the privacy sheet as being able to accept lab results for the patient. You just placed the chart on the provider's desk because the results just came back. The results are normal but the provider is out of the office and will not return until the next day. The policy of the office is that no test results are given to a patient until they have been signed off by the provider.

1. What makes it all right for this particular patient's spouse to receive his wife's lab results?

   _____

   _____

2. Would it be okay to share the results with spouse since the results are normal?

   _____

   _____

3. Are there any other options for giving the spouse the information?

   _____

   _____

   _____

JOURNALING EXERCISE
Assignment 3-9

What content within this chapter was most meaningful to you? Why? List some examples of how you might apply information contained in this chapter, both during your training and after you enter the health care industry.

Fundamentals of Documentation

FIELD RELEVANCY AND BENEFITS

A large percentage of how the medical assistant communicates with other health care professionals is through written documentation. Whether it is documenting in a chart, sending a fax, or corresponding through e-mail, providers and other health care professionals will gauge much of your performance by how well you document information.

If your documentation is incomplete, contains spelling errors, or is ambiguous, it will immediately diminish the receiver's view of your intellect and could be the stumbling block that hinders your ability to succeed in the health care industry and receive promotions; however, superb documentation will assist in spotlighting your "professional worth" and will facilitate forward movement in your professional journey.

The information in this chapter corresponds with all types of practices in which the medical assistant may be employed.

NOTE SHEET

Guidelines for Documenting in the Patient's Chart

_____

_____

_____

_____

Documenting and Sending Faxes

_____

_____

_____

_____

Making Corrections or Addendums to Chart Notes

_____

_____

_____

Writing and Sending E-mails

_____

_____

_____

VOCABULARY REVIEW

Assignment 4-1: Matching

Match the term with its definition and place the corresponding letter in the blank.

____ 1. Joint Commission

____ 2. Participating provider

____ 3. Referral

____ 4. Addendum

____ 5. ISMP

____ 6. Precertification

____ 7. "Do Not Use Abbreviation List"

A. Process in which certain procedures must be approved prior to being performed in order to have them covered by the insurance company

B. An addition or supplement to a previous chart note

C. A list of abbreviations that are commonly misinterpreted and may no longer be used when documenting orders within the patient's medical record, or when writing orders that are to be sent to other healthcare facilities

D. Separate organization that specifically seeks ways to promote medication safety; has also compiled a list which is referred to as "List of Error-Prone Abbreviations, Symbols, and Dose Designations"

E. A process in which one provider recommends the services of another provider (usually a specialist) to oversee certain aspects of the patient's care

F. A facility that contracts with the insurance company to provide laboratory or diagnostic services

G. A national organization that focuses on improving the quality and safety of care provided by health care organizations; published a "Do Not Use List" of medication abbreviations as part of its 2006 National Patient and Safety Goals

Assignment 4-2: Sentence Completion

Fill in the blanks below with Essential Terms from this chapter.

Lisa works for Dr. Beachler who is not seeing patients this afternoon. Lisa is catching up on some paper work. She pulls the charts for tomorrow's patients, completes the callbacks, and prepares the lab specimens for the courier. One of Dr. Beachler's patients, Mark Stevens, had some chest pain last week so Dr. Beachler ordered a heart ultrasound on the patient. In order to get the patient's payer to pay for the testing, Lisa had to obtain a(n) (1) _____ from the insurance company prior to testing. The test came back abnormal so Dr. Beachler now wants Lisa to send the patient to Dr. Wong, a well-respected cardiologist. Because the patient belongs to an HMO plan, Lisa must obtain a(n) (2) _____ from the insurance company in order for the insurance company to pay for the visit to the cardiologist. The cardiology group asks Lisa to call the patient and have him get some blood work performed before his first visit. Lisa looks in the UHC directory to see which lab is a(n) (3) _____. Lisa calls the lab, sets up the testing for the patient, and calls the patient back with the results. She then records the information in the patient's chart. Lisa discovers after signing off the entry that she forgot to list the time of the testing. She makes a(n) (4) _____ to the entry to include the time of the visit.

CHAPTER REVIEW

Assignment 4-3: Acronym Review

Write what the following acronym stands for.

ISMP: _____

Assignment 4-4: Short Answer

1. Fill in the chart below with 11 "Documentation Dos" and four "Documentation Don'ts" when documenting in the medical record.

Dos	
1.	7.
2.	8.
3.	9.
4.	10.
5.	11.
6.	
Don'ts	
1.	3.
2.	4.

2. List the steps that should be taken when making a correction or an addendum to both a paper-based and a paperless record.

Paper-based: _____

_____

_____

Paperless: _____

_____

3. Describe proper etiquette guidelines that should be adhered to when sending professional e-mails.

_____

_____

_____

_____

_____

_____

_____

_____

_____

_____

_____

_____

_____

4. The following chart entry contains nine errors. Many of the errors are the result of using "Do Not Use" abbreviations (see Appendix B). Highlight the errors using a highlighter in the chart entry and transfer the errors to the lines listed below the entry. Describe why each error is incorrect and write in what may be used in place of the error.

> 05/31/2010 9:30 a.m. Allergy serum, 0.5 cc, sub-q, R. arm per Dr. Armstrong. Small
> wheal formed > than the size of a ▮ᵈⁱᵐᵉ (CORR Lisa Brown, RMA 05/31/2010) at the injection
> site follwing the injections. +erythema and edema, pt. states the site is sore and tender to
> the touch. −Resp sx. Appleid ice to area. Informed doctor of reaction. Dr. would like dose to be
> reduced from 0.5 cc to 0.3 ml next visit. LB, RMA ————————————

1. _____

2. _____

3. _____

4. _____

5. _____

6. _____

7. _____

8. _____

9. _____

Assignment 4-5: Certification Practice

Choose the best answer and place the corresponding letter in the blank.

____ 1. When documenting in the medical record, the entry should be:

    A. accurate.

    B. thorough.

    C. typed or written in black ink.

    D. neat and legible.

    E. all of the above.

____ 2. The chief complaint is the reason that the patient is being seen. The complaint should be all of the following *except:*

    A. accurate.

    B. concise.

    C. flow well.

    D. judgmental.

____ 3. The medical office in which you work uses EMR. The provider sends a message to your electronic task box with a high priority symbol asking you to contact Rebecca Harting instructing her to change the way that she is taking her Dilantin. You notify the patient and document the phone call within the electronic progress note. You then complete the entry, locking you out of the progress note. You reopen the progress note and discover that you made an error. What is the correct method for correcting an error or making an addendum in the EMR?

    A. Open a new note and type in the correction.

    B. Click on the addendum or change button and follow the directions.

    C. There is no way to correct an error once the note has been locked.

    D. Notify your clinical supervisor and she will fix the error.

____ 4. The way that a provider discovers the reason for the patient's office visit is by reading:

    A. the patient's H&P.

    B. the patient's lab reports.

    C. the patient's social history.

    D. the patient's chief complaint.

____ 5. One pitfall that should be avoided in regards to documentation is:

    A. procrastination.

    B. initiative.

    C. completeness.

    D. accuracy.

____ 6. Which of the following would be regarded as a "Documentation Don't"?

    A. Use standard abbreviations

    B. Use illegible handwriting

    C. Use correct spelling

    D. Document accurately

____ 7. A follow-up note from a previous visit is a:

    A. chief complaint.

    B. lab report.

    C. patient education.

    D. progress note.

____ 8. Items that should be included when documenting an in-office procedure includes all of the following *except:*

    A. the name of the procedure.

    B. the name of the provider ordering the procedure.

    C. any complications during or following the procedure.

    D. the name and address of the facility.

____ 9. Information that should be included in a medication entry includes all of the following *except:*

   A. the lot number of any syringes that are used to administer the medication.

   B. the name of the medication.

   C. the strength of the medication.

   D. the route of the medication.

____ 10. Information that should be included when documenting an educational session includes all but which of the following?

   A. The date and time of the session

   B. The topic of the session

   C. The patient's highest level of education

   D. Who was present for the session

____ 11. Information that should be included when documenting a prescription includes all but which of the following?

   A. Name of the pharmacy where the prescription was called in

   B. Name of the pharmacist that you spoke with

   C. The pharmacist's license number

   D. Name of the prescribed medication

____ 12. What should be documented in regard to a telephone screening?

   A. The general complaint

   B. Patient's responses to the screening questions

   C. Instructions that were given to the patient

   D. All of the above

____ 13. Information that should be included when documenting a referral within the chart note includes all but which of the following?

   A. The patient's employer's name

   B. Method used to obtain the referral

   C. Name of the referral provider

   D. Name of the referring provider

____ 14. Information that should be included when documenting a hospitalization includes all but which of the following?

   A. Name and location of the hospital

   B. Dates of admission

   C. Reason for admission

   D. The patient's insurance information

____ 15. Information that should be included when documenting a precertification includes:

   A. the date the request was made.

   B. the name of the carrier's representative.

   C. the name of the insurance company.

   D. all of the above.

SKILL APPLICATION CHALLENGES

Assignment 4-6: Flash Card Connection

1. Refer to Appendix A in the back of the textbook. Make up a set of flash cards for each abbreviation. (Helpful hint: Using different colors of flash cards for the different groups of abbreviations may assist in quicker memorization of the abbreviations.)

2. Refer to Appendix B in the back of the textbook. Make up a set of flash cards for the "Do Not Use" abbreviations. These abbreviations should be placed on bright neon flash cards as a reminder not to use them.

Assignment 4-7: Documentation Exercise

Rewrite the following chart note in long hand.

03-15-2010 10:15 am: Pt. C/O R. sided abd pain (7) x 3 days. + N/V, Last BM 4 days

ago. Fever X 2 days (99-102°F) ↓appetite. LMP: 02-14-2010, OTC Med: Tums (-relief) -RX,

NKDA. Colleen Frye, CMA (AAMA) ————————————————————

COMPLETING SPECIAL FORMS

The following assignments are to assist you in completing special forms and in learning how to document information onto a progress note. Each assignment will list which forms are necessary to complete the assignment.

Assignment 4-8: Documenting a Progress Note

Work Form Necessary: FORM 4-1

Directions: Transfer the following information in proper documentation format onto the progress note, Work Form 4-1.

February 08, 2010 10:00 a.m.: Jillian Longfellow, born 03/11/1969, is here for a follow-up appointment from her last visit regarding her UTI. Jillian finished the Macrobid as directed, but still feels the urge to urinate. Pain upon urination; urinating 3 times per hour. Has visible blood in the urine (shows up on tissue paper when she wipes). Patient is complaining of moderate lower back pain (around an 8 on the pain scale). Taking OTC: Aleve 220 mg every four hours (very little relief). Erika Simmons, RMA

Assignment 4-9: Documenting Lab Results onto a Reporting Form and onto a Progress Note

Work Forms Necessary: FORM 4-1, FORM 4-2, and FORM 4-3

Directions: Transfer the following information to Work Forms 4-1, 4-2 and 4-3. (*Note:* You will continue to use Work Form 4-1, which you started in Assignment 4-8.) To learn how to document the full procedure onto a progress note, refer to Table 4-1, Documenting Lab Procedures, in the textbook.

After examining Jillian Longfellow, Dr. Brown asks the medical assistant, Erika Simmons, to perform a physical and chemical urinalysis on the patient's urine. Results to the physical and chemical urinalysis are below. Please transfer the results of the physical and chemical urinalysis to the urine reporting form (Work Form 4-2) and the urinalysis log (Work Form 4-3), and make a note on the progress note. Since the lab result information is already on the lab form you will just need to state that the tests were performed and where to find the results on the progress note, for example, 02/08/2007 10:30 a.m. Physical & Chemical UA per Dr. Brown. Results can be found on the urinalysis reporting form in the lab section of the chart.

02/08/2010 10:30 a.m. Location (Long Street Office)
    Lab results were as follows: Physical & Chemical UA: Color: Amber, Appearance: Cloudy: Odor: Strong Ammonia: Leukocyte (Moderate), Nitrite (Positive), Urobilinogen (Normal), pH (7.5), Protein (30+), Blood (Moderate), Specific Gravity (1.030), Ketones (Negative), Bilirubin (Negative), Glucose (250)
    Tested by Erika Simmons, RMA

Assignment 4-10: Documenting an Outside Appointment onto a Progress Note

Work Form Necessary: FORM 4-1

Directions: Document the information from the phone call onto Work Form 4-1. (*Note:* Again, continue using Work Form 4-1.) Table 4-9 in the textbook lists steps for recording outside procedures, which is very similar for recording outside appointments.

After reviewing the results, Dr. Brown decides to refer Jillian to a urologist. He is concerned that the patient is not responding to treatment. Since Jillian belongs to an HMO plan, Erika (Dr. Brown's medical assistant) needs to set up a referral for the patient. Erika first calls the urologist to make certain that she can get an appointment for the patient.
    Erika contacts Dr. Michael Hale's office, a urologist listed on Jillian's HMO plan and speaks with Terri Kissler (a scheduler for Dr. Hale). The time the call takes place is 10:45 a.m. Terri expresses to Erika that the first appointment available is on Tuesday, February 12, 2010 at 10:00 a.m. Erika pauses for a moment to ask Jillian, who is standing next to the phone, if the date and time works with her schedule. She states that it does. Erika accepts the appointment for the patient and tells Terri that she will send the referral just as soon as she completes it. Erika hangs up the phone and shares all of the information with Jillian who appears to have a clear understanding of the instructions.

Assignment 4-11: Completing a Referral and Documenting the Referral onto a Progress Note

Work Forms Necessary: FORM 4-1, FORM 4-4

Directions: Continuing to use Work Form 4-1, state that you faxed the referral to UHC on February 8, 2010 at 2:00 p.m. Use the Referral Information in the table below to complete Work Form 4-4.

Provider	Dr. Michael Hale (Urologist) NPI # 5487955121
Provider's address	4442 Huber Drive, Suite 111-A Westerville, OH 43081 (614) 872-1988
Insurance information	United Health Care (UHC) Group # 52737
Diagnosis	UTI (599.0 ICD-9 Code; CPT Code 99214)
Referring provider	Darryl J. Brown, M.D. NPI # 4512872571
Referring provider's address	1843 E. Long Street Columbus, OH 43221 (614) 994-9383
Appointment date	February 12, 2010
Patient name	Jillian E. Longfellow

Patient ID number	284-99-0366
Patient's DOB	March 11, 1969
Patient's address	1454 Placid Drive Columbus, OH 43235
Patient's telephone number	Home: 614-487-4585 Cell: 614-203-4481

Assignment 4-12: Completing a Fax Cover Form

Work Form Necessary: FORM 4-5

Directions: Prepare a fax cover sheet (using Work Form 4-5) to be sent to Children's Hospital to the Surgical Floor for PAT. Refer back to the textbook for information on completing a fax lead form.

You work for Drs. Raymond, Shue, and Beachler. You are submitting three pages, *not* including fax cover sheet. Use this information to prepare your fax cover sheet, as well as the information in the table below.

Reports being submitted	• Chest x-ray report • Blood work • History
Date of fax	June 14, 2010
Time of fax	0800
Attention	Joan Keel, RN
Department	Surgery
Children's Hospital fax number	650-420-3146
Children's Hospital telephone number	650-420-3240
Patient's name	LaShonda Baaker
Patient's DOB	04-14-1999
Surgery date	Surgery scheduled for June 20, 2010 at 0800
Name of sender	Your name

Assignment 4-13: Documenting a Medication

Work Form Necessary: FORM 4-6

Directions: Using the information below, document a medication on Work Form 4-6. Refer to Table 4-3 in the textbook for steps for documenting a medication.

Patient's name: Timothy Heller

DOB: 12-10-1968

Doctor's order: Dr. Henderson orders the patient to have a flu immunization.

Today's date: 06/15/12

Time of administration: 0900

The standard adult dose is 0.5 ml.

Name of manufacturer: Prevention Inc

Lot number: 27A119

Exp. date: 06/2013

Route: IM

Location: R. Deltoid

Medical assistant's name and title: Brad Green, RMA

No complications during or following the injection.

Assignment 4-14: Documenting a Procedure

Work Form Necessary: FORM 4-6

Directions: Using the information given below, document the procedure on Work Form 4-6. Refer to Table 4-2 in the textbook for steps for documenting a procedure.

Patient's name: Timothy Heller

Doctor's order: Dr. Henderson ordered a 12-Lead EKG

Today's date: 06/15/12

Time of EKG: 0915

No complications. Gave a copy of the EKG to Dr. Henderson.

Medical assistant's name and title: Brad Green, RMA

Assignment 4-15: Documenting a Prescription

Work Form Necessary: FORM 4-7

Directions: Using the information given below, document the prescription on Work Form 4-7. Refer to Table 4-4 in textbook for steps for documenting prescriptions.

Patient's name: Holly Hatfield

Patient's DOB: 02/15/1989

Provider's name: Chelsie Wong

Date: 03/18/12

Time prescription prepared: 11:15 a.m.

Name of Rx: Paxil CR 12.5 mg Tablets Number Dispensed 30

Instructions: Take 1 daily

0 Refills

Name of medical assistant: Sasha Disorov, CMA (AAMA)

Assignment 4-16: Documenting a Patient Education Session

Work Form Necessary: FORM 4-7

Directions: Using the information given below, document the patient education session, using Work Form 4-7. Refer to Table 4-5 in the textbook for steps for documenting a patient education session.

Patient's name: Holly Hatfield

Provider's name: Chelsie Wong

Date: 03/18/12

Time of session: 11:30 a.m.

Name of session: Living with Anxiety

Mother present for session: Both Holly and mother appeared to comprehend all of the information. The medical assistant explained how to reduce anxiety and provided tips for what to do when anxiety is present. The patient was given several brochures on anxiety and instructed to call the office if symptoms worsen. Both the mother and patient appeared to comprehend the information.

Name of medical assistant: Sasha Disorov, CMA (AAMA)

FIELD APPLICATION CHALLENGES

Assignment 4-17

Read the following Field Application Challenges and respond to the questions following each scenario.

1. You received a fax from Dr. O'Malley's office concerning Dorothy J. Fuller. She is not a patient at your office nor is she on the referral list. What would you do?

    _____

    _____

2. Leslie Gunther is scheduled for surgery today at 1 p.m. The hospital calls this morning to state the PAT information is not in her chart. You retrieve Leslie's chart and see documentation that states the information was faxed to the hospital three days ago. There is also a copy of the fax confirmation verifying that the information was sent out. What would you do?

    _____

    _____

    _____

    _____

    _____

JOURNALING EXERCISE

Assignment 4-18

What content within this chapter was most meaningful to you? Why? List some examples of how you might apply information contained in this chapter, both during your training and after you enter the health care industry.

Work Form 4-1

PROGRESS NOTE		
Patient Name:		DOB:

DATE/TIME	PROGRESS NOTES	ALLERGIES

Work Form 4-2

URINALYSIS REPORTING FORM

Tested by: _____   Time: _____

Doctor: _____ Location: _____ Date: _____

Leukocytes	Negative ☐		Trace ☐	Small+ ☐	Moderate++ ☐	Large+++ ☐
Nitrite	Negative ☐		Positive ☐	(Any degree of pink color is Positive)		
Urobilinogen	Normal ☐	Normal 1 ☐	2 ☐	4 ☐	8 ☐	
Protein	Negative ☐	Trace ☐	30+ ☐	100++ ☐	300+++ ☐	2000 or more ++++ ☐

pH	5.0 ☐	6.0 ☐	6.5 ☐	7.0 ☐	7.5 ☐	8.0 ☐	8.5 ☐
Blood	Negative ☐	Trace ☐ Non-Hemolyzed	Moderate ☐ Non-Hemolyzed	Large ☐ Hemolyzed	+ ☐ Small	++ ☐ Moderate	+++ ☐ Large
Specific Gravity	1.000 ☐	1.005 ☐	1.010 ☐ Trace	1.015 ☐ Small	1.020 ☐ Moderate	1.025 ☐ Large	1.030 ☐ Large
Ketone	Negative ☐	mg/dL	5 ☐ Small	15 ☐ Moderate	40 ☐ Large	50 ☐	150 ☐
Bilirubin	Negative ☐		+ ☐ 1/10 (tr.)	++ ☐ 1/4	+++ ☐ 1/2	☐ 1	☐ 2 or more
Glucose	Negative ☐	g/dL (%) mg/dL	100 ☐	250 ☐	500 ☐	1000 ☐	2000 ☐ or more

Microscopic

WBC _____ /HPF	EPITHELIAL CELLS _____/HPF	APPEARANCE_____
RBC _____ /HPF	TYPE _____	ODOR _____
CASTS _____ /LPF	TRICHOMONAS _____	COMMENTS: _____
TYPE_____	BACTERIA _____	_____
CRYSTALS _____	OTHER _____	_____
YEAST _____	Color _____	_____

Work Form 4-3

Urinalysis Log

Patient Name	Date	Dr	Glu	Bili	Ket	Blo	SG	pH	Pro	Uro	Nit	WBC	MA

Work Form 4-4

MANAGED CARE PLAN
AUTHORIZATION REQUEST

Aetna	☐	Cigna	☐
Medical Mutual	☐	PurCare	☐
UHC	☐	Other	☐

Member Group ID No. _____

TO BE COMPLETED BY PRIMARY CARE PHYSICIAN OR OUTSIDE PROVIDER

Patient Name: _____ Date: _____

M ___ F ___ Birthdate: _____ Home phone number: _____

Address: _____ Cell phone number: _____

Primary Care Physician: _____ NPI #:_____

Referred to : _____ NPI #:_____

Address:_____

Office phone number: _____

Diagnosis Code: _____ Diagnosis: _____

Diagnosis Code: _____ Diagnosis: _____

Authorization Requested for Procedures/Test/Visits:

Procedure Code: _____ Description: _____

Procedure Code: _____ Description: _____

Facility to be used: _____ Estimated length of stay:_____

Office ☐   Outpatient ☐   Inpatient ☐   Other ☐

List of potential consultants (i.e., anesthetist, assistants, or medical/surgical):_____

Physician's signature: _____

TO BE COMPLETED BY PRIMARY CARE PHYSICIAN

PCP Recommendation: _____ PCP Initials: _____

Date eligibility checked: _____ Effective date:_____

TO BE COMPLETED BY UTILIZATION MANAGEMENT

Authorized _____ Not authorized _____

Deferred _____ Modified _____

Authorization Request #_____

Work Form 4-5

FACSIMILE SHEET

DATE: _____   TIME: _____

TO: _____   Company Name: _____

DEPT: _____   No. of Pages (including this page): _____ pages

Fax Number: _____   Phone Number: _____

FROM: _____   PHONE: _____

DEPT: _____

RE: _____

Comments:

_____

_____

_____

_____

_____

NOTE: This transmittal is intended only for the use of the individual or entity to which it is addressed and may contain information that is privileged, confidential and exempt from disclosure by law. If you are not the intended recipient, any dissemination, distribution, or photocopying of this communication is strictly prohibited. If you have received this communication in error, please notify the office stated below immediately by telephone and return the original fax to us at the address below by U.S. Postal Service. Thank you.

If you cannot read this fax or if pages are missing, please contact:

Raymond, Shue & Beachler

4587 North Street ♦ Yourtown, USA 01234
Office: (123) 456-7890 Fax: (123) 456-7891

Work Form 4-6

PROGRESS NOTE

Patient Name: DOB:

DATE/TIME	PROGRESS NOTES	ALLERGIES

Work Form 4-7

PROGRESS NOTE		
Patient Name:		DOB:

DATE/TIME	PROGRESS NOTES	ALLERGIES

C H A P T E R **5**

Conducting a Patient Interview and Developing a Medical History

FIELD RELEVANCY AND BENEFITS

The medical history is one of the most important documents found in the patient's chart. Regardless of whether you work in a specialty practice or a general practice, the majority of new patients will need to have a history developed. Medical assistants who possess good interviewing skills are instrumental in supplying puzzle pieces that aid the provider in making an accurate diagnosis and in predicting future ailments. Possessing these skills will help to confirm your worth to the provider, thus making you a valued employee.

NOTE SHEET

Therapeutic Communications

_____

_____

_____

_____

Incorporating Effective Interviewing Techniques

_____

_____

_____

Stages of the Patient Interview

_____

_____

_____

_____

Tools Used to Collect Medical History Information

_____

_____

_____

Types of Health Histories	**The Comprehensive Medical History**
_____	_____
_____	_____
_____	_____
_____	_____

VOCABULARY REVIEW

Assignment 5-1: Spelling Review

Find the words below that are misspelled; circle them and then correctly spell them in the spaces provided.

Body language

Emerancy health history

Family medical history

Gesture

Past history

Social history

Usual childhood diseases

Comprehensive medical history

Episodec medical history

Genagram

Interval health history

Proximics

Theraputic communication

_____   _____   _____

_____   _____

Assignment 5-2: Sentence Completion

Fill in the blanks below with Essential Terms from this chapter. (*Hint:* Not all the words will be used.)

1. E.T. Hall defines _____ as "the way people use space in their environment."

2. _____ is best described as an exchange of information between the health care worker and patient that leads to the advancement of the patient's physical and emotional well being.

3. Employing _____ along with verbal communication helps to enhance the message that is being sent and is often incorporated during the questioning phase of the patient interview.

4. Chief complaint in combination with the history of the present illness would be an example of a(n) _____ _____.

5. Defined as a complete health history that covers the patient's personal, social, and family history from the time of birth until the time the history is developed, a(n) _____ is usually performed on the initial visit and updated every one to two years thereafter.

6. A(n) _____ is a type of history that provides the triage team with vital information for diagnosing the patient's condition and for prioritizing the order in which patients are seen.

7. A(n) _____ has two components—a family tree and list of familial diseases.

8. _____ is defined as gestures, postures, and facial expressions by which a person manifests various physical, mental, or emotional states and communicates nonverbally with others.

9. The _____ is the reason the patient is being seen.

10. A(n) _____ includes the patient's previous health concerns, current health concerns, and current medication list.

CHAPTER REVIEW

Assignment 5-3: Acronym Review

Write what each of the following acronyms stands for.

1. UCD: _____
2. UCHD: _____
3. PH: _____
4. PHH: _____
5. ROS: _____
6. CC: _____

Assignment 5-4: Short Answer

1. List three components of body language.

   A. _____

   B. _____

   C. _____

2. Describe two types of tools that are used to collect data for the medical history.

   A. _____

   B. _____

3. List the four stages of the patient interview.

   A. _____

   B. _____

   C. _____

   D. _____

4. What is another sense that is used during active listening? Describe how this sense is being used.

   _____

   _____

5. What are the three parts/sections of the comprehensive medical history? Describe what information would be found in each section.

   A. _____

   _____

   _____

   _____

   B. _____

   _____

   _____

   _____

   C. _____

   _____

   _____

   _____

6. Define proxemics.

_____

_____

7. If possible, how many feet apart should the interviewer be from the patient during the patient interview?

_____

8. What is a genogram and how is it used?

_____

_____

_____

Assignment 5-5: Certification Practice

Choose the best answer and place the corresponding letter in the blank.

_____ 1. The distance when giving the patient a hug is described as:
   A. personal distance.
   B. social distance.
   C. public distance.
   D. intimate distance.

_____ 2. A farmer comes into the office today to be seen about a persistent sore on his face that will not go away. What part of his medical history may be especially helpful to the provider in making a diagnosis on this patient?
   A. Episodic medical history
   B. Personal medical history
   C. Family medical history
   D. Social medical history

_____ 3. A 37-year-old white female is scheduled for her annual exam today. She states that her sister who is 32 years old was recently diagnosed with melanoma and her Grandma Helga was diagnosed with breast cancer at the age of 72. This information would be listed within what part of the comprehensive medical history?
   A. Episodic medical history
   B. Personal medical history
   C. Family medical history
   D. Social medical history

_____ 4. Sally is here to today to discuss the status of her depression after being placed on antidepressant therapy. What type of history information would be important for this type of visit?
   A. Comprehensive medical history
   B. Episodic medical history
   C. Interval or follow-up history
   D. Emergency health history

_____ 5. This type of history is often performed in emergency facilities.
   A. Comprehensive medical history
   B. Episodic medical history
   C. Interval or follow-up history
   D. Emergency health history

_____ 6. Repeating or rephrasing the main idea of the sentence is called:
   A. clarification.
   B. restating.
   C. reflecting.
   D. summarizing.

____ 7. This technique is usually incorporated at the conclusion of the interview.

    A. Clarification

    B. Restating

    C. Reflecting

    D. Summarizing

____ 8. "So your mommy says that your tummy hurts. Can you point to the part of your tummy that hurts the most?" What listening technique would this example describe?

    A. Clarification

    B. Restating

    C. Reflecting

    D. Summarizing

____ 9. Which family members would **not** be included in the family medical history?

    A. Siblings

    B. Parents

    C. Cousins

    D. Grandparents (maternal and paternal)

____ 10. You have a patient coming in today who speaks very little English. Whose responsibility is it to arrange for an interpreter?

    A. The patient

    B. The patient's family

    C. The medical staff

    D. The provider

____ 11. Questions regarding each of the major body systems and parts are known as:

    A. ROS.

    B. CC.

    C. FH.

    D. SH.

____ 12. Lifestyles can have a large impact on the prevention or launching of certain diseases or conditions.

    A. True

    B. False

____ 13. "How long has the pain been going on?" is an example of:

    A. an open-ended question.

    B. a closed-ended question.

    C. using a leading question.

    D. demanding an explanation.

____ 14. All of the following are good examples of "asking close-ended questions" *except:*

    A. On a scale of 1 to 10, how would you rate your pain?

    B. How many episodes of diarrhea have you experienced over the last three days?

    C. How many Extra Strength Tylenol did you take?

    D. What is the reason for your visit today?

____ 15. All of the following are examples of ineffective questioning techniques *except:*

    A. clarifying something that the patient stated that was confusing.

    B. advising the patient on what they need to say.

    C. incorporating medical terms within your questioning.

    D. using leading questions.

SKILL APPLICATION CHALLENGE
Assignment 5-6: Documentation Exercise

Complete a genogram for your family. Either use the example in your textbook to guide you in getting started or go to this Web site: *www.hhs.gov/familyhistory*. The family history should go back at least two generations.

COMPLETING SPECIAL FORMS
Assignment 5-7: Completing a Medical History

Work Form Necessary: FORM 5-1

Directions: Interview a friend, neighbor, or family member who has multiple health problems. Complete Work Form 5-1, a medical history form. On a separate sheet of notebook paper, expound on all Yes questions by asking the following: Duration of Condition, Course of Treatment, Current Status of Condition, and Date of Resolve (if applicable).

FIELD APPLICATION CHALLENGE
Assignment 5-8

Read the following Field Application Challenge and respond to the question following the scenario.

Bailey Tanner, a 16-year-old female, is here today for a physical examination. Bailey's mom is also present for the exam. You notice that Bailey's mom answers all of your questions before Bailey has an opportunity to respond. The last part of the history involves sensitive subject matter regarding the patient's sexual history. Should the mother be allowed to stay during this part of the questioning? List the reasons for your response. If your response is that you would ask the mother to leave, what would be an appropriate way to do so?

_____

_____

_____

_____

_____

_____

_____

_____

JOURNALING EXERCISE
Assignment 5-9

What content within this chapter was most meaningful to you? Why? List some examples of how you might apply information contained in this chapter, both during your training and after you enter the health care industry.

Work Form 5-1

CONFIDENTIAL HEALTH HISTORY

Name: _____ Date: _____

Birthdate: _____ Age: _____ Date of last physical examination: _____

Occupation: _____

Reason for visit today: _____

MEDICATIONS List all medications you are currently taking	**ALLERGIES** List all allergies

SYMPTOMS Check [✓] symptoms you currently have or have had in the past year.

GENERAL
- ☐ Chills
- ☐ Depression
- ☐ Dizziness
- ☐ Fainting
- ☐ Fever
- ☐ Forgetfulness
- ☐ Headache
- ☐ Loss of sleep
- ☐ Loss of weight
- ☐ Nervousness
- ☐ Numbness
- ☐ Sweats

MUSCLE/JOINT/BONE
Pain, weakness, numbness in:
- ☐ Arms
- ☐ Back
- ☐ Feet
- ☐ Hands
- ☐ Hips
- ☐ Legs
- ☐ Neck
- ☐ Shoulders

GENITO-URINARY
- ☐ Blood in urine
- ☐ Frequent urination
- ☐ Lack of bladder control
- ☐ Painful urination

GASTROINTESTINAL
- ☐ Appetite poor
- ☐ Bloating
- ☐ Bowel changes
- ☐ Constipation
- ☐ Diarrhea
- ☐ Excessive hunger
- ☐ Excessive thirst
- ☐ Gas
- ☐ Hemorrhoids
- ☐ Indigestion
- ☐ Nausea
- ☐ Rectal bleeding
- ☐ Stomach pain
- ☐ Vomiting
- ☐ Vomiting blood

CARDIOVASCULAR
- ☐ Chest pain
- ☐ High blood pressure
- ☐ Irregular heart beat
- ☐ Low blood pressure
- ☐ Poor circulation
- ☐ Rapid heart beat
- ☐ Swelling of ankles
- ☐ Varicose veins

EYE, EAR, NOSE, THROAT
- ☐ Bleeding gums
- ☐ Blurred vision
- ☐ Crossed eyes
- ☐ Difficulty swallowing
- ☐ Double vision
- ☐ Earache
- ☐ Ear discharge
- ☐ Hay fever
- ☐ Hoarseness
- ☐ Loss of hearing
- ☐ Nosebleeds
- ☐ Persistent cough
- ☐ Ringing in ears
- ☐ Sinus problems
- ☐ Vision - Flashes
- ☐ Vision - Halos

SKIN
- ☐ Bruise easily
- ☐ Hives
- ☐ Itching
- ☐ Change in moles
- ☐ Rash
- ☐ Scars
- ☐ Sores that won't heal

MEN only
- ☐ Breast lump
- ☐ Erection difficulties
- ☐ Lump in testicles
- ☐ Penis discharge
- ☐ Sore on penis
- ☐ Other

WOMEN only
- ☐ Abnormal Pap Smear
- ☐ Bleeding between periods
- ☐ Breast lump
- ☐ Extreme menstrual pain
- ☐ Hot flashes
- ☐ Nipple discharge
- ☐ Painful intercourse
- ☐ Vaginal discharge
- ☐ Other

Date of last menstrual period _____

Date of last Pap Smear _____

Have you had a mammogram? _____

Are you pregnant? _____

Number of children _____

MEDICAL HISTORY Check [✓] the medical conditions you have or have had in the past.

- ☐ AIDS
- ☐ Alcoholism
- ☐ Anemia
- ☐ Anorexia
- ☐ Appendicitis
- ☐ Arthritis
- ☐ Asthma
- ☐ Bleeding Disorders
- ☐ Breast Lump
- ☐ Bronchitis
- ☐ Bulimia
- ☐ Cancer
- ☐ Cataracts

- ☐ Chemical Dependency
- ☐ Chicken Pox
- ☐ Diabetes
- ☐ Emphysema
- ☐ Epilepsy
- ☐ Gall Bladder Disease
- ☐ Glaucoma
- ☐ Goiter
- ☐ Gonorrhea
- ☐ Gout
- ☐ Heart Disease
- ☐ Hepatitis
- ☐ Hernia

- ☐ Herpes
- ☐ High Cholesterol
- ☐ HIV Positive
- ☐ Kidney Disease
- ☐ Liver Disease
- ☐ Measles
- ☐ Migraine Headaches
- ☐ Miscarriage
- ☐ Mononucleosis
- ☐ Multiple Sclerosis
- ☐ Mumps
- ☐ Pacemaker
- ☐ Pneumonia

- ☐ Polio
- ☐ Prostate Problem
- ☐ Psychiatric Care
- ☐ Rheumatic Fever
- ☐ Scarlet Fever
- ☐ Stroke
- ☐ Suicide Attempt
- ☐ Thyroid Problems
- ☐ Tonsillitis
- ☐ Tuberculosis
- ☐ Typhoid Fever
- ☐ Ulcers
- ☐ Vaginal Infections
- ☐ Venereal Disease

CONFIDENTIAL HEALTH HISTORY

continues

Work Form 5-1 *(continued)*

HOSPITALIZATIONS

Year	Hospital	Reason for Hospitalization and Outcome

Have you ever had a blood transfusion? ☐ Yes ☐ No
If yes, please give approximate dates: _____

OCCUPATIONAL CONCERNS Check (✓) if your work exposes you to the following:	HEALTH HABITS Check (✓) which substances you use and indicate how much you use per day/week.	PREGNANCY HISTORY		
		Year of Birth	Sex of Birth	Complications if any
☐ Stress	☐ Caffeine			
☐ Hazardous Substances	☐ Tobacco			
☐ Heavy Lifting	☐ Drugs			
☐ Other	☐ Alcohol			

SERIOUS ILLNESS/INJURIES	DATE	OUTCOME

FAMILY HISTORY Fill in health information about your family.

Relation	Age	State of Health	Age at Death	Cause of Death	Check (✓) if your blood relatives had any of the following Disease	Relationship to you
Father					☐ Arthritis, Gout	
Mother					☐ Asthma, Hay Fever	
Brothers					☐ Cancer	
					☐ Chemical Dependency	
					☐ Diabetes	
					☐ Heart Disease, Strokes	
Sisters					☐ High Blood Pressure	
					☐ Kidney Disease	
					☐ Tuberculosis	
					☐ Other	

I certify that the above information is correct to the best of my knowledge. I will not hold my doctor or any members of his/her staff responsible for any errors or ommisions that I may have made in the completion of this form.

_____   _____
Signature   Date

_____   _____
Reviewed By   Date

C H A P T E R **6**

Developing In-Office Screening Skills

FIELD RELEVANCY AND BENEFITS

One of the most frequent tasks that medical assistants perform is rooming patients and obtaining the patient's chief complaint. Medical assistants need to develop patient complaints so that that they can properly prepare the patient and set up the room for the examination. The screening skills of the assistant will also help to prepare the provider for the examination by providing insight regarding the patient's symptoms before the provider enters the room. Good screening and anticipation skills are necessary to take your career to the next level.

Medical assistants who possess good screening and anticipation skills will be invaluable to the provider, thus making their "market worth" more, which translates into a higher salary for the medical assistant.

NOTE SHEET

Establishing Boundaries

_____

_____

_____

_____

Improving Anticipation Skills and Following Office Protocol

_____

_____

_____

_____

The Role of the Medical Assistant during In-Office Screenings

_____

_____

_____

The Provider's Role during the Assessment Process

_____

_____

_____

The Follow-Up Appointment/Progress Note

_____

_____

_____

_____

VOCABULARY REVIEW

Assignment 6-1: Matching

Match the term with its definition and place the corresponding letter in the blank.

____ 1. Anticipation skills

____ 2. Duration

____ 3. History of the present illness (HPI)

____ 4. Standing orders

____ 5. Subjective information

____ 6. Symptoms

A. Period of time that the patient has experienced symptoms

B. Information that is supplied by the patient

C. A list of written orders developed by the provider for procedures that are to be performed when the patient complains of specific symptoms (not used much today)

D. A list of signals or signs experienced by the patient which are indicative of a specific disease or condition

E. Ability to know what the provider needs before having to ask

F. A series of symptoms or signs that are related to the patient's complaint

Assignment 6-2: Sentence Completion

Fill in the blanks below with Essential Terms from this chapter.

1. The medical assistant will ask the patient about her _____ (signs or signals) to write the chief complaint.

2. The patient states "I feel like I have been hit by a dump truck. My body aches when I move and my head is pounding." This would be an example of _____.

3. The provider will need to complete her own _____ for reimbursement purposes.

4. _____ will develop over time. These are skills that assist the medical assistant in knowing how to set up the room and patient for the exam.

5. OB-GYN offices are examples of offices that have one set price in place for prenatal visits, the delivery of the baby, and follow-up visits. _____ in this type of practice may include performing a chemical urinalysis on all pregnant patients.

CHAPTER REVIEW

Assignment 6-3: Acronym Review

Write what each of the following acronyms stands for.

1. HPI: _____

2. CC: _____

3. WT: _____

4. HT: _____

5. TPR: _____

6. HA: _____

7. OTC: _____

8. PCN: _____

Assignment 6-4: True or False

Fill in the blank with a "T" for true statements and an "F" for false statements. Rewrite the false statements to make them true.

____ 1. Documenting chief complaint is also known as the reason for the visit.

_____

_____

____ 2. Drug allergies should be written in green so that they stand out.

_____

_____

____ 3. The medical assistant is always responsible for recording both the chief complaint and HPI information.

_____

_____

____ 4. The chief complaint that prompted the patient to seek medical attention is referred to as objective information.

_____

_____

____ 5. The reason military time is used often in medical establishments is that it is more concise and less ambiguous than standard time.

_____

_____

Assignment 6-5: Short Answer

1. What are three parts an in-office screening that may be recorded by the provider?

_____

2. Information that should be recorded during a follow-up interview includes:

_____

_____

3. Information that should be available during a follow-up interview includes:

_____

_____

4. List at least four activities that are part of the provider's role during the assessment process:

_____

_____

_____

5. Give two examples of instances in which global billing may be in place.

_____

6. When working with pediatric patients, it is assumed that their vocabulary is not fully developed. What tool can be used to help establish a child's level of pain? What other types of patients may benefit from this method?

_____

_____

7. Give at least four in-office screening responsibilities of the medical assistant.

_____

_____

_____

_____

Assignment 6-6: Matching

Military time uses the numbers 00 to 23 to identify each of the hours within its system. Match the Standard Time to the Military Time:

Answer	Standard Time	Military Time
____	1. 4:00 p.m.	A. 0130 hours
____	2. 1:00 a.m.	B. 1200 hours
____	3. 8:00 p.m.	C. 1800 hours
____	4. 2:00 a.m.	D. 0200 hours
____	5. 12:00 p.m.	E. 1637 hours
____	6. 1:30 p.m.	F. 0710 hours
____	7. 6:00 p.m.	G. 1330 hours
____	8. 1:30 a.m.	H. 1600 hours
____	9. 7:10 a.m.	I. 0100 hours
____	10. 4:37 p.m.	J. 2000 hours

Assignment 6-7: Certification Practice

Choose the best answer and place the corresponding letter in the blank.

____ 1. When dating a chief complaint or progress note, which format should be used when documenting the date?

   A. Day/month/year

   B. Month/year/day

   C. Month/day/year

   D. Day/year/month

____ 2. What instruments or items should be available for patients complaining of ear symptoms? (Items may be on the tray or off to the side.)

   A. Ophthalmoscope, sterile swabs, pen light, irrigation solution

   B. Pen light, warmed laryngeal mirror

   C. Cautery unit, biopsy container, anesthetic

   D. Otoscope, audiometer, irrigation equipment (4x4s, irrigating solution)

____ 3. A patient complains of urinary symptoms. She states that over the weekend she developed some pain during urination and she has a "burning feeling" when she goes to the bathroom. What might the medical assistant do prior to physician examination?

    A. Perform a chemical urinalysis on the patient.

    B. Perform a microscopic urinalysis on the patient.

    C. Send out a urine specimen for a culture and sensitivity.

    D. If office policy: Collect a clean catch urine specimen from the patient and wait for orders from the provider before doing anything with the urine. (Preserve urine if it is going to be a while by placing it in the refrigerator.)

____ 4. All of the following are part of the provider's role during the assessment process *except:*

    A. performing ROS.

    B. forming a diagnosis.

    C. collecting the chief complaint.

    D. performing an examination of the patient.

____ 5. When the provider or medical assistant questions a patient about the duration of a symptom(s), what are they asking the patient to do?

    A. Describe the symptoms.

    B. List associated symptoms that commonly are associated with the complaint.

    C. Describe how long the symptoms have been present.

    D. None of the above

____ 6. Which question is not associated with a headache?

    A. Visual disturbances?

    B. N/V present?

    C. Coughing episodes?

    D. Location of headache and severity?

____ 7. Which question is not commonly associated with abdominal pain?

    A. N/V present?

    B. Last BM and texture?

    C. Any fever?

    D. Edema in ankles?

____ 8. All would be examples of subjective information *except:*

    A. BP: 120/86

    B. "I feel like a dump truck hit me."

    C. "My head aches."

    D. "I caught my hand in the hedge trimmer."

____ 9. Which information would not be included in a progress note?

    A. Record of patient's compliance for home care instructions

    B. Today's date and time

    C. Drug allergies

    D. How symptoms have been since the patient's last visit

____ 10. Martha is in for a follow-up visit regarding a mole that was removed from her back. The pathology report came back this week. Where should this information be placed to make it easier for the provider to find the results for Martha's visit?

    A. Under the corresponding tabs in the chart (pathology and labs)

    B. Special folder marked labs

    C. Should be attached to the front inside cover of the chart

    D. Should be attached to the rear cover of the chart

___ 11. This center dictates that providers must now show medical necessity for all procedures performed for patients that have Medicare or Medicaid coverage; no procedure can be performed until the provider has had an opportunity to thoroughly examine the patient to determine if the test is medically necessary.

   A. CDC

   B. CMS

   C. NCCAM

   D. NPSG

___ 12. Dr. Leaderman likes her medical assistants to use military time when charting/documenting. Which of the times would indicate 2:30 p.m.?

   A. 0230 hours

   B. 2:30pm

   C. 2230 hours

   D. 1430 hours

___ 13. What is the correct way to record the date and time in a patient's chart?

   A. Begin with date, then time

   B. Patient's chief complaint, then date and time

   C. At the end of the progress note

   D. Date and time are not needed

___ 14. What is the preferred method for signing off a note in the patient's chart?

   A. List initials of your first and last name only.

   B. List first and last name only.

   C. List the initials of your first and last name followed by your credential.

   D. List both your first and last name, followed by your credential.

___ 15. The patient complains of general shortness of breath with no other symptoms. What procedure(s) may be performed?

   A. Respiration

   B. Pulse oximetry

   C. Oxygen therapy

   D. All of the above

SKILL APPLICATION CHALLENGE

Assignment 6-8: Project

Working in pairs, one student should play the part of the patient and the other student should play the part of the medical assistant. (Switch back and forth.) Practice taking the following chief complaints. Practice developing the complaints using Table 6-2 in the textbook. (Keep in mind, you will probably not fully develop the complaint in the field, but learning what questions to ask will help you know how to set up the room for the exam.) At the bottom of each complaint, list what instruments and supplies you would prepare for the provider, how you would have the patient disrobe, and any comfort measures you would provide for the patient.

* 5-year-old complaining of a splinter in his left foot

* 80-year-old female's annual physical with multiple symptoms to report

* Construction worker complaining of debris in his left eye

* 33-year-old male with a migraine

* 30-year-old female complaining of N/V, diarrhea for the past two days

Assignment 6-9: Reading Chart Notes

Decode the following chart note. Put all the information into lay terms. Define the abbreviations and listed medical terms.

Subjective Information

   A. 02-12-2011
      1530 hours

   B. CC: "I think I have a cold" x 5 days.

   C. +Sore throat (10) +R ear pain (7) −Headache. +productive cough (yellow-green phlegm). −fever. Self treatment: 2 Regular Strength Tylenol Cold Tabs q 6 hours × 2 days. (Little Relief). −other OTC medications, −Rx

   D. Allergies: Penicillin and latex

Objective Information

   E. WT: 125 lbs. HT 5'7" T: 99.1-1/4 F R 20 P 76 reg. BP 118/76 $^{L. Arm}$

A. _____

B. _____

C. _____

   _____

   _____

   _____

D. _____

E. _____

   _____

COMPLETING SPECIAL FORMS

Assignment 6-10: Documenting/Charting Exercise

Work Form Necessary: FORM 6-1

Directions: Rewrite the information onto a progress note (Work Form 6-1), using common abbreviations (refer to Appendix A in the textbook).

The patient's name is Shea Mullinar and her date of birth is 10/10/1984. The date of the appointment is November 23, 2011, and the time of the appointment is 1:00 p.m. You are to use military time when recording the time. Patient is here to have sutures removed on her L. thumb. Patient denied any pain at this time. Patient states that she took all of the prescribed antibiotic and followed all home care instructions. The dressing appeared to be clean and dry upon removal and there were no signs of drainage on the bandage. Use your name in the closing signature followed by the initials SMA (for student medical assistant).

FIELD APPLICATION CHALLENGES
Assignment 6-11

Read the following Field Application Challenges and respond to the questions following each scenario.

1. A 32-year-old male patient comes into the office complaining of back pain. He states that he injured his back while lifting a heavy box at work two days ago but didn't think that the injury was serious. He states that the back pain is getting worse and that he now has a burning pain running down his left leg. What additional form(s) will need to be completed for this patient? Why is charting extra-sensitive in these types of cases?

_____

_____

_____

_____

2. You work for one of the most well-respected providers in town. The provider sees over 100 patients each day and relies heavily on her medical assistants. The provider lately has been asking you to do things that are beyond the scope of a medical assistant. You continually tell her that you do not feel comfortable performing the skills she is asking you to perform. She gets very irritated and asks one of the other medical assistants to perform these controversial tasks. The other medical assistant appears to have no problem with performing these tasks. What might you do to help the provider understand your stance on performing these controversial tasks? What should you do if the provider does not agree with your position on performing these tasks?

_____

_____

_____

_____

_____

_____

_____

_____

_____

_____

JOURNALING EXERCISE
Assignment 6-12

What content within this chapter was most meaningful to you? Why? List some examples of how you might apply information contained in this chapter, both during your training and after you enter the health care industry.

Work Form 6-1

PROGRESS NOTE		
Patient Name:		DOB:

DATE/TIME	PROGRESS NOTES	ALLERGIES

C H A P T E R **7**

Conducting Telephone Screenings

FIELD RELEVANCY AND BENEFITS

The telephone is the lifeline of the office. Even though the clinical medical assistant may not be responsible for answering the phone, the medical assistant may have responsibilities for screening patient calls, setting up outside appointments, calling patients with test results, and calling in prescriptions. Learning how to properly screen patients and use various forms of telecommunications technology are skills that should be developed during your medical assisting training program. Technological advances have given us many more options for communicating with patients outside the office including the use of computers, fax machines, and text messaging equipment. Medical assistants who are familiar with proper patient screening techniques and know how to properly use each component of telecommunications technology will be a valuable asset to all types of medical offices.

NOTE SHEET

Customer Service and Telecommunications

_____
_____
_____
_____

Telephone Medicine

_____
_____
_____
_____

Triaging

_____
_____
_____

Screening Patient Test Results

_____
_____
_____

Calling in Prescriptions

_____

_____

_____

Working with TDD or TTY Devices

_____

_____

_____

Sending Faxes

_____

_____

_____

Video Conferencing

_____

_____

_____

Electronic Mail (E-mail)

_____

_____

_____

VOCABULARY REVIEW

Assignment 7-1: Matching

Match the term with its definition and place the corresponding letter in the blank. (Some definitions may be used more than once.)

____ 1. Algorithm

____ 2. Appointment grid

____ 3. Emergency medical service or EMS

____ 4. Panic lab value

____ 5. Telecommunications

____ 6. Telecommunications device for the deaf (TDD)

____ 7. Teletypewriter (TTY)

____ 8. Telephone triage

____ 9. Telephone screener

____ 10. Triaging

A. A value which requires the immediate attention of a qualified provider; it may or may not be considered life-threatening but usually is quite serious

B. Sending electromagnet signals through such devices as the telephone, television, radio, and computer modem

C. Specially trained to use a telephone screening manual that lists common types of concerns that patients call about for that particular practice. The person giving instructions never makes any decision without the aid of a screening manual or provider.

D. Sorting patients according to the extent of their injuries or illnesses

E. Lists specific symptoms under a list of appointment actions

F. Listens to the patient's symptoms and determines what action to take as a result; may be considered practicing medicine over the phone.

G. Devices which allow deaf patients to type messages between the medical office staff and the patient

H. Decision tree; includes step-by-step protocol which states an action that should be taken based on the patient's response

I. A service providing prehospital care to patients who are acutely ill or who have life-threatening injuries or illnesses

Assignment 7-2: Sentence Completion

Fill in the blanks below with Essential Terms from this chapter.

1. The clinical medical assistant may use either of these two devices to communicate messages to deaf patients regarding lab results or prescription information: _____.

2. _____ is defined as: a value which requires the immediate attention of a qualified practitioner.

3. This is a role that the medical assistant can perform on patients who call into the office with symptoms:

   _____.

4. Sorting patients according to the extent of injuries or illnesses. Patients who have life-threatening illnesses or injuries are seen before patients with milder symptoms. This process is called: _____.

CHAPTER REVIEW

Assignment 7-3: Acronym Review

Write what each of the following acronyms stands for.

1. EMS: _____

2. TTY: _____

3. TDD: _____

Assignment 7-4: True or False

Fill in the blank with a "T" for true statements and an "F" for false statements. Rewrite the false statements to make them true.

____ 1. A technique that can help you remember to smile is to place a mirror in front of the telephone.

   _____

   _____

____ 2. Patients with acute symptoms are always scheduled for a same-day appointment.

   _____

   _____

____ 3. Patients calling in with life-threatening symptoms should be encouraged to come in immediately to be seen by the provider.

   _____

   _____

____ 4. A medical assistant performing the functions of a telephone screener should not perform screenings unless the practitioner is on-site.

   _____

   _____

____ 5. The documentation of telephone encounters is just as important as the telephone screening itself.

   _____

   _____

____ 6. It is not important to correct a patient who refers to you as the physician's nurse.

   _____

   _____

Assignment 7-5: Short Answer

1. What are five types of life-threatening emergencies?

   _____

   _____

   _____

2. Why are patients today more prone to seek the services of several physicians throughout their life span?

   _____

   _____

   _____

3. Name at least two components of an effective telephone screening program.

   _____

   _____

   _____

   _____

4. What three attributes are essential for someone taking on the role of a telephone screener?

   _____

   _____

   _____

5. Before the screening process begins, medical assistants should perform what steps?

   A. _____

   _____

   B. _____

   _____

   C. _____

   _____

6. Why should panic values be handled as soon as possible?

   _____

   _____

7. Audrey has tried to reach Dr. Rich's patient by phone regarding her blood work for the past two days. The blood work is normal and there are no concerns. The patient does not have voice mail or answering machine. What are some other options for Audrey?

   _____

   _____

8. Elizabeth has reached the answering machine at the Rose's residence. The office's "notice of privacy" states that the office may leave limited information on the patient's answering machine unless the patient requests that no information be left on the answering machine. The patient has not requested that "no information be left on the answering machine." What information can Elizabeth leave on the answering machine?

   _____

   _____

9. What information should be given to the pharmacist when requesting a prescription?

_____

_____

_____

_____

10. Name at least three instances in which a medical assistant may use e-mail.

_____

_____

_____

_____

Assignment 7-6: Certification Practice

Choose the best answer and place the corresponding letter in the blank.

_____ 1. All are nonlife-threatening emergencies *except:*

A. strep throat.

B. fever.

C. SOB.

D. N/V.

_____ 2. If the medical assistant is going to handle sick calls from patients, he should take on the role of a:

A. screener.

B. nurse.

C. triager.

D. interpreter.

_____ 3. When may a medical assistant give out test results?

A. Any time a lab sends the report over

B. After the provider reviews the report and releases the medical assistant to give out the information

C. When the patient calls in to ask for lab results

D. When another medical assistant states that you can give the patient the lab results

_____ 4. You are a floater for the cardiology office. You are filling in today to assist with the front desk. A call comes in from a relay operator. Who is likely to be on the other line?

A. Another provider

B. Deaf patient

C. Limited English patient

D. Patient rescheduling an appointment

_____ 5. A pharmacist calls requesting approval to refill a patient's medication. You should:

A. take a message and tell the pharmacist that you will give the information to the patient's provider.

B. tell the pharmacy that all patients need to see their provider before any refills are given.

C. check the chart to see if any refills have been approved; if not check with the provider.

D. transfer the call directly to the provider.

_____ 6. Video conferencing may be used for all of the following *except:*

A. to discuss health-related information with a patient with limited English or who is deaf.

B. to teach students how to perform various surgeries and other procedures.

C. to talk with friends who have a video camera hooked up to their computers.

D. to monitor patients who are chronically ill and unable to visit the provider.

____ 7. What types of calls can a medical assistant handle without checking with the provider first?

    A. Unsatisfactory progress reports from patients

    B. A patient requesting x-ray results

    C. A request for a prescription refill that has been approved in the patient's chart

    D. A call from the hospital wanting to discuss a patient's progress

____ 8. If a caller asks for medical advice from a medical assistant, the medical assistant should:

    A. put the patient on hold and call 911.

    B. offer advice.

    C. explain why he cannot give out medical advice and urge the patient to set up an appointment with the provider or transfer the call to the provider.

    D. hang up on the patient.

____ 9. After speaking with the patient on the telephone, a medical assistant must always:

    A. schedule an appointment for the patient.

    B. document the conversation.

    C. meet with the health care team to discuss the call.

    D. bill the patient for the telephone call.

____ 10. Which item(s) should be included on a fax cover sheet?

    A. The person for whom the fax is intended

    B. Phone and fax number of the receiving party

    C. Confidentiality statement

    D. All of the above

SKILL APPLICATION CHALLENGES

Assignment 7-7: Documentation Exercise

Mrs. Lemmon calls to update the physician regarding how well a new sleeping medication is working. The medical assistant wrote the message shown below. Provide the missing components on the lines provided after the message form.

Message Form	
To: Dr. Morgan	Date and Time: 08/12/2012
From: Mrs. Lemmon	
Phone Number:	
Message: Following up with you after being placed on Ambien. Patient states she is	
sleeping much better now ("5-7 hours per night"). The only problem is that patient	
states that she is feeling jittery throughout the day. Also having problems with	
memory. Wants to know if these symptoms will go away.	
Action to be taken: Please call patient back.	
Message taken by: Melinda Parker, CMA	

Missing information: _____

_____

Assignment 7-8: Project

Using numbers from your local phonebook, make a list of telephone numbers that would be commonly used when working in a medical facility.

Organization	Telephone Number
Poison control center	_____
Hospitals (with emergency numbers)	_____
Police (nonemergency)	_____
Fire department (nonemergency)	_____
Public health facilities:	
Urgent Care	_____
American Red Cross	_____
Medicaid agencies	_____
Family health services:	
Psychologists	_____
Social services	_____
St. Vincent DePaul Society	_____
Meals on Wheels	_____
Other	_____
WIC program and services	_____
Associations:	
American Cancer Society	_____
American Lung Association	_____
Easter Seals	_____
Other	_____

COMPLETING SPECIAL FORMS

Assignment 7-9: Completing a Telephone Message Form

Work Forms Necessary: FORM 7-1, FORM 7-2

Directions: Using the scenario information below, arrange the information onto the telephone message form, using Work Form 7-1. Then, put the same information onto a Progress Note (Work Form 7-2). Use military time when documenting the time.

On May 17, 2012, Paige Robinson calls the office at 10:30 a.m. to state her daughter, Lauren (DOB 11/11/2011), woke up with tiny bumps all over her body; has a temperature of 101.2°F; is cranky; and has not taken a bottle since 9:00 p.m. last evening. Lauren was seen yesterday for her 6-month check-up. She received the following immunizations: Rota, DTaP, Hib, and PCV. Mom gave Lauren Infant Tylenol two hours ago, but there is no change in her temperature. The number where Paige can be reached is 412-335-7845. Lauren's provider is Dr. Bailey. (Paige has no known drug allergies.)

FIELD APPLICATION CHALLENGES

Assignment 7-10

Read the following Field Application Challenges and respond to the questions following each scenario.

1. A patient calls the office stating that he has chest pain that is radiating down his left arm, neck, and jaw, and that he is having problems breathing. The patient is alone. What should the medical assistant do next?

   _____

   _____

   _____

   _____

2. In the space below, write an away message that you would leave on your e-mail stating that you will be out of the office to attend a conference for one week.

   _____

   _____

   _____

JOURNALING EXERCISE

Assignment 7-11

What content within this chapter was most meaningful to you? Why? List some examples of how you might apply information contained in this chapter, both during your training and after you enter the health care industry.

Work Form 7-1

Message Form
To: Date and Time:
From:
Phone Number:
Message:
Action to be taken:
Message taken by:

Work Form 7-2

PROGRESS NOTE		
Patient Name:		DOB:

DATE/TIME	PROGRESS NOTES	ALLERGIES

C H A P T E R **8**

Assisting Patients with Special Needs

FIELD RELEVANCY AND BENEFITS

Working in the health care industry presents many challenges due to the many types of patients that you will serve. Illness and injury do not discriminate. The medical assistant must be prepared to work with patients from all cultures and all age groups and must be properly prepared to assist patients with physical and mental disabilities.

Working with such a diverse group of patients may be a bit awkward and challenging if you have not been properly prepared to do so. The contents of this chapter will enlighten you of the laws that protect special populations and will provide you with tips on how to improve communication with special needs patients. Information within this chapter is applicable to the majority of practices in which medical assistants work.

NOTE SHEET

Legal Issues and Special Needs Patients

_____

_____

_____

_____

Working with Patients with Special Needs

_____

_____

_____

_____

VOCABULARY REVIEW

Assignment 8-1: Matching

Match the term with its definition and place the corresponding letter in the blank.

____ 1. ADA Standards for Accessible Design

____ 2. Auxiliary services

____ 3. Civil Rights Act

____ 4. Guide dogs

____ 5. Limited English proficiency (LEP)

____ 6. Mental health

____ 7. Mental illness

____ 8. Mental impairment

____ 9. Mentally challenged

____ 10. Postlingual

____ 11. Prelingual

____ 12. Sighted guide assistance

A. English is not the primary language and the individual has a difficult time reading, speaking, or comprehending English

B. Patient who became deaf after she started talking

C. How people look at themselves, their lives, and the other people in their lives; evaluate their challenges and problems; and explore choices

D. Sighted individual who gives a blind individual assistance in walking

E. Brain functions at a subnormal intellectual level

F. Disorder that disrupts a person's ability to think, feel, and relate to others

G. Aids that will help to ensure effective communication when working with deaf patients

H. Prohibits discrimination against someone because of race, color, sex, national origin, or religion

I. Patient who became deaf before she started talking

J. Dogs specially trained to guide their visually impaired or blind owners

K. Condition or illness which impairs the mind's ability to process information in a "normal" fashion

L. Mandates construction companies to design buildings that are accessible to all persons, including those who have dexterity and limited mobility problems

Assignment 8-2: Misspelled Words

Underline the correctly spelled term.

1. Demenita   Dementia   Dimentia

2. mental ilness   mantal illness   mental illness

3. fiscal disablity physical disbility physical disability

4. diversity   diverisity   divercity

5. culuture   culture   calture

6. singed English   signed Enlish   signed English

7. Telecommuniciation Telecommunicaiton Telecommunication

8. Assistance   Assistanse   Asistance

CHAPTER REVIEW

Assignment 8-3: Acronym Review

Write what each of the following acronyms stands for.

1. ADA: _____
2. ADAAG: _____
3. ASL: _____
4. CASE: _____
5. SEE: _____
6. TTY: _____
7. TRS: _____
8. TDD: _____

Assignment 8-4: True or False

Fill in the blank with a "T" for true statements and an "F" for false statements. Rewrite the false statements to make them true.

____ 1. Pediatric offices are usually slow-paced.

_____

_____

____ 2. Patients with dementia usually only experience difficulty with large tasks.

_____

_____

____ 3. Body language is an integral part of the communication process.

_____

_____

____ 4. The ADA accommodates only disabled veterans.

_____

_____

____ 5. Whenever a guide dog is wearing a harness, it means the dog is "working."

_____

_____

____ 6. Brochures should state that interpreting services are available for patients with LEP at no extra charge.

_____

_____

____ 7. You should show a child the needle and syringe so that she can prepare herself mentally for the injection.

_____

_____

____ 8. All seniors become distressed when health care workers have body piercings and tattoos in unusual places.

_____

_____

___ 9. When leading a blind person, you should reach out and grasp the person's arm.

___ 10. Be careful what you say in front of a deaf person, because she may be able to read lips.

Assignment 8-5: Short Answer

1. What is the most common sign language used in the United States and parts of Canada?

2. List three tips that can be used when performing invasive procedures on a pediatric patient.

3. What are the proper steps for providing sighted guide assistance to a blind patient?

4. Why might a senior adult state a sentence like, "You are so rough"?

5. What is the purpose of the Americans with Disabilities Act (ADA)?

6. Name at least four population groups that are included in the ADA provision.

7. New building codes require Braille plates for identification purposes. Name at least three locations where the plates should be placed.

8. Why is it better to use a professional interpreter as opposed to a family member or friend during a patient office visit?

_____

_____

_____

_____

_____

9. List four examples of auxiliary aids and services that can be used to assist hearing-impaired and deaf patients.

_____

_____

_____

10. How should a medical assistant navigate a blind patient up the stairs?

_____

_____

_____

11. List three examples of "accessible design" features that can accommodate patient with disabilities.

_____

_____

_____

_____

_____

Assignment 8-6: Certification Practice

Choose the best answer and place the corresponding letter in the blank.

____ 1. Which culture believes that blood is the source of life and that it isn't regenerated? The patient might be apprehensive about having blood drawn.
   A. Western population
   B. Latin American population
   C. Asian population
   D. Middle Eastern population

____ 2. Which culture usually opposes male health care providers from examining female patients?
   A. Western population
   B. Latin American population
   C. Asian population
   D. Middle Eastern population

____ 3. The average life expectancy today is what age?
   A. 65 years
   B. 75 years
   C. 80 years
   D. 85 years

____ 4. What is the name that most seniors prefer to be addressed as?

    A. First name

    B. Honey, Sweetie

    C. Last name

    D. Mr. or Mrs.

____ 5. What color leash would a hearing guide dog be wearing?

    A. Orange

    B. Yellow

    C. Blue

    D. Red

____ 6. All gestures do not mean the same thing to all cultures. What gesture would be considered acceptable by most people?

    A. Direct eye contact

    B. Proxemics

    C. Warm smile

    D. Pointing a finger

____ 7. Who would be responsible for arranging for an interpreter during an office visit for an LEP patient?

    A. The provider's office

    B. The patient

    C. The family of the patient

    D. The government

____ 8. When assisting blind patients, all would be correct procedures *except:*

    A. Introduce "new" people as they enter the area and let the patient know where people are positioned in reference to the patient.

    B. Use sight words.

    C. Use verbal cues.

    D. Move the patient's personal belongings without their knowledge.

____ 9. When working with an interpreter, the correct room arrangement would be:

    A. Place the chairs in a row.

    B. Set the room up in circular pattern.

    C. Set the room up in triangular pattern.

    D. Set the room up so the medical assistant is beside the patient.

____ 10. Speech reading is also known as which of the following?

    A. Tongue movement

    B. Facial gestures

    C. Reading lips

    D. Listening

____ 11. What is paramount in the eyes of most seniors?

    A. Professionalism

    B. Work ethic

    C. Articulation of medical terminology

    D. Compliments and the nice gestures

____ 12. Impairment that restricts or prevents normal functioning of a particular limb or group of limbs would be termed:

    A. mental illness.

    B. dementia.

    C. mental impairment.

    D. physical disability.

____ 13. Mental impairment may be brought on by:

    A. mental illness.

    B. brain damage.

    C. senility.

    D. all of the above.

____ 14. The National Institute of Mental Health states that one in five adults suffers from:

    A. mental disorder.

    B. dementia.

    C. physical disability.

    D. culture diversity.

____ 15. Contributing factors of dementia include all of the following *except:*

    A. income level.

    B. Alzheimer's disease.

    C. alcoholism.

    D. traumatic brain injury.

____ 16. Which of the following would be the ideal person to use as an interpreter for a patient with limited English?

    A. Spouse of the patient that speaks English

    B. A coworker that has taken some courses in the native language of the patient

    C. An interpreter who has a complete understanding of the patient's native language and is trained to do medical interpreting

    D. None of the above

____ 17. Touching is usually practiced more in what population(s)?

    A. Asian population

    B. Russian population

    C. Latin population

    D. Both B and C

SKILL APPLICATION CHALLENGES

Assignment 8-7: Projects

1. Select your own culture group or one in which you are interested (Japanese, Greek, Irish, etc.) and do an Internet search for issues related to aging in that group using "____-elderly." Write a half-page summary on your findings.

2. Contact an interpreting company and find out how much it would cost to have an interpreter come out to your location and provide interpreting services for one hour for the following: an Arabic interpreter, a blind interpreter, and a Spanish interpreter.

FIELD APPLICATION CHALLENGE

Assignment 8-8

Read the following Field Application Challenge and respond to the question following the scenario.

You work for a family practice. Joshua, an 11-year-old MRDD patient, is here with his mother. He needs to have his blood drawn and have his MMR shot today. For the most part, Joshua does a good job of sitting still, but has a history of moving during invasive procedures. How will you approach Joshua?

_____

_____

_____

_____

JOURNALING EXERCISE
Assignment 8-9

What content within this chapter was most meaningful to you? Why? List some examples of how you might apply information contained in this chapter, both during your training and after you enter the health care industry.

C H A P T E R **9**

Patient Education

FIELD RELEVANCY AND BENEFITS

Patient education is an essential component of the health care process and usually includes topics related to health maintenance, disease management, and preparation instructions for diagnostic procedures. The medical assistant must be prepared to provide the patient with current instructional information and a list of available resources that will assist the patient in overall compliance. The information in this chapter is applicable to a variety of different practices, especially specialty practices.

NOTE SHEET

Adult Education Principles

_____
_____
_____
_____

Stimulating Patient Compliance

_____
_____
_____
_____

Settings and Procedures

_____
_____
_____
_____

Topics for Education

_____
_____
_____
_____

Communication

_____
_____
_____
_____

Conducting Educational Sessions over the Telephone

_____
_____
_____
_____

Identifying Community Resources for the Patient

_____

_____

_____

_____

VOCABULARY REVIEW

Assignment 9-1: Matching

Match the term with its definition and place the corresponding letter in the blank.

____ 1. Active listening

A. Learns more by reading or looking at pictures

____ 2. Audio learner

B. Involves focusing on the information at hand, not allowing your mind to wander, and observing the patient for additional cues other than what they are stating verbally.

____ 3. Echoing

C. Learns more by listening to information

____ 4. Tactile learner

D. Involves simple repetition of the material

____ 5. Visual learner

E. Learns most by touching, holding, or by doing

Assignment 9-2: Sentence Completion

Fill in the blanks below with Essential Terms from this chapter.

1. _____ is an effective technique in verbal communication. This technique helps alleviate the patient's stress

   and anxiety.

2. _____ means to let the patient know you consider his feelings legitimate.

3. _____ is a summary of the learning session. It serves two purposes. First, it restates the material that is to

   be reviewed and learned. Secondly, it tells the patient that you have also been listening to their input.

4. _____ is a way to identify the patient's feelings and respond with understanding.

5. _____ includes a variety of questions. These questions then draw the patient into the conversation,

   which is a key principle of adult education.

CHAPTER REVIEW

Assignment 9-3: Short Answer

1. Name five characteristics of an adult learner.

   A. _____

   B. _____

   C. _____

   D. _____

   E. _____

2. Name the three types of learners and describe the way each learns best.

   A. _____

   B. _____

   C. _____

3. Describe at least two common educational topics presented over the phone.

_____

_____

_____

4. List five barriers that can impede the educational process.

_____

Assignment 9-4: Matching

Match the term with its definition and place the corresponding letter in the blank.

____ 1. Adaptive questioning

____ 2. Echoing

____ 3. Empathy

____ 4. Validation

____ 5. Reassurance

____ 6. Summarization

A. Way to identify the patient's feelings and respond with understanding. Used to strengthen rapport with the patient.

B. Restates the material reviewed and learned. You have listened to the patient's input.

C. Helps to alleviate the stress that the patient might be experiencing.

D. Repeating of the material. Promotes interaction and clarification.

E. To let the patient know you consider his feelings legitimate.

F. Questions that draw the patient into the conversation. Allows the educator to evaluate the patient's understanding.

Assignment 9-5: True or False

Fill in the blank with a "T" for true statements and an "F" for false statements. Rewrite the false statements to make them true.

____ 1. Nonverbal communication includes the use of body language, eye contact, and active listening.

_____

_____

____ 2. When conducting a patient education session regarding how to take medication, there is no need to document the session or have the patient repeat back the information.

_____

_____

____ 3. The highest level of patient education occurs when the health care worker is cognizant of learning theories and strategies and has a basic understanding of educational principles.

_____

_____

____ 4. A highly motivated patient is more likely to be a noncompliant patient because they feel like they know more than the educator.

_____

_____

____ 5. The more senses used in learning, the more material will be retained.

_____

_____

____ 6. Begin each patient education session by setting goals together of what each party wants to obtain from the session.

_____

_____

____ 7. Active listening usually employs good eye contact.

_____

_____

Assignment 9-6: Certification Practice

Choose the best answer and place the corresponding letter in the blank.

____ 1. This type of verbal communication involves simple repetition of the material.

   A. Adaptive questioning

   B. Echoing

   C. Empathy

   D. Validation

____ 2. The first step in the development of a patient education session is to:

   A. document it in the patient's chart.

   B. evaluate the effectiveness of the education session.

   C. decide which tool you will use for the session.

   D. identify the purpose and topic of the education session.

____ 3. The term noncompliance means:

   A. refusing to follow prescribed orders.

   B. patient only half-listens to what is stated during the educational session.

   C. patient doesn't like the physician.

   D. none of the above.

____ 4. This type of verbal communication involves letting the patient know you consider his feelings legitimate.

   A. Adaptive questioning

   B. Echoing

   C. Empathy

   D. Validation

____ 5. Ways to stimulate patient compliance include:

   A. Include family members in the session.

   B. Follow up each session with written material.

   C. Call the patient, one to two days after the session.

   D. Be a role model.

   E. all of the above.

____ 6. All are common topics for patient education *except:*

   A. smoking cessation.

   B. Medicare and Medicaid new reimbursement procedures.

   C. diabetes management.

   D. heart health.

____ 7. All are examples of patient community resources *except:*

    A. social service organizations.

    B. interpreting services.

    C. Chamber of Commerce.

    D. public health and human services.

____ 8. Barriers that may prohibit patient compliance include:

    A. transportation.

    B. interest.

    C. time.

    D. all of the above.

____ 9. Lecture, presentation, CDs, and audio tapes are excellent tools for which of the following learning styles?

    A. Visual

    B. Audio

    C. Tactile

    D. All of the above

____ 10. The overall purpose of patient education is to:

    A. involve patients in volunteer work.

    B. provide patient with the latest news in medicine.

    C. promote health.

    D. meet with the patient one-on-one.

____ 11. Examples of educational sessions over the telephone would include all of the following *except:*

    A. self exams.

    B. introduction of new medication.

    C. special dietary changes.

    D. instructions for the patient to see a specialist.

____ 12. All are theories regarding adult education *except:*

    A. Increasing *self-esteem* is a strong motivator for the adult patient.

    B. Adults prefer to *set the pace* for their learning, controlling start and stop times.

    C. Adults prefer group activities over self-directed activities.

    D. Adults often *seek out information,* which assists in understanding and coping with disease and treatment.

____ 13. If a patient is hearing impaired, what would be the best tools to be incorporated into the educational session?

    A. Videotapes

    B. Handouts

    C. Taped lecture

    D. CDs

____ 14. Tools that would be helpful for blind patients during a patient education session include:

    A. pamphlets and brochures.

    B. videotapes.

    C. posters.

    D. Braille materials.

____ 15. Illustrating the value of the educational session would help to nurture what adult learner characteristic?

    A. Autonomous

    B. Extensive life experience

    C. Goal-oriented

    D. Practical

    E. Need for respect

_____ 16. Illustrating why a patient education session is useful would help to nurture what adult learner characteristic?

    A. Autonomous

    B. Extensive life experience

    C. Goal-oriented

    D. Practical

    E. Need for respect

_____ 17. Involving the patient in the learning process, rather than just supplying facts, would help to nurture which adult learner characteristic?

    A. Autonomous

    B. Extensive life experience

    C. Goal-oriented

    D. Practical

    E. Need for respect

SKILL APPLICATION CHALLENGES

Assignment 9-7: Projects

1. Select a disease or disorder about which to educate the students in your class. You can deliver a presentation using PowerPoint, or you may give a speech in regards to your topic. You should use a variety of visual aids. Key points should include the following: The name of the disease or condition, symptoms of the disease, risk factors for the disease, diagnostic tools used to diagnose the disease, treatment options, and tips for living with the disease. Consider the members of your audience. How would they learn best? Do you have access to audiovisual equipment or the Internet? Who can provide you with additional information?

2. As a medical assistant in a pediatric office, you are given the task of updating the patient education files. The file contains handouts on immunizations, nutrition, and healthy/exercise lifestyles. Many of the handouts are old. Do an Internet search and review the top diseases that are plaguing pediatric patients today. List five new educational topics you would include and provide materials for each one.

3. Make up a list of support groups along with their contact information that are available in your community. Look in the phone book, on Web sites, in local hospital directories, or in local newspapers. Be prepared to share this information with class members. Once all of the class has shared their findings, merge the lists so that one new list contains everyone's information. Display the list somewhere in the classroom so that it can be used as a reference when teaching patient education sessions.

FIELD APPLICATION CHALLENGES

Assignment 9-8

Read the following Field Application Challenges and respond to the questions following each scenario. Utilize the Internet to help you answer some of the questions.

1. You work for a dermatology office. What advice might you give to an 11-year-old fair-skinned girl who is planning to visit her grandparents in Florida for the summer?

_____

_____

_____

_____

2. You work for an orthopedic office. One of your patients is a child who just had a cast put on his arm. What would be helpful information for this patient and his parents?

_____

_____

_____

_____

_____

_____

_____

JOURNALING EXERCISE
Assignment 9-9

What content within this chapter was most meaningful to you? Why? List some examples of how you might apply information contained in this chapter, both during your training and after you enter the health care industry.

CHAPTER **10**

Principles of Infection Control and OSHA Standards

FIELD RELEVANCY AND BENEFITS

Being familiar with OSHA guidelines and other infection control principles is important, regardless of the type of practice in which you work. As a medical assistant, you will encounter infection control issues in all practices and you will be expected to adhere to OSHA standards in any and all specialty practices. Some practices will present more hazards and exposure risks than others. The implementation of good infection control techniques will help to reduce the risk of transmitting diseases such as AIDS, hepatitis, and other infectious diseases from one patient to another and from the patient to the health care worker.

NOTE SHEET

The Infection Process

_____
_____
_____
_____

The Chain of Infection

_____
_____
_____
_____

Environmental Requirements for Microorganisms

_____
_____
_____
_____

Stages of Infection

_____
_____
_____
_____

The Body's Mechanisms of Defense

_____

_____

_____

_____

Infection Control

_____

_____

_____

_____

Universal Blood and Body Fluid Precautions

_____

_____

_____

_____

Commonly Transmitted Bloodborne Diseases

_____

_____

_____

_____

OSHA Regulations

_____

_____

_____

_____

Exposure to Hazardous Chemicals

_____

_____

_____

_____

Safeguards in the Educational Environment

_____

_____

_____

_____

VOCABULARY REVIEW

Assignment 10-1: Matching

Match the term with its definition and place the corresponding letter in the blank.

____ 1. Antigen

____ 2. Antibody

____ 3. Biohazard

____ 4. Engineering controls

____ 5. Fomite

____ 6. Normal flora

____ 7. Seroconversion

____ 8. Sharps

____ 9. Bloodborne pathogen

____ 10. Epidemiology

____ 11. Immunity

____ 12. Pathogen

____ 13. Medical asepsis

____ 14. Opportunistic infection

____ 15. Vector

A. Inanimate (nonliving) object contaminated with infectious material, capable of transmitting disease

B. Microorganisms usually present in different parts of the body that do not pose a threat to the host

C. The point that detectable antibodies are present in the serum, causing a positive antibody test.

D. A protein particle capable of neutralizing or controlling a specific antigen

E. Invading organism such as a bacteria or virus, that stimulates antibody production within the body

F. Devices such as needles, slides, and such that could cause puncture wounds or other injuries to the skin

G. Any substance contaminated with blood or body fluids that could transmit disease

H. Devices and practices used to separate employees from workplace hazards

I. Microorganisms that cause disease

J. Carriers of microorganisms such as insects or rodents

K. Destruction of microorganisms after they leave the body

L. Infections that do not normally occur unless the infected individual has a weakened immune system

M. The study of infectious disease

N. Protection from disease

O. A pathogen that can be transmitted through blood or OPIM

Assignment 10-2: Misspelled Words

Underline the correctly spelled term.

1. epidemiology   epedemiology   epademiology

2. immunosupresed   imunosupresed   immunosuppressed

3. resistence   resistance   resistince

4. immunoglobulen   immunoglobulin   imunoglobulin

5. sanitization   sanitazation   sanatization

CHAPTER REVIEW

Assignment 10-3: Acronym Review

Write what each of the following acronyms stands for.

1. HIV: _____

2. AIDS: _____

3. OPIM: _____

4. OSHA: _____

5. PPE: _____

6. MSDS: _____

Assignment 10-4: True or False

Fill in the blank with a "T" for true statements and an "F" for false statements. Rewrite the false statements to make them true.

____ 1. Each step in the chain of infection must occur to spread an infectious disease.

_____

_____

____ 2. Bacteria are multicelled organisms that lack a nucleus.

_____

_____

____ 3. Almost anything can serve as a reservoir in the chain of infection.

_____

_____

____ 4. Medical asepsis is the destruction of microorganisms after they leave the body.

_____

_____

____ 5. The terms inflammation and infection are synonymous with one another.

_____

_____

____ 6. Administration of a vaccine would be an example of artificial active immunity.

_____

_____

____ 7. BSI is a component of universal precautions and is practiced in all health care facilities.

_____

_____

____ 8. A patient with HIV will definitely develop AIDS.

_____

_____

____ 9. Hepatitis C can be contracted through an organ transplant.

_____

_____

____ 10. The Bloodborne Pathogens Standard was developed to reduce the risk of needlestick injuries.

_____

_____

____ 11. PPE provides a protective barrier between the health care worker and infectious body fluids such as blood or OPIM.

_____

_____

____ 12. A sharps container would fall under the category of engineering controls.

_____

_____

____ 13. The stage of an HIV infection in which seroconversion takes place is during the primary stage of infection.

_____

_____

____ 14. Diagnostic criteria for HIV include: a positive confirmatory test for HIV and one of the following: CD4 count < 200 or < 14% of total lymphocyte count, or the presence of an opportunistic infection.

_____

_____

____ 15. Examples of opportunistic infections include: candida infections, cytomegalovirus, and *Pneumocystis carinii* pneumonia.

_____

_____

____ 16. The use of chemical agents to destroy microorganisms is termed as sterilization.

_____

_____

____ 17. All employees must receive OSHA training within 90 days of their first day of employment.

_____

_____

____ 18. Water temperature at the eyewash station should not exceed 100°F or 37°C.

_____

_____

____ 19. Medical records associated with an exposure incident must be kept separate from the employee's personnel record and must be on file for the length of employment plus 30 years.

_____

_____

____ 20. A 5% bleach solution is an effective disinfectant to use when cleaning surfaces contaminated with blood or OPIM.

_____

_____

Assignment 10-5: Short Answer

1. List the five classifications of pathogenic organisms.

   _____

2. List and describe the six stages of infection.

   _____

   _____

   _____

   _____

   _____

3. Describe the purpose of the inflammatory response.

   _____

   _____

4. List both local and systemic signs of inflammation.

   _____

   _____

5. Place the appropriate letter (B=biohazard container, S=sharps container, R=regular trash) beside each type of medical waste that corresponds with proper disposal of biohazardous wastes when following OSHA guidelines.

   A. Microbiology specimens   _____

   B. Dressing that contains blood or OPIM   _____

   C. Cover slips   _____

   D. Empty urine container   _____

   E. Surgical pathology specimens   _____

   F. Used gloves with no visible blood or OPIM   _____

   G. Used needles   _____

   H. Fecal specimen container   _____

   I. Drapes with vaginal secretions   _____

   J. Empty containers that held semen samples   _____

6. Under what circumstances might a health care facility dispose of items contaminated with all types of body fluids—including urine, saliva, and stool—into the biohazardous trash?

   _____

7. List and describe the environmental factors or conditions that must be present in order for a microorganism to grow and prosper.

   _____

   _____

   _____

   _____

   _____

   _____

8. List some ways that you can prevent or reduce microbial growth in the office.

_____

_____

_____

_____

9. What two classifications of workers must be included when considering employees at risk of exposure incidents? Give examples of the types of employees that may fit into these categories.

_____

_____

_____

_____

Assignment 10-6: Certification Practice

Choose the best answer and place the corresponding letter in the blank.

____ 1. Which of the following would not be considered to be a threat to the host?

    A. Bacteria

    B. Fungi

    C. Rickettsiae

    D. Normal flora

____ 2. Choose the final step in the chain of infection.

    A. Portal of exit

    B. Reservoir

    C. Susceptible host

    D. Means of transmission

____ 3. Yeasts and molds would fall under the classification of:

    A. bacteria.

    B. fungi.

    C. rickettsiae.

    D. none of the above.

____ 4. In which of the following ways can a pathogen enter a susceptible host?

    A. Inhalation

    B. Ingestion

    C. Sexual transmission

    D. All of the above

____ 5. In which stage of infection would a patient be if presenting with a general complaint of malaise?

    A. Incubation

    B. Acute

    C. Prodromal

    D. Invasion and multiplication

____ 6. Which of the following would be considered a systemic sign of inflammation?

    A. Fever

    B. Pain

    C. Redness

    D. Heat

____ 7. Which of the following are components that participate in the immune response?

    A. T-cells

    B. B-cells

    C. Antibodies

    D. All of the above

____ 8. During which type of immunity are T-cells present?

    A. Humoral

    B. Cell-mediated

    C. Passive

    D. Natural

____ 9. Immunity that is produced by administering a vaccine containing an antibody would be classified as:

    A. artificial active.

    B. artificial passive.

    C. natural active.

    D. natural passive.

____ 10. Which of the following has been shown to be more effective for removing transient flora from the hands than regular soap and water?

    A. Surgical soap

    B. Alcohol-based hand rubs

    C. Hand sanitizers

    D. Double handwashing

____ 11. Gloves should be worn during all of the following activities except:

    A. administering an injection.

    B. performing a venipuncture.

    C. documenting in the chart.

    D. handling a urine specimen.

____ 12. Which of the following precautions were developed primarily to help control the transmission of HIV and hepatitis B?

    A. PPE

    B. Universal precautions

    C. OPIM

    D. Pathogens Standard

____ 13. When following standard precautions, which of the following should be considered as potentially infectious?

    A. All body fluids

    B. Tissue specimens

    C. Mucous membranes

    D. All of the above

____ 14. What precautions were developed in 1996 as a counterpart to standard precautions that should be used when working with patients who have a known highly infectious disease?

    A. Universal Precautions

    B. General Precautions

    C. Transmission-Based Precautions

    D. Bloodborne Pathogens Standard

____ 15. Which of the following are means of transmission for HIV?

A. Puncture with used needle

B. Touching dried blood, then touching the eyes

C. Receiving a tattoo with unsterile equipment

D. All of the above

____ 16. Which of the following administrations established the Bloodborne Pathogens Standard?

A. OSHA

B. CDC

C. HHS

D. MMR

____ 17. Which of the following would be an example of an engineering control?

A. Sharps container

B. Shielded needle devices

C. Plastic capillary tubes

D. Only A and B

E. All of the above

____ 18. Applying lipstick in the laboratory would be a breach of:

A. engineering controls.

B. work practice controls.

C. facility controls.

D. PPE controls.

____ 19. All of the following are true statements regarding the biohazard label *except:*

A. The label is fluorescent orange or red in color.

B. The label must be displayed on refrigerators used to store blood, blood products, OPIM, and body fluids.

C. Clear plastic bags may be used in place of the biohazard label.

D. The label must be secured to all containers that hold contaminated materials.

____ 20. Which of the following must be available to all employees regarding the use of hazardous chemicals used in the facility?

A. MSDS forms

B. Biohazard trash cans

C. Ventilation hoods

D. None of the above

____ 21. What type of flora is generally found on the hands?

A. Resident flora

B. Transient flora

C. Normal flora

D. All of the above

____ 22. What type of flora is considered pathogenic and needs to be removed from the skin in order to prevent transmission to other patients?

A. Resident flora

B. Transient flora

C. Normal flora

D. None of the above

SKILL APPLICATION CHALLENGE
Assignment 10-7: Case Study

Today's date is October 10, 2011. Kelly L. Leonard, CMA (AAMA), is working in Dr. Pendleton's general practice. Kelly is preparing to perform an ESR on a patient sample from Grace Beavers. She is wearing gloves and her lab coat. While opening the lavender top tube of blood, some of the blood splashes in Kelly's L. eye. Kelly immediately flushes her left eye, using the eyewash station for 20 minutes and reports the incident to her supervisor, Janet Vick, RN. What PPE or other precautions should Kelly have taken to prevent this exposure from occurring in the first place?

_____

_____

_____

COMPLETING SPECIAL FORMS
Assignment 10-8: Exposure Incident Report Exercise

Work Form Necessary: FORM 10-1

Directions: Using the Case Study in Assignment 10-7 and the information below, fill out Work Form 10-1 (Employee Bloodborne Pathogen Exposure Incident Report).

Kelly's social security number is 123-45-6789 and her home address is 1234 Carter Lane, Toddler, OH, 14458. Home phone number: 222-333-5858, work phone number: 222-345-2323. Dates of her HepB vaccines are 01-10-07, 02-10-07, and 07-10-07. The source individual gave permission for her blood to be tested for HIV and HBV and Kelly also gave permission to have her blood tested. The source individual tested positive for HBV and negative for HIV. Kelly tested negative for both. Gamma globulin was administered to Kelly on 10-10-2011 by Dr. Connor James with recommended follow-up testing in six months.

FIELD APPLICATION CHALLENGE
Assignment 10-9

Read the following Field Application Challenge and respond to the questions following the scenario.

The OSHA inspector drops by the medical facility for an impromptu inspection. While observing in the phlebotomy area, he notices that the medical assistant is not wearing a lab coat and is wearing only one glove on the hand used for drawing the sample. The medical assistant has also removed the index finger of the glove for better palpation of the vein. After cleansing the site, the medical assistant palpates the site again and then performs the venipuncture.

1. List the errors made by the medical assistant in the above scenario.

   _____

   _____

   _____

   _____

2. The OSHA inspector may issue the medical office _____ as a result of the medical assistant not following the

   proper precautions, which may result in _____.

JOURNALING EXERCISE
Assignment 10-10

What content within this chapter was most meaningful to you? Why? List some examples of how you might apply information contained in this chapter, both during your training and after you enter the health care industry.

Work Form 10-1

EMPLOYEE POST-EXPOSURE INCIDENT REPORT

Today's Date:	
Employee's Full Name:	Social Security No:

Employee's Address:	Home Phone No.:	Work Phone No:

Date of Exposure:

Type of Exposure: (check one of the following)

	Needle stick with contaminated needle
	Mucosal splashing/spraying of blood or OPIM
	Skin piercing/abrasion with contaminated sharps
	Other

Employee Vaccinated Against Hepatitis B Virus: _____ Yes _____ No

Dates of Vaccinations: 1. _____ 2. _____ 3. _____

Supervisor's Name and Signature:

Source Name:

Permission for HBV and HIV Testing: _____ Yes _____ No

Source Test Results: HBV:_____ Positive _____ Negative
HIV: _____ Positive _____ Negative

Employee Test Results: HBV:_____ Positive _____ Negative
HIV: _____ Positive _____ Negative

Name and Signature of Treating Physician:	Date of Treatment:

Type of Treatment Given:

Recommended Follow-Up Treatment:

C H A P T E R **11**

Basic Vital Signs and Measurements

FIELD RELEVANCY AND BENEFITS

The medical assistant is instrumental in collecting vital signs and other body measurements from the patient in preparation for an examination by the provider. Initial patient screening involves obtaining vital signs along with other health assessment questions. Today's modern medicine dictates efficient use of time and the medical assistant must be able to obtain accurate vital signs and other measurements in a limited time frame. Accuracy when performing these skills is crucial in order to provide the practitioner with the correct information on which to base his diagnosis.

NOTE SHEET

Introduction to the Patient

_____

_____

_____

_____

Height and Weight

_____

_____

_____

_____

Vital Signs

_____

_____

_____

_____

VOCABULARY REVIEW

Assignment 11-1: Matching

Match the term with its definition and place the corresponding letter in the blank.

____ 1. Hyperpnea

____ 2. Dysrhythmia

____ 3. Afebrile

____ 4. Pyrexia

____ 5. Metabolism

____ 6. Baseline

____ 7. Calipers

____ 8. Pulse rhythm

____ 9. Pulse pressure

____ 10. Arrhythmia

A. Without fever

B. A known or initial value with which further determinations are compared

C. The regularity of pulse beats

D. Another name for dysrhythmia

E. The difference between the systolic and diastolic pressure

F. Abnormal or disturbed heart rhythm

G. A condition of being feverish

H. Occurs as nutrients are processed in the body; cells produce energy and heat is produced

I. An instrument used for measuring percentages of body fat

J. Increased respiratory rate and breathing that is deeper than normal

Assignment 11-2: Definitions

Define the following terms.

1. Diastole: _____

2. Korotkoff sounds: _____

3. Pulse volume: _____

    _____

4. Systolic pressure: _____

    _____

5. Vasodilation: _____

6. Metabolism: _____

    _____

7. Bradycardia: _____

Assignment 11-3: Sentence Completion

Fill in the blanks below with Essential Terms from this chapter.

1. An abnormally high heart rate of more than 100 beats per minute is known as _____.

2. A(n) _____ is an instrument used to determine arterial blood pressure.

3. _____ is a decrease in the diameter of the blood vessels.

4. Also known as the centigrade scale, _____ is the official scientific measurement of temperature.

5. _____ is the standard grade of measurement generally used for temperatures in the United States.

6. A person who has an elevated body temperature is said to be _____.

7. An individual who is 20 to 30 percent above his normal weight is said to be suffering from _____.

8. _____ is breathing which is easiest while in a sitting or standing position.

9. The act of breathing is referred to as _____.

10. Deep breathing followed by periods of apnea, usually observed while the patient is sleeping is termed as

_____.

CHAPTER REVIEW
Assignment 11-4: Short Answer

1. Complete the information requested in the table below. Refer to the first line as an example.

Route	Location	Accuracy	Variables and Suggestions for Obtaining the Most Accurate Temperature and Avoiding Injury	Normal Temperature
Mouth/oral cavity	Under the tongue, beside the frenulum linguae	Considered accurate if patient can close mouth completely and keep mouth closed throughout the procedure.	Should not be used when the patient has recently eaten, had something to drink, or smoked. Caution the patient about biting down on the thermometer.	98.6°F (37°C)
Rectal				
Aural/ tympanic membrane				
Axillary				
Temporal				

2. Identify the pulse points on the following figure.

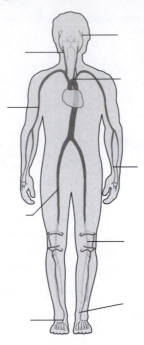

3. List the four standard vital signs and the normal adult reading for each one.

_____

_____

_____

4. List 12 factors that can cause changes in blood pressure. (Hint: Some factors are combined when referring to Table 11-9 in the textbook.)

_____

_____

Assignment 11-5: Certification Practice

Choose the best answer and place the corresponding letter in the blank.

____ 1. Which of the following measurements is not considered to be a vital sign?

   A. Temperature

   B. Pulse

   C. Respiration

   D. Height

____ 2. Which of the following could cause an inaccurate blood pressure reading?

   A. Needle of aneroid dial at zero

   B. Diaphragm of stethoscope placed below the cuff

   C. Using a cuff that is too large

   D. Diaphragm of stethoscope placed over the brachial artery

____ 3. A pulse rate of 50 in an adult would be indicated as:

   A. normal rate.

   B. bradycardia.

   C. tachycardia.

   D. bradypnea.

____ 4. When taking a radial pulse on a patient you note some irregularity in the rhythm. For how long should you count the pulse?

    A. One full minute

    B. 30 seconds

    C. 45 seconds

    D. 15 seconds

____ 5. Blood pressure that is lower than normal would be classified as:

    A. hypertension.

    B. hypotension.

    C. orthostatic hypotension.

    D. both A and B.

____ 6. Which of the following can affect the respiratory rate?

    A. Emotions

    B. Physical activity

    C. Medications

    D. All of the above

____ 7. At what location is the diaphragm of the stethoscope placed when taking an apical pulse?

    A. At the fourth intercostal space to the left of the sternum

    B. To the right at midsternum level

    C. Over the apex of the heart at the fifth intercostal space

    D. At the third intercostal space to the left of the sternum

____ 8. The difference between an oral temperature reading and a temporal temperature reading is:

    A. no difference.

    B. 1 degree.

    C. 2 degrees.

    D. one-half of a degree.

____ 9. A rapid respiration rate with normal or shallow respirations would be termed as:

    A. hyperpnea.

    B. tachypnea.

    C. bradypnea.

    D. both A and B.

    E. none of the above.

____ 10. Which of the following would be a contraindication for an oral temperature?

    A. An 8-year-old child

    B. A patient with a nasal obstruction

    C. A 75-year-old patient

    D. All the above

____ 11. Which of the following is the best indicator of weight-related health?

    A. Desirable weight chart

    B. BSA

    C. BMI

    D. Provider's opinion

____ 12. A patient with a BMI of 35 would be considered:

    A. at an acceptable weight.

    B. obese.

    C. overweight.

    D. normal.

____ 13. A patient with a temporal temperature reading of 100.3°F would be considered:

    A. febrile.

    B. afebrile.

    C. normal.

    D. average.

____ 14. A normal rectal temperature reading would be:

    A. 99.6°F.

    B. 98.6°F.

    C. 97.6°F.

    D. 99.8°F.

____ 15. When taking an aural temperature on an adult, the ear canal should be pulled:

    A. straight down.

    B. up and back.

    C. down and back.

    D. straight out.

____ 16. In comparison to a normal rectal temperature reading, a normal axillary temperature reading would be:

    A. one degree lower.

    B. the same.

    C. one degree higher.

    D. two degrees lower.

____ 17. A fever of 100.4°F to 102.2°F would be considered:

    A. high.

    B. low-grade.

    C. slightly elevated.

    D. fatal.

____ 18. When obtaining a pulse rate, which of the following should also be evaluated?

    A. Rhythm

    B. Strength

    C. Pattern

    D. Both A and B

    E. All of the above

____ 19. In order for an adult pulse rate to be considered tachycardic, it must be above:

    A. 100 BPM.

    B. 120 BPM.

    C. 115 BPM.

    D. 110 BPM.

____ 20. Calculate the pulse deficit if the radial pulse is 68 and the apical pulse is 80.

    A. 15

    B. 12

    C. 10

    D. 22

____ 21. The blood pressure phase when ventricles are relaxed is referred to as:

    A. systole.

    B. diastole.

    C. systole.

    D. apole.

___ 22. If 57-year-old Mr. Leonard has a blood pressure reading of 160/100, he is considered to have:

    A. normal or ideal blood pressure.

    B. stage I hypertension.

    C. stage II hypertension.

    D. prehypertension.

___ 23. During which phase of Korotkoff sounds do the pulsation sounds become softer and more muffled?

    A. Phase two

    B. Phase three

    C. Phase four

    D. Phase five

___ 24. At what percent does oxygen intervention usually become necessary?

    A. 95%

    B. 86% in a COPD patient

    C. 88%

    D. 90%

___ 25. What is an additional reading that may be measured as part of the vital signs?

    A. Pain rating

    B. Oxygen saturation

    C. Height and weight

    D. Both A and B

___ 26. Blood pressure that drops upon standing is referred to as:

    A. standing hypertension.

    B. standing hypotension.

    C. orthostatic hypotension.

    D. orthostatic hypertension.

___ 27. The bladder of the blood pressure cuff should be placed directly over the patient's:

    A. radial artery.

    B. femoral artery.

    C. brachial artery.

    D. carotid artery.

___ 28. While preparing to take a patient's blood pressure, you notice that the patient has a difficult time rolling up his sleeve—the sleeve is constricting blood flow to the area. You should do which of the following before taking the patient's blood pressure?

    A. Have the patient remove his arm from his sleeve or his entire shirt.

    B. Have the patient roll the sleeve back down and take the blood pressure through his clothing.

    C. Take the blood pressure with the sleeve rolled up.

    D. None of the above

___ 29. You notice that the needle on the aneroid sphygmomanometer is not centered on zero when the cuff is completely deflated. Which of the following applies?

    A. The cuff is not properly calibrated.

    B. The cuff should not be used again until it is properly calibrated.

    C. Using the cuff the way it is may produce inaccurate results.

    D. All of the above

___ 30. Which of the following applies to an aneroid reading?

    A. Results are recorded as odd numbers.

    B. Results are recorded as even numbers.

    C. Results are recorded as either odd or even numbers.

    D. None of the above

____ 31. Patients should always be asked about which of the following prior to taking an oral temperature reading?

   A. When the patient ate last

   B. When the patient drank last

   C. If the patient is a smoker, when they last smoked

   D. All of the above

____ 32. Patients that have had a mastectomy should not have a blood pressure taken on the side that the mastectomy was performed because it may lead to a condition known as lymphedema (a backup of lymph fluid in the area due to the removal of lymph glands in the area). What would you do if the patient had both breasts removed?

   A. Record a note in the chart explaining why you didn't take the reading.

   B. Take a reading at a different site such as the thigh or wrist with an appropriate cuff.

   C. Consult with the physician if no alternative equipment is available.

   D. Both B and C

____ 33. According to the AAFP, a large adult cuff should be selected:

   A. when the diameter of the patient's upper arm is over 13 inches.

   B. when the diameter of the patient's upper arm is over 15 inches.

   C. when the diameter of the patient's upper arm is over 17 inches.

   D. when the diameter of the patient's upper arm is over 20 inches.

____ 34. The structure within the brain that controls breathing is the:

   A. cerebrum.

   B. medulla oblongata.

   C. cerebellum.

   D. pons.

____ 35. The artery that is palpated during adult CPR is the:

   A. brachial.

   B. radial.

   C. carotid.

   D. femoral.

SKILL APPLICATION CHALLENGES
Assignment 11-6: Project

1. Choose another student to be your patient and obtain and record blood pressure readings after the following:

   A. Climbing a flight of stairs: _____

   B. Being seated for 10 minutes: _____

   C. Immediately upon standing: _____

   D. Immediately upon lying down: _____

2. Explain the possible reasons for the differences in the readings.

   _____

   _____

   _____

Assignment 11-7: Plotting Activities

1. Plot the following height measurements on the height bar by drawing a line at the correct mark and placing the corresponding letter on the line.

   A. 5 feet, 5 inches

   B. 5 feet, 4½ inches

   C. 5 feet, 3 inches

   D. 5 feet, 2¼ inches

   E. 5 feet, ½ inch

```
152 ── ── 5FT
153 ── ──
154 ── ──
155 ── ── 1
156 ── ──
157 ── ── 2
158 ── ──
159 ── ──
160 ── ── 3
161 ── ──
162 ── ── 4
163 ── ──
164 ── ──
165 ── ── 5
166 ── ──
167 ── ── 6
168 ── ──
```

2. Plot the following weight measurements on the weight bar by drawing a line on the correct mark and placing the corresponding letter on the line.

   A. 11¼ pounds

   B. 12½ pounds

   C. 15 pounds

   D. 18¾ pounds

   E. 21¼ pounds

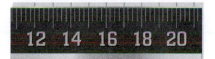

3. Plot the following blood pressure readings on the aneroid dial by placing a line on the correct mark for the systolic pressure (mark line with corresponding letter and an "S") and the correct mark for the diastolic pressure (mark the line with the corresponding letter of the reading and a "D").

A. 98/66

B. 104/78

C. 120/80

D. 146/88

E. 180/102

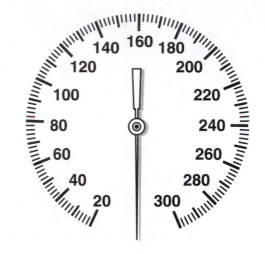

Assignment 11-8: Documentation Exercise

10/10/2012 9:00 a.m. Mr. Anthony is a new patient and is here for a complete physical examination. You obtain his height (73 inches) and weight (175 pounds). He tells you that he is concerned about his blood pressure and wants to be certain that it is OK. Vital sign measurements include: temperature taken by the temporal artery method (99.6°F), pulse rate of 110, a respiration rate of 20, and a blood pressure rate of 138/86. Document the information into the following chart note.

FIELD APPLICATION CHALLENGE

Assignment 11-9

Read the following Field Application Challenge and respond to the questions following the scenario.

You have been asked to take a pulse and a blood pressure reading on 80-year-old Mrs. Leonard who is very frail and thin. The provider is running ahead of schedule and is waiting on you so that he can examine the patient so you have to work rather quickly. You take the patient's pulse rate which is 96 beats per minute. You notice that that the patient's heart appears to skip a few beats. The patient's blood pressure is 152/94.

1. What type of blood pressure cuff would work best on this patient? _____

2. After reading about variables that can affect blood pressure readings in the chapter, what may be a contributor to the patient's pulse rate being so high?

_____

3. What stage of hypertension does the patient have?

_____

4. The patient's heart rhythm would be termed as what?

_____

JOURNALING EXERCISE
Assignment 11-10

What content within this chapter was most meaningful to you? Why? List some examples of how you might apply information contained in this chapter, both during your training and after you enter the health care industry.

C H A P T E R **12**

The Physical Exam

FIELD RELEVANCY AND BENEFITS

The medical assistant is instrumental in preparing the room and the patient for the complete physical examination. Following the patient interview, the medical assistant must be able to determine how the provider will want the patient disrobed and what supplies and instruments will be necessary for the exam. Duties during the exam may include: positioning and draping of the patient, handing items to the provider, collecting specimens, and continuous monitoring of the patient. Medical assistants with good "anticipation skills" will be highly regarded by providers and supervisors. Information in this chapter may be applied to all kinds of practices, and is especially relevant for those working in general or family practice.

NOTE SHEET

The Examination Room

_____

_____

_____

_____

Patient Preparation

_____

_____

_____

_____

Patient Positioning and Draping

_____

_____

_____

_____

Patient Assessment

_____

_____

_____

_____

VOCABULARY REVIEW

Assignment 12-1: Matching

Match the term with its definition and place the corresponding letter in the blank.

____ 1. Palpation

____ 2. Posture

____ 3. Inspection

____ 4. Auscultation

____ 5. Vertigo

____ 6. Mensuration

____ 7. Manipulation

____ 8. Percussion

____ 9. Tympany

____ 10. Examination

A. Checking the extension or flexion of a joint by applying forceful movement

B. Position of the body, whether standing, sitting, or lying down

C. Disturbance in the equilibrium of the body and balance or another name for dizziness

D. The process of measuring

E. The process of observing the patient for scars, lesions, and other pathological signs

G. Touching the body to evaluate pain and tenderness, and organ size

H. Using the fingertips to tap the body slightly but sharply to determine position, size, and consistency of underlying structures or cavities

I. Process of listening to sounds within the body with the aid of a Stethoscope

J. A hollow drum sound

K. A process in which the body is inspected to determine the presence or absence of disease.

CHAPTER REVIEW

Assignment 12-2: True or False

Fill in the blank with a "T" for true statements and an "F" for false statements. Rewrite the false statements to make them true.

____ 1. The exam table paper only needs to be changed if it is visibly soiled.

_____

_____

____ 2. The Sims' position may be used for rectal examinations and enemas.

_____

_____

____ 3. The lithotomy position is used when inserting a catheter.

_____

_____

____ 4. The knee-chest position may be used to examine the rectum and anus.

_____

_____

_____ 5. The supine position is used to examine the back and vertebrae.

_____

_____

_____ 6. Disinfecting spray should be used before rooming the next patient if the previous patient had a contagious respiratory infection.

_____

_____

_____ 7. The medical assistant's duty *during* the HEENT portion of the physical exam is to perform visual acuity testing.

_____

_____

Assignment 12-3: Certification Practice

Choose the best answer and place the corresponding letter in the blank.

_____ 1. For an evaluation of the head, neck, and shoulders, which of the following positions would be used?
   A. Sitting
   B. Supine
   C. Dorsal recumbent
   D. Sims'

_____ 2. In which of the following examination techniques are sounds evaluated by tapping the body with the fingers?
   A. Palpation
   B. Inspection
   C. Manipulation
   D. Percussion

_____ 3. Which of the following components of the physical exam is either completely or partially performed by the medical assistant?
   A. General survey
   B. Vital signs
   C. Skin
   D. Both A and B
   E. All of the above

_____ 4. Which of the following examination techniques would be used to evaluate the cardiovascular system?
   A. Auscultation
   B. Inspection
   C. Palpation
   D. All of the above

_____ 5. The Sims' position would be used for which of the following types of exams?
   A. Rectal or prostate
   B. Abdominal
   C. Vaginal
   D. Genitalia

____ 6. A patient becomes very dizzy after getting down from the exam table. If at all possible the patient should be escorted back up onto the exam table and placed in which of the following positions?

    A. Prone

    B. Supine

    C. Trendelenburg

    D. Semi-Fowler's

____ 7. Which of the following positions would be used for a patient having a colon exam?

    A. Sims'

    B. Knee-chest

    C. Lithotomy

    D. Both A and B

____ 8. Of the following instruments, which one would be used to examine the ear?

    A. Aural speculum

    B. Otoscope

    C. Ophthalmoscope

    D. Pen light

____ 9. Which of the following would not be routinely used during a physical exam?

    A. Percussion hammer

    B. Stethoscope

    C. Hemostat

    D. Tongue depressor

____ 10. For which types of exams and procedures could the dorsal recumbent position be used?

    A. Abdominal

    B. Rectal

    C. Catheterization

    D. All of the above

____ 11. A patient presents with shortness of breath and chest pains; which position would assist the patient with breathing?

    A. Supine

    B. Prone

    C. Semi-Fowler's

    D. Lithotomy

____ 12. Which examination technique(s) is(are) primarily used during the HEENT portion of the physical exam?

    A. Auscultation

    B. Inspection

    C. Palpation

    D. Only B and C

____ 13. Percussion is mainly used to evaluate:

    A. the thorax and lungs.

    B. the pelvic region.

    C. the abdominal region.

    D. the carotid artery.

___ 14. Which of the following examination techniques would the medical assistant utilize during the prescreening process?

A. Inspection

B. Palpation

C. Mensuration

D. Both A and C

___ 15. While preparing the examination room for the next patient, the medical assistant notices that the exam table paper is wet. What important steps should be taken to ensure the cleanliness of the exam table?

A. Change the exam table paper.

B. Dry the surface of the exam table with a paper towel and replace the table paper.

C. Disinfect the area that is wet and replace the table paper.

D. Disinfect the entire surface of the exam table and replace the table paper.

___ 16. Choose the primary rationale behind draping the patient.

A. Privacy and dignity

B. Visualization

C. Accessibility

D. None of the above

___ 17. Which of the following examination techniques would be used to measure the circumference of a swollen ankle and leg in a patient with congestive heart failure?

A. Inspection

B. Mensuration

C. Palpation

D. Percussion

___ 18. Patients should be allowed to rest a moment before being escorted off of the table because some patients suffer from _____ and can become very dizzy with swift position changes.

A. Vomiting

B. Pain

C. Vertigo

D. Both A and C

___ 19. Patients should be encouraged to do which of the following prior to examination?

A. Empty their bladder

B. Turn off their cell phone

C. Remove the appropriate clothing

D. All of the above

___ 20. A small cardboard testing card along with a bottle of developer used to evaluate blood in the stool is referred to as a(n):

A. fecal occult blood test.

B. fecal Pap test.

C. occult bowel test.

D. all of the above.

SKILL APPLICATION CHALLENGES

Assignment 12-4: Project

Complete a tray setup for a complete physical examination. In the space below, list each instrument on your tray and the rationale for its use.

1. _____

2. _____

3. _____

4. _____

5. _____

6. _____

7. _____

8. _____

9. _____

10. _____

11. _____

12. _____

13. _____

14. _____

15. _____

16. _____

17. _____

Assignment 12-5: Patient Position Labeling

Identify the following patient positions and list one example for which the position is used.

	Position	Position Name	Example
1.			
2.			
3.			
4.			
5.			
6.			
7.			

FIELD APPLICATION CHALLENGE
Assignment 12-6

Read the following Field Application Challenge and respond to the questions following the scenario.

Mrs. Price is being seen in the office today for an assessment of her lower back pain and urinary symptoms. She appears to be very agitated and nervous. She is reluctant to get on the scales and later hesitates to give a urine specimen following the physician's examination. .

1. What can you do as the medical assistant to convince the patient to step on the scales?

   _____

   _____

2. How might you prompt the patient to give you the needed urine specimen?

   _____

   _____

   _____

3. What can the medical assistant do to help reduce the patient's anxiety?

   _____

   _____

   _____

   _____

JOURNALING EXERCISE
Assignment 12-7

What content within this chapter was most meaningful to you? Why? List some examples of how you might apply information contained in this chapter, both during your training and after you enter the health care industry.

C H A P T E R **13**

Eye and Ear Exams and Procedures

FIELD RELEVANCY AND BENEFITS

Familiarity with basic specialty procedures is vital to the well-trained medical assistant. The days of the general practitioner treating all that ails the patient are gone and the field of medicine has become the world of the specialist.

NOTE SHEET

Types of Providers Who Specialize in Treating Eye Disorders

_____

_____

_____

_____

Patient Screening for the Eyes

_____

_____

_____

_____

Visual Acuity Testing

_____

_____

_____

_____

Eye Instillation

_____

_____

_____

_____

Eye Irrigation

_____

_____

_____

_____

Types of Providers Who Treat Conditions of the Ear

_____

_____

_____

_____

Hearing Defects

_____

_____

_____

_____

Ear Instillation

_____

_____

_____

_____

The Ear

_____

_____

_____

_____

Patient Screening for the Ear

_____

_____

_____

_____

Hearing Acuity

_____

_____

_____

_____

Ear Irrigation

_____

_____

_____

_____

VOCABULARY REVIEW
Assignment 13-1: Matching
Match the term with its definition and place the corresponding letter in the blank.

____ 1. Hyperopia

____ 2. Auricle

____ 3. Cerumen

____ 4. Instillation

____ 5. Glaucoma

____ 6. Astigmatism

____ 7. Conjunctivitis

____ 8. Snellen chart

____ 9. Ophthalmic

____ 10. Audiometer

____ 11. Optician

____ 12. Otoscope

____ 13. Visual acuity

____ 14. Tympanometer

____ 15. Otic

A. Pertaining to the ear

B. Chart used to test distance visual acuity

C. Farsightedness

D. Fills prescriptions for eye glasses

E. Screening procedure used to detect errors in refraction

F. A device used to measure the patency and mobility of the ear drum

G. Device used to measure hearing acuity at different sound frequencies

H. Pertaining to the eye

I. Instrument used to visualize the external ear canal and tympanic membrane

J. Inserting liquid, such as medication, into a body cavity such as the eye or ear

K. Ear wax

L. Abnormal curvature of the cornea causing blurred vision

M. Eye disease usually characterized by an increase in intraocular pressure resulting in possible blindness

N. External ear or visible part of the ear

O. Inflammation of the mucous membrane that lines the eyelid

Assignment 13-2: Sentence Completion

Fill in the blanks below with Essential Terms from this chapter.

1. A(n) _____ is an instrument used to visualize the external ear canal and the tympanic membrane.

2. The medical doctor who specializes in diagnosis and treatment of diseases and disorders of the eye is a(n) _____.

3. The device used to measure hearing acuity at different sound frequencies is an _____.

4. _____ is an eye disease characterized by an increase in intraocular pressure resulting in possible blindness.

5. A foreign body can be flushed from the eye by performing a(n) _____.

6. A(n) _____ is a professional licensed to measure visual acuity and prescribe corrective lenses.

7. The instrument used to visualize the interior of the eye is the _____.

CHAPTER REVIEW
Assignment 13-3: True or False

Fill in the blank with a "T" for true statements and an "F" for false statements. Rewrite the false statements to make them true.

_____ 1. Visual acuity testing can determine if the patient has an eye disease.

_____

_____ 2. A common screening test for color vision is the Ishihara test.

_____

_____ 3. The Pelli-Robson chart is a testing tool used to detect astigmatism.

_____

_____ 4. A refractive disorder is a condition in which the lens and cornea do not bend light correctly resulting in visual defects.

_____

_____ 5. Presbyopia is a congenital condition of farsightedness due to abnormal curvature of the cornea.

_____

_____ 6. The abbreviations OD, OS, and OU should be used when documenting procedures that involve the eye.

_____

_____ 7. NVA stands for near visual acuity.

_____

_____ 8. A test that compares air conduction to bone conduction is the Rinne Test.

_____

_____ 9. A child under the age of five should stand 20 feet away from the chart during visual acuity testing.

_____

_____ 10. The HOTV eye chart is a chart that can be used with patients that have limited English.

_____

Assignment 13-4: Short Answer

1. Explain the difference between a conduction hearing loss and nerve deafness.

   _____

   _____

   _____

   _____

   _____

2. List three types of irrigation solutions used for eye injuries and conditions.

   _____

3. List and describe four types of ear irrigation systems.

   A. _____

   B. _____

   C. _____

   _____

   D. _____

   _____

4. List the two types of gross hearing tests that utilize a tuning fork.

   _____

5. Describe the medical assistant's role during visual acuity testing.

   _____

   _____

   _____

   _____

   _____

   _____

   _____

   _____

   _____

Assignment 13-5: Certification Practice

Choose the best answer and place the corresponding letter in the blank.

_____ 1. Which of the following disorders is usually associated with increased intraocular pressure?

   A. Cataract

   B. Stye

   C. Hyperopia

   D. Glaucoma

_____ 2. Another name for the eardrum is the:

   A. auricle.

   B. pinna.

   C. tympanic membrane.

   D. eustachian tube.

____ 3. Choose the instrument that measures hearing acuity at different frequencies.

   A. Tympanometer

   B. Audiometer

   C. Tuning fork

   D. Weber test

____ 4. Irrigation fluid should be flushed through the eye from:

   A. the outer canthus to the inner canthus.

   B. the inner canthus to the outer canthus.

   C. the middle of the eye.

   D. the upper eyelid.

____ 5. Interpret the following results of a visual acuity test: R. eye 20/10.

   A. The patient sees at 20 feet what most people are able to see from 10 feet.

   B. The patient sees at 10 feet what most people are able to see from 20 feet.

   C. The patient's vision is poor in the right eye.

   D. The patient's vision is excellent in the right eye.

____ 6. Which of the following connects the auricle to the tympanic membrane?

   A. Pinna

   B. Eustachian tube

   C. External auditory canal

   D. Ossicle

____ 7. When screening a patient for any disorders or problems with the eyes, the medical assistant should ask which of the following questions?

   A. Do you have any visual disturbances, double vision, or light sensitivity?

   B. Do you experience excessive tearing?

   C. Do you see blind spots or halos around objects?

   D. All of the above

____ 8. Which of the following conditions may be indicated when a patient complains of an inability to see objects up close?

   A. Myopia

   B. Astigmatism

   C. Hyperopia

   D. Cataract

____ 9. Which of the following eye specialists would perform cataract surgery?

   A. Optometrist

   B. Optician

   C. Ophthalmologist

   D. General surgeon

____ 10. Which of the following steps should be completed after a visual acuity screening?

   A. Place eye drops in the patient's eyes.

   B. Clean the occluder with alcohol.

   C. Perform an eye irrigation.

   D. Instruct the patient to rub his eyes.

____ 11. The medical name for an ENT is an:

   A. otorhinolaryngologist.

   B. eye, ear, nose, and throat specialist.

   C. otopharyngologist.

   D. ototympanologist.

_____ 12. Which chart is used to conduct contrast sensitivity testing?

A. Snellen

B. Ishihara

C. Pelli-Robson

D. Amsler grid

_____ 13. Which of the following degrees of hearing loss can affect language development?

A. Mild

B. Moderate

C. Moderate-severe

D. Severe

_____ 14. During an eye instillation, the upper eyelid is pulled up and the patient is instructed to look:

A. down.

B. up.

C. to the right.

D. to the left.

_____ 15. When performing an eye irrigation, the medical assistant would do all of following *except:*

A. place the patient in a supine or sitting position with head turned toward the affected eye.

B. check the expiration date of the solution.

C. irrigate the eye from the outer canthus to the inner canthus.

D. warm irrigating solution to body temperature.

_____ 16. When irrigating the ear in children over the age of three and adults, the auricle should be pulled:

A. up and back.

B. down and back.

C. straight back.

D. straight down.

_____ 17. Sound amplitude is measured in:

A. Zs.

B. percent.

C. decibels.

D. hertz.

_____ 18. Sound frequency is measured in:

A. Zs.

B. percent.

C. decibels.

D. hertz.

_____ 19. Which of the following tests is used for near visual acuity?

A. Contrast Sensitivity

B. Jaeger

C. Pelli-Robson

D. Ishihara

_____ 20. Which of the following charts are used during pediatric screenings?

A. Tumbling E

B. Tumbling C chart

C. LEA chart

D. All of the above

SKILL APPLICATION CHALLENGES
Assignment 13-6: Documentation Exercise

Correctly chart the following information regarding a visual acuity screening using the Snellen chart as ordered by Dr. Leonard. The date is 10/10/2010 and it is 12:30 p.m. The patient read the line marked 20/40 with his right eye, 20/20 with his left eye, and 20/20 with both eyes. The patient was wearing eyeglasses and appeared to be squinting at times. Sign your name followed by the initials SMA.

Assignment 13-7: Project

Research the topics of macular degeneration and retinal detachment and prepare a short report on these disorders. Include treatments used to correct or improve these conditions, including any new experimental treatments being used along with statistics on success.

FIELD APPLICATION CHALLENGE
Assignment 13-8

Read the following Field Application Challenge and respond to the questions following the scenario.

The provider orders an ear irrigation on a patient due to a buildup of cerumen. The medical assistant is in a hurry and places the irrigating solution into a bulb syringe without warming it. The patient begins to complain of pressure and dizziness during the irrigation, but the medical assistant reassures the patient that the procedure will be over within just a few minutes, and that it is common to feel a bit of pressure and dizziness, and continues the irrigation. There was no cerumen in the return basin.

1. What things did the medical assistant do incorrectly in the above scenario?

_____

_____

2. Why should the ear irrigation solution be warmed?

_____

_____

3. When the patient complained of pressure and dizziness what should the medical assistant have done?

_____

_____

JOURNALING EXERCISE
Assignment 13-9

What content within this chapter was most meaningful to you? Why? List some examples of how you might apply information contained in this chapter, both during your training and after you enter the health care industry.

C H A P T E R **14**

Gastrointestinal Evaluations and Procedures

FIELD RELEVANCY AND BENEFITS

Following a physical examination in the primary physician's office, further evaluation in a specialist's facility for a gastrointestinal illness or disorder may be indicated. The medical assistant may participate in the office exam, prepare and educate the patient for a GI procedure, or assist in a diagnostic test or procedure. Understanding the structure and function of the GI system along with the examinations, procedures, and associated pathology will allow for the highest standard of care for the gastrointestinal patient. Information in this chapter is applicable when working in family practice, general practice, internal medicine, and especially in gastroenterology practices.

NOTE SHEET

Types of Physicians Who Specialize in Treating Gastrointestinal and Liver Disorders

_____

_____

_____

_____

Patient Screening for the Gastrointestinal System

_____

_____

_____

_____

GI Examinations Performed in the Medical Office

_____

_____

_____

_____

Diagnostic Procedures

_____

_____

_____

_____

Nutrition

_____

_____

_____

_____

Exercise

_____

_____

_____

_____

Eating Disorders

_____

_____

_____

_____

VOCABULARY REVIEW

Assignment 14-1: Matching

Match the term with its definition and place the corresponding letter in the blank.

____ 1. Hepatologist

____ 2. Proctologist

____ 3. Anorexia nervosa

____ 4. Proctoscope

____ 5. Referred pain

____ 6. Gastroenterologist

____ 7. Defecate

____ 8. Anoscope

____ 9. Fecal occult blood

____ 10. Stool culture

____ 11. Bulimia nervosa

____ 12. Fissure

____ 13. Parietal pain

____ 14. Ova and parasites

____ 15. Hemorrhoids

____ 16. Visceral pain

____ 17. USDA

____ 18. Sigmoidoscopy

____ 19. Colonoscopy

A. Examination of the sigmoid colon with a lighted scope

B. Eating disorder characterized by binging and purging

C. A provider who specializes in treating diseases and disorders of the liver

D. Eating disorder in which the patient drastically reduces food intake in an effort to minimize body weight

E. Occurs when organs in the GI tract contract and distend

F. A pain that is felt at a location other than the original pain site

G. A test that looks for microorganisms in the stool

H. Department of the government which is responsible for executing policies on agriculture, farming, and food

I. A type of speculum used to visualize the anus

J. Testing to identify intestinal parasites and their eggs

K. Instrument used to visually inspect the anus and rectum

L. Pain in the abdominal wall

M. The act of evacuating or emptying the bowels

N. A doctor who specializes in treating gastrointestinal disorders

O. Painful, swollen, and bleeding veins in the anal region

P. A linear ulcer located on the edge of the anus

Q. Hidden blood found in the stool

R. A provider who specializes in treating diseases and disorders of the colon, rectum, and anus

S. Examination of the colon with a lighted scope

CHAPTER REVIEW

Assignment 14-2: Acronym Review

Write what each of the following acronyms stands for.

1. GI: _____

2. EGD: _____

3. ERCP: _____

4. C-DIFF: _____

5. ACS: _____

6. USDA: _____

7. O&P: _____

8. MUFA: _____

Assignment 14-3: Short Answer

1. Compare and contrast the eating disorders anorexia nervosa, bulimia nervosa, compulsive overeating, and night eating syndrome.

   A. Anorexia nervosa: _____

   _____

   _____

   B. Bulimia nervosa: _____

   _____

   _____

   C. Compulsive overeating: _____

   _____

   _____

   D. Night eating syndrome: _____

   _____

   _____

2. Explain the importance of good nutrition as it relates to health and disease.

   _____

   _____

   _____

   _____

3. Describe the following procedures that are performed by a gastroenterologist.

   A. Sigmoidoscopy: _____

   _____

   B. Capsule endoscopy: _____

   _____

C. 24-hour pH monitoring: _____

_____

D. Hydrogen breath test: _____

_____

E. Colonoscopy: _____

_____

F. Esophagogastroduodenoscopy (EGD): _____

_____

G. Endoscopic retrograde cholangiopancreatography (ERCP): _____

_____

_____

H. Enteroscopy: _____

_____

I. Endoscopic ultrasound: _____

_____

Assignment 14-4: Certification Practice

Choose the best answer and place the corresponding letter in the blank.

____ 1. Which of the following would be a role of the medical assistant working in a gastroenterology practice?

  A. To provide patient education regarding a colonoscopy

  B. To perform fecal occult blood testing

  C. To help with insertion of the sigmoidoscope

  D. All of the above

____ 2. A burning, cramping, aching pain is characterized as:

  A. referred pain.

  B. parietal pain.

  C. abdominal pain.

  D. visceral pain.

____ 3. When instructing a patient regarding preparation for collecting a fecal occult blood test sample, you would include all of the following *except:*

  A. Avoid red meat, raw vegetables, fruits, and rectal suppositories for three days prior to collection.

  B. Do not consume alcoholic beverages for three days prior to collection.

  C. Avoid NSAIDs for seven days prior to collection.

  D. Collect samples on three different days.

____ 4. What organism is responsible for the condition known as pseudomembranous colitis?

  A. *Helicobacter pylori*

  B. *Clostridium difficile*

  C. *Streptococcus pyogenes*

  D. *Vibrio cholerae*

____ 5. Pasta would be an example from which of the following food groups?

  A. Carbohydrates

  B. Fats

  C. Dairy

  D. Grains

____ 6. Which of the following would not be a health benefit from the vegetable food group?

    A. No cholesterol

    B. Vitamin A

    C. Iron transport

    D. Vitamin C

____ 7. Which of the following would be the best indicator of a patient's nutritional habits?

    A. Food diary

    B. Weight loss

    C. Skin tone

    D. Muscle tone

____ 8. All of the following are recommendations regarding physical activity *except:*

    A. Engage in at least 30 minutes of moderate activity daily.

    B. Include stretching exercises for flexibility.

    C. Weight loss requires a minimum of 90 minutes of exercise daily.

    D. Longer duration of exercise is more beneficial.

____ 9. Discretionary calories are related to:

    A. fruits.

    B. vegetables.

    C. proteins.

    D. "extras."

____ 10. When instructing a patient on how to collect a fecal sample, all of the following are true *except:*

    A. The patient may use a tongue depressor to collect a small portion of the stool.

    B. Instruct the patient to collect the sample in a wide-mouth jar.

    C. Instruct the patient not to contaminate the specimen with urine.

    D. Refrigerate the specimen if it cannot be taken directly to the lab following defecation.

____ 11. Which of the following minerals helps to maintain blood pressure?

    A. Iron

    B. Zinc

    C. Potassium

    D. All of the above

____ 12. Which food group helps to build and maintain bones?

    A. Grains

    B. Fruits and vegetables

    C. Milk and dairy

    D. Meats and oils

____ 13. Which food group is high in fiber and helps to reduce the risk of coronary disease?

    A. Grains

    B. Fruits and vegetables

    C. Milk and dairy

    D. Meats and oils

____ 14. Which mineral helps to transport oxygen around the body?

    A. Calcium

    B. Iron

    C. Sodium

    D. Magnesium

____ 15. Which food group's leader nutrients include folate, iron, and magnesium?

    A. Grains

    B. Fruits and vegetables

    C. Milk and dairy

    D. Meats and oils

____ 16. What vitamin is important for good eye health?

    A. Vitamin A

    B. Vitamin B

    C. Vitamin C

    D. Vitamin D

____ 17. The major nutrients in this food group include calcium, phosphorous, potassium, and vitamin K.

    A. Grains

    B. Fruits and vegetables

    C. Milk and dairy

    D. Meats and oils

____ 18. This vitamin is important for energy and the formation of blood cells.

    A. Vitamin A

    B. Vitamin B

    C. Vitamin C

    D. Vitamin D

____ 19. Vitamins A, D, E, and K all have something in common. What is it?

    A. They are all important for good skin.

    B. They are all water-soluble.

    C. They are all fat-soluble.

    D. They are all important for cardiac health.

____ 20. Which of the following nutrients helps to reduce the risk of cardiovascular disease?

    A. Proteins

    B. Oils

    C. Vitamins

    D. Omega-3 fatty acids

____ 21. Which of the following vitamins is important for healing wounds and also assists with iron distribution?

    A. Vitamin A

    B. Vitamin B

    C. Vitamin C

    D. Vitamin D

____ 22. Which of the following vitamins assists with immunity and is considered an antioxidant?

    A. Vitamin A

    B. Vitamin E

    C. B Complex

    D. Vitamin C

____ 23. Which of the following are considered risk factors for colon cancer?

    A. A family history of colon cancer

    B. A personal history of colon polyps

    C. A high fat diet

    D. All of the above

SKILL APPLICATION CHALLENGES

Assignment 14-6: Projects

1. Construct a three-day diet that contains high-fiber content for a patient suffering from IBS. Include breakfast, lunch, dinner, and snacks.

2. Design informational pamphlets to be given to patients that explain the following procedures and include special preparation instructions:

   A. Fecal occult blood test

   B. Sigmoidoscopy

   C. Colonoscopy

   D. EGD

FIELD APPLICATION CHALLENGE

Assignment 14-7

Read the following Field Application Challenge and respond to the questions following the scenario.

A 55-year-old male is sent to your office to have an esophagogastroduodenoscopy. He is a heavy drinker and smoker who also consumes spicy foods on a daily basis. He is quite anxious about having the procedure performed and is afraid he might choke during insertion of the scope. His father and younger brother were both diagnosed with esophageal cancer. His father died, but the brother was just recently diagnosed and is taking chemotherapy.

1. List the risk factors the patient has for developing esophageal cancer.

   _____

   _____

2. How might you calm the patient's fears about the procedure?

   _____

   _____

JOURNALING EXERCISE

Assignment 14-8

What content within this chapter was most meaningful to you? Why? List some examples of how you might apply information contained in this chapter, both during your training and after you enter the health care industry.

C H A P T E R **15**

Cardiovascular Exams and Procedures

FIELD RELEVANCY AND BENEFITS

The medical assistant must be able to perform an accurate EKG recording. The medical assistant does not interpret the EKG tracing, but should be able to recognize artifacts and abnormal rhythms so that proper adjustments can be made during the testing. EKGs are performed in several types of medical practices including family practice, cardiology, urgent care, and internal medicine.

NOTE SHEET

Types of Physicians Who Specialize in Treating Cardiovascular System Diseases and Disorders

_____

_____

_____

_____

Patient Screening for the Cardiovascular System

_____

_____

_____

_____

Anatomy of the Heart

_____

_____

_____

The Heart's Electrical Conduction System

_____

_____

_____

The Cardiac Cycle

_____

_____

_____

_____

EKG Equipment and Supplies

_____

_____

_____

_____

Rhythm Strip

_____

_____

_____

_____

Performing the Resting 12-Lead EKG

_____

_____

_____

_____

Artifacts

_____

_____

_____

_____

Defibrillation

_____

_____

_____

_____

Types of EKG Units

_____

_____

_____

_____

EKG Lead Placement

_____

_____

_____

_____

Standardizing the EKG

_____

_____

_____

_____

Mounting the EKG Tracing

_____

_____

_____

_____

Cardiac Arrhythmias

_____

_____

_____

_____

Miscellaneous Cardiac Diagnostic Testing

_____

_____

_____

_____

VOCABULARY REVIEW
Assignment 15-1: Matching I

Match the term with its definition and place the corresponding letter in the blank.

____ 1. Cardiac catheterization

____ 2. Premature ventricular contractions

____ 3. Repolarization

____ 4. Baseline

____ 5. Bipolar leads

____ 6. Rhythm strip

____ 7. Cardiac cycle

____ 8. Paroxysmal atrial tachycardia

____ 9. Cardioversion

____ 10. Tachycardia

A. Sudden onslaught of increased heart rate ranging from 150 to 250 BPM

B. The process of restoring normal sinus rhythm through the use of medications or electrical current

C. Contractions that occur early in the cycle; they are characterized by the absence of the P wave, a wide QRS complex, and a T wave that deflects opposite the QRS complex.

D. An additional 10- to 12-inch tracing of limb lead II that is used to check for arrhythmias and other cardiac occurrences

E. Period of relaxation of the heart

F. Heart rate above 100 BPM

G. Procedure in which the coronary arteries are visualized to determine the percentage of blockage

H. Flat horizontal line that separates the waves of the EKG cycle

I. EKG limb leads I, II, and III

J. One complete heart beat

Assignment 15-2: Matching II

Match the term with its definition and place the corresponding letter in the blank.

____ 1. Electrocardiogram

____ 2. Depolarization

____ 3. Precordial

____ 4. Normal sinus rhythm

____ 5. Isoelectric

____ 6. Holter monitor

____ 7. Lead

____ 8. Artifact

____ 9. Augmented leads

____ 10. Premature atrial contractions

K. Interference that causes irregularities on the EKG tracing

L. EKG leads aVR, aVL, and aVF

M. Recording or tracing of the electrical activity of the heart

N. Flat horizontal line on the EKG tracing; baseline

O. Discharge of electrical activity that causes the heart to contract

P. The heart's rhythm within normal limits

Q. Premature contractions of the atria of the heart; sometimes seen in healthy individuals but also may be seen in patients with heart problems

R. Portable ambulatory EKG worn by the patient for 24 hours to detect cardiac abnormalities

S. The six chest leads of a standard 12-lead EKG

T. May refer to the different recordings taken of the electrical impulses coming from the heart at different angles or to the electrodes or sensors that are placed on the body during an EKG

Assignment 15-3: Misspelled Words

Underline the correctly spelled term.

1. ahrrhythmia   arrhythmia   arrhythemia

2. cardioversion   cardeovertion   cardioveartion

3. difibrillation   difibrallation   defibrillation

4. ischemia   iscemia   eschemia

5. galvinometer   galvanometer   gallvenometer

6. standardization   standardazation   standardizasion

7. stylis   stilus   stylus

8. isoelectric   iso-electric   isoeelectric

CHAPTER REVIEW

Assignment 15-4: Acronym Review

Write what each of the following acronyms stands for.

1. MI: _____

2. PACs: _____

3. EKG: _____

4. ECG: _____

5. PVCs: _____

6. PAT: _____

7. BPM: _____

8. V-tach: _____

9. V-fib: _____

Assignment 15-5: True or False

Fill in the blank with a "T" for true statements and an "F" for false statements. Rewrite the false statements to make them true.

____ 1. A single-channel EKG machine records all limb leads at once.

_____

_____

____ 2. All EKG machines automatically mark each lead for identification.

_____

_____

____ 3. The EKG tracing is made as a result of the heat from the stylus melting the plastic covering on the paper.

_____

_____

____ 4. Because skin is a poor conductor of electricity, an electrolyte solution is used.

_____

_____

____ 5. Lead I traces the electrical activity between the left arm and the left leg.

_____

_____

____ 6. A Holter monitor has four to five leads.

_____

_____

____ 7. Lead aVL records the difference in voltage between the right arm and a midpoint between the left arm and left leg.

_____

_____

____ 8. Standardization serves as quality assurance that the machine is working properly..

_____

_____

____ 9. It is okay to use leads from a different manufacturer if you have run out of leads for the unit you are using.

_____

_____

____ 10. If the patient's QRS wave is going off the graphing lines, you should turn the sensitivity control or "gain" down to 5.

_____

_____

Assignment 15-6: Short Answer

1. Trace the circulation of blood through the heart to the tissues of the body by completing the chart below. The first structure(s) is provided for you.

A. Superior and inferior vena cava	H.
B.	I.
C.	J.
D.	K.
E.	L.
F.	M.
G.	N.

2. Trace the heart's electrical system by filling in the diagram below.

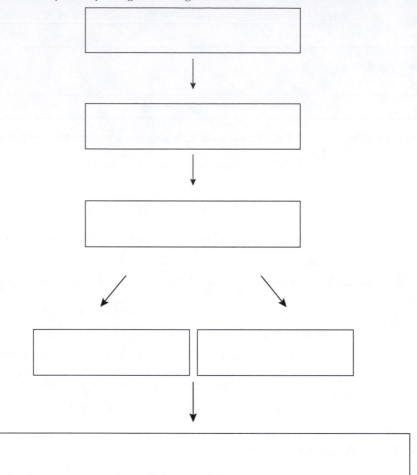

3. The firing of the SA node causes the _____ to contract. The firing of the AV node and its branches causes the _____ to contract.

4. Why is cardiac defibrillation sometimes necessary?

_____

_____

_____

5. Describe the following miscellaneous cardiac diagnostic tests.

   A. Holter monitor: _____

   _____

   _____

   B. Treadmill stress test: _____

   _____

   _____

   C. Echocardiography: _____

   _____

   _____

D. Cardiac catheterization: _____

_____

_____

_____

E. Noninvasive heart scan: _____

_____

_____

6. Explain the purpose of the graphing lines on the EKG paper.

_____

_____

_____

Assignment 15-7: Certification Practice

Choose the best answer and place the corresponding letter in the blank.

____ 1. Which of the following structures in the electrical conduction system of the heart is known as the "natural pacemaker"?

A. AV node

B. SA node

C. Bundle of His

D. Purkinje fibers

____ 2. Which of the following waves appears after the T wave?

A. P wave

B. R wave

C. S wave

D. U wave

____ 3. Which of the following statements is true regarding the isoelectric line?

A. It is a flat horizontal line.

B. It is the line that separates EKG cycles.

C. It is used as a reference point when vertically centering the tracing.

D. All of the above

____ 4. Which of the following provides not only the EKG tracing but an analysis of the tracing as well?

A. Multichannel EKG unit

B. Interpretive EKG unit

C. Automatic EKG unit

D. Facsimile

____ 5. How many electrodes are placed on the body when recording a 12-lead EKG?

A. 12

B. 10

C. 8

D. 7

____ 6. What occurs during depolarization?

A. Discharge of electrical energy

B. The heart is recharging

C. The heart is resting

D. None of the above

____ 7. Large squares on the EKG paper measure:

    A. 1 mm × 1 mm.

    B. 2 mm × 2 mm.

    C. 0.5 mm × 0.5 mm.

    D. 5 mm × 5 mm.

____ 8. What do the horizontal lines on the EKG paper measure?

    A. Amplitude

    B. Timing

    C. Interval between complexes

    D. Height of the complexes

____ 9. Which of the following limb wires is not used other than for grounding purposes?

    A. LA

    B. LL

    C. RL

    D. RA

____ 10. The purpose of including this in an EKG is to detect abnormalities in the patient's heart rhythm that may not be detectable in the standard leads due to the shorter representations of each lead.

    A. Standardization

    B. Markings

    C. Rhythm strip

    D. None of the above

____ 11. The letters aV on leads aVR, aVL, and aVF stand for which of the following?

    A. Anion volt

    B. Assisted voltage

    C. Augmented voltage

    D. Allocated voltage

____ 12. What is the location of lead V4?

    A. Fourth intercostal space at the left of the sternum

    B. Fifth intercostal space at the midclavicular line

    C. Fifth intercostal space at the midaxillary line

    D. Fourth intercostal space to the right of the sternum

____ 13. What is the purpose of the standardization mark on an EKG tracing?

    A. To ensure that the machine is working correctly

    B. To ensure that the stylus is hot enough

    C. To illustrate the height of the average complex

    D. None of the above

____ 14. What step should be taken by the medical assistant if the standardization is greater than 10 mm high?

    A. Adjust the sensitivity control to 5.

    B. Adjust the heat to the stylus.

    C. Stop the tracing and start over.

    D. Follow manufacturer's guidelines in the owner's manual and seek technical assistance if necessary.

____ 15. While performing an EKG, you notice that the patient's heart rate is approximately 200 BPM. What can you do to make the tracing easier to read and interpret?

    A. Adjust the stylus speed.

    B. Adjust the paper speed to 50 mm/sec.

    C. Adjust the paper speed to 20 mm/sec.

    D. No action is required.

____ 16. While performing an EKG on a patient you notice what looks like electrical interference. What steps may assist in correcting the problem?

    A. Make certain that the AC filter is turned on.

    B. Make certain that the cable and lead wires are not crossed or bent.

    C. Turn off electrical units that may be the cause of the interference.

    D. All of the above

____ 17. Mr. Leonard is very apprehensive about having an EKG for his employment physical because he is fearful that an abnormality may appear on the tracing that may cost him the position. What steps should be taken by the medical assistant?

    A. Try to put the patient at ease by addressing his concern.

    B. Ask the patient if he has a personal or family history of heart problems or current symptoms that are causing him to be concerned.

    C. Share the patient's concern with the physician.

    D. All of the above

____ 18. All of the following are medical assisting duties regarding Holter monitoring *except:*

    A. explaining how to fill out the patient diary.

    B. attaching the monitor.

    C. interpreting the tracing.

    D. removing the monitor.

____ 19. All of the following instructions should be given to the patient regarding the Holter monitor *except:*

    A. Do not touch or move electrodes.

    B. Press the event marker when you experience any related symptoms.

    C. It is OK to take a bath as long as the unit does not get wet.

    D. List all activities in the patient diary.

____ 20. Which of the following cardiac diagnostic procedures evaluates and measures plaque in the coronary arteries?

    A. Echocardiogram

    B. Holter monitor application

    C. Dobutamine test

    D. Noninvasive heart scan

____ 21. Which of the following leads records the difference in voltage between the left arm (+ pole) and a midpoint between the RA and LL (negative reference point)?

    A. aVR

    B. aVL

    C. aVF

    D. V-3

____ 22. Which of the following leads records the difference in voltage between the left leg (+ pole) and a midpoint between the right arm and the left arm (negative reference point)?

    A. aVR

    B. aVL

    C. aVF

    D. V-3

____ 23. Which of the following leads records the voltage between the RA and LA?

    A. Lead I

    B. Lead II

    C. Lead III

    D. aVL

___ 24. You notice that the QRS waves are very large and deflecting above the graphing lines on the tracing paper. You should:

    A. turn paper speed up to 50 mm/sec.

    B. turn down paper speed to 10 mm/sec.

    C. turn the gain or sensitivity down to 1/2 (or 5, depending on the unit).

    D. turn the gain or sensitivity up to 2 (or 20, depending on the unit).

___ 25. Prior to performing the EKG, an elderly male patient tells you that he is unable to lie flat due to a neck injury. Which of the following would be the best action to take based on the patient's complaint?

    A. Place the patient in a semi-Fowler's position.

    B. Tell the patient that EKGs are performed with the patient lying down and that you will hurry so that he doesn't have to be in the position very long.

    C. Have the patient stand during the EKG.

    D. Have the patient sit during the EKG.

SKILL APPLICATION CHALLENGES

Assignment 15-8: Labeling

1. Label the different types of interference.

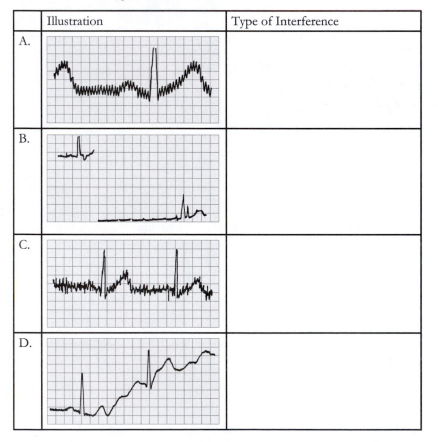

	Illustration	Type of Interference
A.		
B.		
C.		
D.		

2. On the diagram below, draw a circle where each chest lead should be placed.

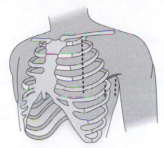

3. On the diagram below, draw squares where each limb lead should be placed.

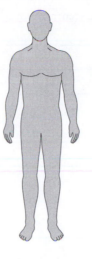

4. Label the following EKG cycle.

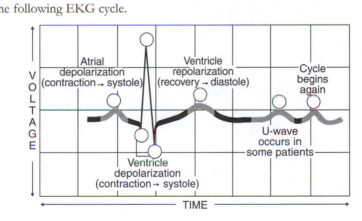

FIELD APPLICATION CHALLENGE
Assignment 15-9

Read the following Field Application Challenge and respond to the questions following the scenario.

The medical assistant is performing an EKG on a 79-year-old male who has a history of cardiac arrhythmias. The provider orders a standard 12-lead tracing along with a rhythm strip. The waves are barely visible on the tracing and there appears to be an interrupted base line only in leads I, II, and AVR.

1. What can be done to the unit to increase the amplitude of the waves?

   _____

   _____

2. Which lead wire(s) may have a problem based on the scenario above?

   _____

   _____

   _____

3. What may be the cause of the interrupted baseline?

   _____

   _____

JOURNALING EXERCISE
Assignment 15-10

What content within this chapter was most meaningful to you? Why? List some examples of how you might apply information contained in this chapter, both during your training and after you enter the health care industry.

C H A P T E R **16**

Pulmonary Examinations and Procedures

FIELD RELEVANCY AND BENEFITS

Respiratory disorders may be identified in any medical facility, from a general practice to a thoracic specialist. The medical assistant must be able to assist in procedures that evaluate lung capacity and respiratory health. Equally important, the medical assistant should be capable of identifying a respiratory crisis and promoting medical intervention. Respiration is an essential component of life. An understanding of the anatomy and physiology of the respiratory system is essential for communication and patient education. You will be able to utilize the skills taught within this chapter in a variety of practices including a general practitioner's office, an urgent care center, and a pulmonology practice.

NOTE SHEET

Types of Physicians Who Specialize in Treating Pulmonary Disorders

_____

_____

_____

_____

Respiratory Health Screening Questions

_____

_____

_____

_____

Factors That May Increase the Patient's Risk for Respiratory Disease

_____

_____

_____

Diagnostic Testing

_____

_____

_____

Medication Inhalation Therapy

_____

_____

_____

_____

Oxygen Administration

_____

_____

_____

_____

VOCABULARY REVIEW

Assignment 16-1: Misspelled Words

Underline the correctly spelled term.

1. Apna   Apne   Apnea

2. Pulmonology   Polmonology   Pulmonlogy

3. Spirmetry   Sprometry   Spirometry

4. Thoracenteses   Thoracentesis   Thrococentsis

5. Tubirculosis   Tuberculosis   Teberculosis

Assignment 16-2: Matching

Match the term with its definition and place the corresponding letter in the blank.

____ 1. Atelectasis

____ 2. Brochoscopy

____ 3. Carcinogens

____ 4. Multidrug-resistant TB (MDR-TB)

____ 5. Pleural effusion

____ 6. Hypoxic

____ 7. Induration

____ 8. Inhaler

____ 9. Mantoux skin test

____ 10. Nebulizer

____ 11. Peak flow meter

____ 12. Pulmonary function test

____ 13. Purified protein derivative (PPD)

____ 14. Pulmonologist

____ 15. Sputum

____ 16. Pulse oximetry

____ 17. Vital capacity

____ 18. QuantiFERON- TB Gold Test (QFT-G)

A. Maximum amount of air the patient can inhale and exhale

B. A common screening test for tuberculosis

C. Handheld portable device that delivers oxygen directly into the lungs

D. Small handheld device that measures the fastest speed air can be blown out of the lungs; is also a great tool for the patient to monitor lung ailments such as asthma while at home.

E. A small premeasured amount of TB antigen which is used for TB testing

F. Indirect test that is used to measure pulse rate and oxygen saturation levels in the blood

G. Units that change liquid medications into an aerosol mist so that they can be inhaled through a mouthpiece or facemask

H. A collapse of the alveoli (air sacs within the lungs)

I. A noninvasive test that checks lung function

J. Describing a patient who has a low oxygen level

K. Strains of tuberculosis that are resistant to medications normally used to treat TB

L. This rather recent screening test for TB is a blood test

M. Fluid or matter that is produced in the lungs and bronchi

N. A degree of hardening of normally soft tissue in the area

O. A physician who specializes in respiratory care

P. Cancer-causing agents

Q. Buildup of excess fluids in the pleural space

R. A procedure used to examine bronchial tubes and related structures

CHAPTER REVIEW

Assignment 16-3: Acronym Review

Write what each of the following acronyms stands for.

1. MDI: _____

2. MDR-TB: _____

3. PEF: _____

4. PPD: _____

5. TB: _____

6. VC: _____

Assignment 16-4: Short Answer

1. What factors that may increase the patient's risk for respiratory disease?

   _____

2. What is the common screening test for tuberculosis?

   _____

3. Arterial blood gases, ABGs, are ordered and studied for what two general purposes?

   A. _____

   B. _____

4. Results of the ABGs will measure what three items?

   A. _____

   B. _____

   C. _____

5. Where are arterial blood gases drawn from?

   _____

6. Why should ABG levels be performed on smokers, in addition to pulse oximetry testing?

   _____

   _____

   _____

7. List at least four benefits that come with smoking cessation.

   _____

   _____

   _____

   _____

   _____

Assignment 16-5: Certification Practice

Choose the best answer and place the corresponding letter in the blank.

____ 1. A test that uses spirometry before and after strenuous activity such as walking on a treadmill or riding a stationary bike is called a(n):

    A. exercise challenge test.

    B. PEF.

    C. PFT.

    D. peak flow meter.

____ 2. Which of the following communicable diseases is not spread through direct or indirect contact with infected individuals?

    A. Influenza

    B. Tuberculosis

    C. Asthma

    D. Pneumonia

____ 3. Which of the following tests is considered to be more accurate when measuring oxygen saturation?

    A. Pulse oximetry

    B. ABGs

    C. Spirometry

    D. PFT

____ 4. Abnormal ABGs might indicate all of the following *except:*

    A. head injury.

    B. respiratory stress.

    C. renal disorders.

    D. gastrointestinal disorders.

____ 5. Which of the following roles should the medical assistant assume when performing pulmonary function testing?

    A. Teacher

    B. Coach

    C. Nurse

    D. Friend

____ 6. The most common type of sleep apnea is:

    A. central.

    B. mixed.

    C. local.

    D. obstructive.

____ 7. Conditions in which SaO2 levels are significant include all of the following *except:*

    A. asthma.

    B. monitoring oxygen therapy.

    C. histoplasmosis.

    D. a possible heart attack.

____ 8. Which of the following diseases or disorders may be diagnosed with the aid of a KOH smear?

    A. Pneumonia

    B. Bronchitis

    C. Tuberculosis

    D. Coccidiodomycosis

___ 9. Which of the following radiological exams is typically performed to view the lung?

    A. Chest x-ray

    B. CT scan

    C. MRI

    D. Bronchoscopy

___ 10. Which of the following radiological exams is noninvasive and gives clearer pictures than traditional x-rays, but may be difficult for patients who are claustrophobic?

    A. Chest x-ray

    B. CT scan

    C. MRI scan

    D. Bronchoscopy

___ 11. All of the following are common medications used in a nebulizer *except:*

    A. anticholinergics.

    B. bronchodilators.

    C. antibiotics.

    D. Corticosteroids

___ 12. All of the following are symptoms for TB *except:*

    A. night sweats.

    B. tachycardia.

    C. cough with bloody sputum.

    D. tonsillitis.

___ 13. The leading cause of cancer death for both males and females according to the American Cancer Society is:

    A. colon cancer.

    B. lung cancer.

    C. breast cancer.

    D. prostate cancer.

___ 14. A test that detects the lungs' ability to function by measuring how rapidly a patient can move air in and out of the lungs is called:

    A. spirometry.

    B. bronchoscopy.

    C. PEF.

    D. nebulizer.

___ 15. Normal oxygen saturation levels are:

    A. 80% to 90%.

    B. 90% to 95%.

    C. 96% to 100%.

    D. over 100%.

___ 16. A test that is performed by wrapping a small strap around the patient's nail bed on a finger or toe is called:

    A. PFT.

    B. pulse oximetry.

    C. ABG.

    D. nebulizer.

___ 17. A spirometer should be calibrated:

    A. once a week.

    B. once a month.

    C. quarterly.

    D. on any day that testing is performed.

____ 18. How many liters of air should be injected into the unit when calibrating the spirometer?

    A. One liter

    B. Two liters

    C. Three liters

    D. Four liters

____ 19. Normal PFTs should fall within what percentage of the predicted value?

    A. 35%

    B. 45%

    C. 75%

    D. 85%

____ 20. The following are all guidelines for using a peak flow meter *except:*

    A. The pointer on the flow meter should start on the number 10.

    B. Remove all candy, food, or gum from mouth before starting the test.

    C. Breathe out as hard and fast as possible.

    D. Record the highest reading of three attempts.

____ 21. Following TB skin testing, the patient should return to the office:

    A. one to two days following testing.

    B. two to three days following testing.

    C. three to four days following testing.

    D. one week following testing.

____ 22. Which of the following secretions may be required when checking the lungs for infections?

    A. Nasal secretions

    B. Mucus secretions

    C. Saliva

    D. Sputum

____ 23. If patients test positive for tuberculosis, they should also have which of the following procedures or tests performed to see if they have an active case of tuberculosis?

    A. Chest x-ray

    B. PPD test

    C. Mantoux test

    D. None of the above

____ 24. Components of a nebulizer include:

    A. compressor.

    B. nebulizer tubing.

    C. medicine cup.

    D. all of the above.

____ 25. Which of the following variables would not affect pulse oximetry testing?

    A. Calluses on the digit being used

    B. Having unusually short digits

    C. Nail polish on the digit being used

    D. Ambient lighting in the area

COMPLETING SPECIAL FORMS

Assignment 16-6: Completing a Lab Requisition Form for a Sputum Culture

Work Form Necessary: FORM 16-1

Directions: Using the scenario information below, complete the lab requisition form (Work Form 16-1).

Sandy B. Bell needs to have a sputum culture done today, July 7, 2010. Her provider, Dr. Thomas Weston, thinks that she may have pneumonia.

> Patient's address: 111 Guthrie Road, Douglasville, NY 01234
> Patient's DOB: 08-11-55
> Patient's telephone number: (123) 858-9989
> Provider's number: 25698745
> Provider's address: Douglasville Medicine Associates, 5076 Brand Blvd, Douglasville, NY 01234
> Provider's telephone number: (123) 456-7890
> Test code: 45213
> Test name: Sputum Culture
> Specimen type: Sputum
> Tube type/collection container: Nonsterile specimen container
> ICD-9: 481.0
> CPT: 87070

FIELD APPLICATION CHALLENGE

Assignment 16-7

Read the following Field Application Challenge and respond to the questions following the scenario.

It is Monday morning and Maria Santias calls to state that she is not feeling well. While on the phone with her, you hear her wheezing. Maria states that she is having trouble breathing. She has a history of asthma and has an asthma inhaler at home. She states that she took the recommended number of puffs from her inhaler but has not gotten any relief.

1. Based on this information, what should you have Mary do?

_____

_____

2. Document the phone call and your instructions to the patient on the following chart note. Use today's date and your name and SMA in the closing signature.

JOURNALING EXERCISE
Assignment 16-8

What content within this chapter was most meaningful to you? Why? List some examples of how you might apply information contained in this chapter, both during your training and after you enter the health care industry.

Work Form 16-1

ABC Laboratory	
Patient's Name	**Patient's Address**
Patient's Date of Birth:	**Patient's Telephone Number**
Provider Name: **Provider Number:**	**Provider Address & Phone:**

Testing Information

Test Date:	
Test Code:	
Test Name:	
Specimen Type:	
Tube Type/ Collection Container:	
ICD-9 Code:	
CPT Code(s):	

C H A P T E R **17**

Women's Health Issues: Obstetrics and Gynecology

FIELD RELEVANCY AND BENEFITS

The field of obstetrics and gynecology (OB-GYN) presents some unique challenges for the medical assistant that are not found in other medical specialty practices. This specialty requires the medical assistant to have a thorough knowledge of the female reproductive system and how it functions, as well as a general knowledge of diseases and disorders that are unique to females.

The medical assistant must be able to prepare the patient for the OB-GYN or prenatal exam and must obtain and document all necessary information related to the type of exam being performed. A thorough OB-GYN history must be obtained to be used as a reference base. Patient education plays an important role in this specialty, and it also helps to promote good health for women before, during, and after pregnancy. The medical assistant must possess a basic knowledge of highly specialized laboratory and diagnostic tests that are related to OB-GYN and be familiar with any special patient preparation guidelines to help ensure accurate results. Information in this chapter will be useful for those working in family practice, general practice, internal medicine, and OB-GYN offices.

NOTE SHEET

Types of Physicians Who Specialize in Treating Diseases and Disorders of the Female Reproductive System

_____

_____

_____

_____

Gynecology

_____

_____

_____

_____

Patient Screening for the Female Reproductive System

_____

_____

_____

_____

The Menstrual Cycle

_____

_____

_____

_____

The Gynecological Exam

_____

_____

_____

_____

Gynecological Diagnostic Tests and Procedures

_____

_____

_____

_____

Sexually Transmitted Diseases

_____

_____

_____

_____

Obstetrics

_____

_____

_____

_____

Prenatal Care

_____

_____

_____

_____

Prenatal Diagnostic Tests and Procedures

_____

_____

_____

_____

Pregnancy Complications

_____

_____

_____

_____

Labor and Delivery

_____

_____

_____

_____

The Postnatal or Postpartum Period

_____

_____

_____

_____

VOCABULARY REVIEW

Assignment 17-1: Matching

Match the term with its definition and place the corresponding letter in the blank.

____ 1. Abortion

____ 2. Braxton-Hicks

____ 3. Amniocentesis

____ 4. Dysmenorrhea

____ 5. Colposcopy

____ 6. Metrorrhagia

____ 7. Ectopic

____ 8. Effacement

____ 9. Gravida

____ 10. Meconium

____ 11. Eclampsia

____ 12. Toxemia

____ 13. Parturition

____ 14. Puerperium

____ 15. Trimester

A. Another term for preeclampsia

B. Another name for labor

C. Term for the three-month intervals that a pregnancy is divided into

D. Another name for the postpartum period

E. Periods of bleeding that occur in addition to the regular monthly cycles

F. A progression of preeclampsia in which all of the same symptoms are present as seen in preeclampsia but with the addition of seizures or convulsions

G. Total number of pregnancies including the present one

H. Pregnancy occurs outside the uterus; tubal pregnancy

I. First stools of the newborn

J. Thinning and shortening of the cervix to permit the fetus/baby to pass through

K. Examination of the vagina and cervix with the aid of a lighted scope

L. Difficult or painful menstruation

M. Removal or expulsion of an embryo or fetus from the uterus, resulting in death

N. Periodic and painless irregular uterine contractions that usually occur 10 to 20 minutes apart (false labor)

O. Procedure to withdraw amniotic fluid from the amniotic sac for testing purposes (usually genetic testing)

Assignment 17-2: Sentence Completion

Fill in the blanks below with Essential Terms from this chapter.

1. _____ is the expansion of the cervix during labor to facilitate the passage of the fetus.

2. _____ is the period of time from conception to birth.

3. A(n) _____ is also known as a spontaneous abortion.

4. The vaginal discharge of blood, mucous, and tissue coming from the uterus following delivery is known as _____.

5. The period of time before birth is called the _____ period.

6. _____ is the period of time before or around menopause characterized by irregular menses and amenorrhea.

7. A(n) _____ is a procedure in which a surgical incision is made into the abdominal wall to remove the baby from the mother's uterus.

8. _____ refers to the number of live births that a patient has had.

CHAPTER REVIEW

Assignment 17-3: Acronym Review

Write what each of the following acronyms stands for.

1. LMP: _____

2. EDD: _____

3. EDC: _____

4. OB-GYN: _____

5. HPV: _____

6. D and C: _____

7. HRT: _____

8. FAS: _____

9. AFP: _____

10. CVS: _____

Assignment 17-4: True or False

Fill in the blank with a "T" for true statements and an "F" for false statements. Rewrite the false statements to make them true.

____ 1. The fastest rise in STD percentages in the past few years has been among the "senior" population.

_____

_____

____ 2. The endometrium is the muscle layer of the uterus that contracts during labor and delivery.

_____

_____

____ 3. Women who have a normal baseline mammogram at age 40 should have follow-up readings every three years until age 50.

_____

_____

____ 4. The bimanual exam is a pelvic exam conducted by the provider by inserting the fingers of one hand into the vagina and using the other hand to palpate the pelvic organs from the outside.

_____

_____

____ 5. All menopausal women should receive HRT to alleviate the symptoms of menopause.

_____

_____

____ 6. An infertility specialist assists patients who are having problems conceiving.

_____

_____

____ 7. Amniocentesis is often performed to verify the sex of the fetus.

_____

_____

____ 8. An abdominal exam is the part of the initial prenatal exam conducted to detect lumps or swellings that are not part of normal fetal development.

_____

_____

____ 9. A group B strep screening is a normal screening performed on patients who are pregnant because this particular species of bacteria can be life-threatening to the developing fetus.

_____

_____

____ 10. HPV is the most common sexually transmitted disease in the United States.

_____

_____

Assignment 17-5: Short Answer

1. List the three parts of the Bethesda System for Reporting Pap Results and describe the purpose of each section.

   A. _____

   _____

   B. _____

   _____

   C. _____

   _____

2. Provide the recommended schedule for prenatal visits.

   _____

   _____

   _____

3. Describe at what points ultrasound testing is performed during pregnancy and what is evaluated during each ultrasound.

   _____

   _____

   _____

   _____

   _____

   _____

4. List and explain the stages of labor.

    1. _____

       _____

    2. _____

       _____

    3. _____

       _____

5. Discuss the importance of the postpartum exam and what is performed during the exam..

    _____

    _____

    _____

    _____

    _____

    _____

6. List and describe the components of the GYN exam.

    1. _____

    2. _____

    3. _____

    4. _____

    5. _____

Assignment 17-6: Certification Practice

Choose the best answer and place the corresponding letter in the blank.

____ 1. Which of the following medical terms is used when a patient is in labor?

    A. Parity

    B. Puerperium

    C. Parturition

    D. Postpartum

____ 2. From which of the following tests could a diagnosis of endometrial cancer be made?

    A. Pap test

    B. Endometrial biopsy

    C. Maturation index

    D. Hormone level

____ 3. Another name for Braxton-Hicks contractions is:

    A. preterm labor.

    B. false labor.

    C. true labor.

    D. early labor.

____ 4. A pregnant patient considered to be full term at:

    A. 10 months.

    B. 9 months.

    C. 35 weeks.

    D. 36 to 40 weeks.

___ 5. It has been determined that a patient has some atypical cells on her cervix that could potentially become cancerous. Which of the following procedures would the provider perform to freeze the atypical cells?

    A. Electrosurgery

    B. Nitrosurgery

    C. LEEP

    D. Cryosurgery

___ 6. Which of the following hormones is responsible for the flow of milk following delivery of the baby?

    A. Estrogen

    B. Oxytocin

    C. Insulin

    D. Progesterone

___ 7. A patient is in the office today for her yearly GYN exam. You get her blood pressure and weight and update her medical history. You give her disrobing instructions and then leave the room. Which of the following additional steps should have been performed to promote patient comfort during the exam?

    A. Asking the patient to empty her bladder

    B. Telling the patient to sit in the chair until the provider comes in

    C. Asking the patient if she is warm enough

    D. Asking the patient if she has any questions

___ 8. Which of the following statements about breast cancer is true?

    A. Only women with a family history of the disease are at risk.

    B. Men can develop breast cancer.

    C. You are only at risk if you have a palpable lump in your breast.

    D. None of the above

___ 9. Which of the following advantages of the liquid prep method makes it more desirable than conventional Pap tests?

    A. Only a small portion of cells are used.

    B. It eliminates debris and evenly distributes a thin layer of cells on the slide.

    C. It needs to be performed five days after the LMP.

    D. The test is less expensive.

___ 10. Which of the following abnormalities might the provider be looking for during a rectal exam?

    A. Hemorrhoids

    B. Fistulas

    C. Fissures

    D. All of the above

___ 11. Which of the following is the purpose for an endometrial ablation?

    A. Removal of leiomyomas

    B. Removal or destruction of the entire thickness of the endometrium

    C. To freeze cells on the cervix

    D. To view the interior of the uterus

___ 12. The term *para* stands for:

    A. the number of pregnancies.

    B. the number of premature births.

    C. the number of full term births.

    D. the number of live births.

___ 13. Which of the following actions would you take when a patient who is scheduled for her Pap test tells you that she just finished her period and douched last night?

    A. Share the information with the provider.

    B. Reschedule her appointment.

    C. Prepare three slides instead of two.

    D. Lubricate the speculum.

___ 14. Which of the following is a rapid test for the detection of chlamydia and gonorrhea?

    A. Amplified DNA probe

    B. LEEP

    C. VDRL

    D. RPR

___ 15. Which of the following would be considered medical assisting duties during the first prenatal exam?

    A. Vital signs

    B. Weight

    C. Draw blood and collect urine for testing

    D. All of the above

___ 16. A patient at 28 weeks gestation phones the office complaining of cramping, pelvic pressure, low-back pain, and regular contractions. Which of the following might be a possible explanation for her symptoms?

    A. Preeclampsia

    B. Toxemia

    C. Preterm labor

    D. Placenta previa

___ 17. Which of the following is the usual gestational age when fetal heart tones can be heard?

    A. 15 to 20 weeks

    B. 10 to 12 weeks

    C. 6 to 8 weeks

    D. 20 to 22 weeks

___ 18. The AFP test is performed to detect which of the following defects?

    A. Gestational diabetes

    B. Fetal gender

    C. Fetal blood type

    D. Neural tube defects

___ 19. Which of the following is a mild form of diabetes that develops in the second or third trimester?

    A. Type I

    B. Type II

    C. Diabetes mellitus

    D. Gestational

___ 20. The correct term for the vaginal discharge that can last for up to six weeks after delivery is:

    A. Lochia rubra

    B. Lochia alba

    C. Lochia serosa

    D. Lochia melanin

SKILL APPLICATION CHALLENGES

Assignment 17-7: Application Activity

Using Naegle's Rule, calculate the following EDDs.

1. LMP: 01-11-08:   EDD: _____

2. LMP: 05-06-09:   EDD: _____

3. LMP: 02-17-11:   EDD: _____

Assignment 17-8: Documentation Exercise

Interpret the following documentations.

1. G:3 P:2 A:1 _____

2. G:1 P:1 A:0 _____

3. G:5 P:3 A:2 _____

Assignment 17-9: Projects

1. Look up the latest methods of birth control and prepare a PowerPoint presentation that illustrates the advantages and disadvantages of each type.
2. Research the topic of new advances in intrauterine surgery to correct fetal abnormalities and write a paper which includes photos to present to the class.
3. Interview an OB-GYN specialist in your area and gather statistics on how many babies the physician has delivered, whether or not the physician's practice uses a midwife, how many multiple births the physician has performed, how many C-sections, etc. Include any interesting information provided by the physician about difficult or unusual births.

FIELD APPLICATION CHALLENGE

Assignment 17-10

Read the following Field Application Challenge and respond to the questions following the scenario.

A 28-year-old female at 20 weeks gestation is in the office today for an ultrasound. She is very excited about the procedure and is anxious to find out the baby's sex but she also states that she is a bit nervous because she has not felt any movement over the past couple of days. You set the patient up for her exam and leave the room to alert the physician about the information provided by the patient. The physician asks you to remain in the exam room during the ultrasound just in case there are any problems. Upon ultrasound examination, the physician cannot see any signs that the heart is beating nor were there any heart tones picked up by the fetal monitor.

1. What do these findings mean?

_____

2. The physician leaves the room after explaining to the patient the progression plan that will be followed from this point forward. The physician was very caring and nurturing but the patient falls apart emotionally after the physician leaves the room. What can you do to assist the patient during this difficult encounter?

_____

_____

_____

JOURNALING EXERCISE

Assignment 17-11

What content within this chapter was most meaningful to you? Why? List some examples of how you might apply information contained in this chapter, both during your training and after you enter the health care industry.

C H A P T E R   **18**

Urology and Male Reproductive Examinations and Procedures

FIELD RELEVANCY AND BENEFITS

Because urological evaluations involve the urinary system of males and the females as well as the male reproductive system, it is important for the medical assistant to be knowledgeable regarding the systems involved along with associated diseases and disorders. The medical assistant must also be knowledgeable about the diagnostic tests performed in a urology practice and be able to educate the patient on proper preparation for these procedures. The skills and knowledge gained by studying the information in this chapter can be used in urology and nephrology practices. Some of the information can also be applied to family practice, pediatrics, and internal medicine practices.

NOTE SHEET

Types of Physicians Who Specialize in Treating Diseases and Disorders of the Urinary and Male Reproductive Systems

_____

_____

_____

_____

Patient Screening for the Urinary System

_____

_____

_____

_____

Diagnostic Testing

_____

_____

_____

Treatments Involving the Urinary Structures

_____

_____

_____

Patient Screening for the Male Reproductive System

_____

_____

_____

_____

Diagnostic Testing Associated with the Male Reproductive System

_____

_____

_____

_____

Lab Work Associated with Male Reproductive Organs

_____

_____

_____

_____

Common Procedures Performed Involving Male Reproductive Organs

_____

_____

_____

_____

Erectile Dysfunction

_____

_____

_____

_____

VOCABULARY REVIEW

Assignment 18-1: Matching

Match the term with its definition and place the corresponding letter in the blank.

____ 1. Benign prostatic hypertrophy

____ 2. Catheterization

____ 3. Circumcision

____ 4. Cystoscopy

____ 5. Dialysis

____ 6. Digital rectal exam

____ 7. Erectile dysfunction (ED)

____ 8. Foley catheter

____ 9. Hemodialysis

____ 10. Urology

A. The provider places a gloved finger into the patient's rectum to examine the prostate for enlargement, lumps, and other abnormalities

B. Insertion of a lighted scope into the bladder

C. Dialysis in which the patient is hooked up to a dialysis unit through tubes that connect to the patient's blood vessels

D. The study of the urinary system and male reproductive system

E. A catheter that includes a balloon so that the catheter can stay in place for prolonged periods of time

F. Enlarged prostate that is not related to cancer of the prostate

G. Removal of the foreskin of the penis

H. Filtering waste products from the blood with the aid of a machine

I. The insertion of a sterile tube directly into the bladder through the urethra to obtain a sterile specimen

J. The inability to achieve or maintain an erection during sexual relations.

Assignment 18-2: Definitions

Define the following terms.

1. Hernia: _____

_____

2. Extracorporeal shock wave lithotripsy (ESWL): _____

_____

3. Intravenous pyelography (IVP): _____

_____

4. Nephrologist: _____

_____

5. Peritoneal dialysis: _____

_____

6. Testicular self-examination: _____

_____

7. Transrectal ultrasound: _____

_____

8. Transurethral resection procedure (TURP): _____

_____

9. Urethral dilatation: _____

_____

10. Vasography: _____

_____

CHAPTER REVIEW

Assignment 18-3: Acronym Review

Write what each of the following acronyms stands for.

1. TURP: _____
2. TRUS: _____
3. TSE: _____
4. BUN: _____
5. CAPD: _____
6. IVP: _____
7. BPH: _____
8. ED: _____

Assignment 18-4: Short Answer

1. What is the medical assistant's role in diagnostic examinations of the urinary system?

_____

2. List and describe three types of access for hemodialysis.

A. _____

_____

B. _____

_____

C. _____

_____

3. What blood tests are performed to determine the health/function of the kidneys?

_____

4. Name the two common types of catheters and describe when each would be used.

A. _____

_____

_____

B. _____

_____

_____

5. List some criteria that must be met prior to receiving a kidney transplant.

_____

_____

_____

Assignment 18-5: Certification Practice

Choose the best answer and place the corresponding letter in the blank.

____ 1. Which of the following types of hemodialysis access is considered the most durable?

A. Graft

B. Fistula

C. Venous catheter/port

D. Peritoneal

____ 2. The best way to diagnose prostate cancer is through:

A. blood test PSA.

B. biopsy.

C. TURP.

D. vasectomy.

____ 3. The process that involves the insertion of a sterile tube directly into the bladder through the urethra using strict sterile technique is called:

A. catheterization.

B. cystoscopy.

C. IVP.

D. ultrasound.

____ 4. A procedure during which the provider can examine both the urethra and bladder is called:

A. catheterization.

B. cystoscopy.

C. IVP.

D. ultrasound.

____ 5. Which of the following terms means excessive urination?

    A. Hematuria

    B. Nocturia

    C. Polyuria

    D. Dysuria

____ 6. Which of the following procedures relieves the symptoms of BPH?

    A. Vasectomy

    B. TURP

    C. TSE

    D. ED

____ 7. The sudden urge to void is referred to as:

    A. polyuria.

    B. frequency.

    C. oliguria.

    D. urgency.

____ 8. The medical term for scanty urination is:

    A. polyuria.

    B. dysuria.

    C. oliguria.

    D. frequency.

____ 9. A radiographic procedure in which contrast dye is injected into the patient through an IV to examine the internal structures of the kidneys and urinary tract is called:

    A. cystoscopy.

    B. IVP.

    C. KUB.

    D. none of the above.

____ 10. A word meaning a narrowing is:

    A. stricture.

    B. stasis.

    C. narrosis.

    D. stent.

____ 11. The term that means crushing of kidney stones is:

    A. lithostasis.

    B. lithotomy.

    C. lithotripsy.

    D. triptolithiasis.

____ 12. Which of the following terms means the inability to control urine flow?

    A. Urgency

    B. Incontinence

    C. Dysuria

    D. Polyuria

____ 13. Which of the following terms means an overgrowth of tissue?

    A. Hyperplasia

    B. Hyperhistia

    C. Hyperplegia

    D. Supraplasia

___ 14. The radiological procedure that is used to evaluate patency of the vas deferens and ejaculatory ducts is called:

    A. TURP.

    B. TRUS.

    C. biopsy.

    D. vasography.

___ 15. Women are often prone to cystitis (inflammation of the bladder). Symptoms of cystitis include urinary frequency, urgency, and dysuria. Which of the following educational tips would *not* be helpful for preventing future infections?

    A. Stay away from cotton underwear; use nylon instead.

    B. Avoid fragranced soaps and bubble baths that may irritate the urethra.

    C. Woman should wipe from front to back.

    D. Urinate frequently and empty entire bladder.

SKILL APPLICATION CHALLENGES

Assignment 18-7: Labeling

    1. Label the parts of the male urinary system.

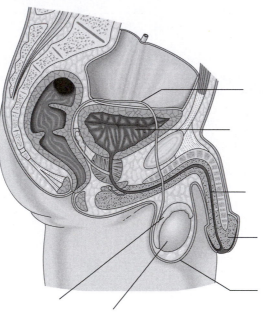

    2. Label the parts of the female urinary system.

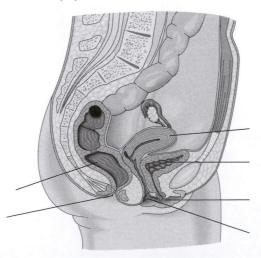

3. Label the parts of the female external genitalia.

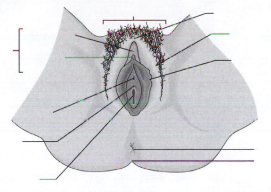

Assignment 18-8: Project

Look up the term "kidney transplant" using your preferred Internet search browser.

1. On the lines below, make a list of people that may be potential donors for someone needing a kidney.

   A. _____

   B. _____

   C. _____

2. How long is a patient's stay in the hospital following a kidney transplant?

   _____

3. What is the length of time a kidney may be out of the donor's body before placing it into recipient's body? How is the kidney preserved?

   _____

   _____

   _____

4. What types of patients would not be considered as suitable for a kidney transplant?

   _____

   _____

   _____

Assignment 18-9: Case Study

Part I: A patient calls on the phone complaining of excruciating pain in his lower back and abdomen on the left side. The pain came on suddenly and the patient now has blood in his urine. The symptoms started approximately one hour ago. Answer the following questions based on this scenario.

1. What might be a likely cause of the patient's symptoms?

   _____

   _____

   _____

   _____

2. What would be typical instructions for a patient with the above symptoms and what forms of treatment are available if the patient does, in fact, have a kidney stone?

_____

_____

_____

_____

_____

_____

Part II: You decide to develop the complaint a bit by asking the patient about his urinary history. The patient denies a history of any urinary tract or kidney problems. Because of the distress the patient is in, you decide to transfer the call to Dr. Roy. Dr. Roy instructs the patient to go to the ER and directs you to call the ER to let them know that he is on his way. Using all of the information presented in Parts I and II, create a chart note that describes the call and the instructions given to the patient (use today's date, the current time, and list yourself as the medical assistant).

FIELD APPLICATION CHALLENGE

Assignment 18-10

Read the following Field Application Challenge and respond to the questions following the scenario.

Mr. Honeycutt is diagnosed with an enlarged prostate. The provider asks you to provide education to the patient regarding his condition. Using a computer search engine, create a list of Web sites that will assist the patient in learning about his condition. Try to include at least one reference that includes an animation. Make a list of Web sites the patient can go to and provide reference information beside each Web site that describes what the patient should click on once they get to the Web site as well as the outstanding features of each Web site. Items of interest for this presentation include: how the size of the prostate affects urine flow; tests that are performed initially and for monitoring purposes thereafter; and procedures that can be performed to correct the condition.

_____

_____

_____

_____

JOURNALING EXERCISE
Assignment 18-11

What content within this chapter was most meaningful to you? Why? List some examples of how you might apply information contained in this chapter, both during your training and after you enter the health care industry?

C H A P T E R **19**

Evaluation and Care of the Pediatric Patient

FIELD RELEVANCY AND BENEFITS

The climate of medicine has changed dramatically over the past several years. The traditional reactive approach to medicine which emphasized treatment has changed to a more proactive approach which focuses on prevention and maintenance.

Years of research have confirmed that illness can be related to a person's lifestyle. Many cancers, heart disease, and other chronic illnesses such as diabetes are triggered by lifestyle choices that begin early in life. Pediatric health care is becoming much more focused on education while still continuing to treat childhood and adolescent disorders. Teaching parents to immunize their children, to make wise dietary and exercise choices for their children, and to keep their children away from pollutants that can wake up dormant cancer cells is the latest emphasis in pediatric health care. Medical assistants must empower themselves with education so that they can instruct young patients and their parents on how to prevent illness as well as to avoid needless injuries by taking a more proactive approach.

Having knowledge about pediatric wellness schedules and immunizations as well as being familiar with common diseases and disorders that children acquire will assist those working in pediatric clinics. The information in this chapter will be beneficial for anyone desiring to work in a pediatric or family practice clinic, or any specialty practices that serve pediatric clients.

NOTE SHEET

Pediatric Age Classifications

_____

_____

_____

_____

Age-Appropriate Communication

_____

_____

_____

_____

Infant/Toddler Measurements

_____

_____

_____

_____

Pediatric Development

_____

_____

_____

_____

Screenings

_____

_____

_____

_____

Vaccinations

_____

_____

_____

_____

Pediatric Injections

_____

_____

_____

_____

Blood Screenings of the Newborn

_____

_____

_____

_____

Circumcision

_____

_____

_____

_____

Adolescent Care

_____

_____

_____

_____

Behavioral and Mental Health Issues

_____

_____

_____

_____

VOCABULARY REVIEW

Assignment 19-1: Sentence Completion

Fill in the blanks below with Essential Terms from this chapter.

1. _____ is the name for an eating disorder in which an individual limits food intake or does not eat at all to the point of starvation.

2. Height or body type that occurs within a family is called _____.

3. A child in the first year of his life is called a(n) _____.

4. _____ is a condition in which the head is abnormally small.

5. _____ development is an area of growth that includes reflexes, gross motor skills, and fine motor skills.

6. Activities that indicate acceptable growth and development patterns are known as _____.

7. The term _____ refers to a child in his first month of life.

8. _____ patients can range from the newborn to the young adult.

9. A teenager is the same as a(n) _____.

10. The term that refers to the initial period following birth is _____.

Assignment 19-2: Misspelled Words

Underline the correctly spelled term.

1. adolesent   adolescent   addolescent
2. circumcision   circumsion   circumscition
3. macrocephale   macrochephaly   macrocephaly
4. familial   famielial   famileal
5. buliemia nervosa   bulemia nervosa   bulimia nervosa
6. chest circumference   chest circumfrence   chest circumferance
7. immunizaitions   immunizations   immunizasions
8. neonat   neonate   kneonate

CHAPTER REVIEW

Assignment 19-3: Acronym Review

Write what each of the following acronyms stands for.

1. IRT: _____
2. DTaP: _____
3. PCV: _____
4. IPV: _____
5. HepB: _____
6. Hib: _____

Assignment 19-4: True or False

Fill in the blank with a "T" for true statements and an "F" for false statements. Rewrite the false statements to make them true.

____ 1. When communicating with a child who has not yet developed language skills, using facial expressions and body motions will help him understand the message you are trying to convey.

_____

_____

____ 2. Breathing, sucking, and rooting are common reflexes in infants.

_____

_____

____ 3. A six-month-old should be able to stand without support.

_____

_____

____ 4. A nine-month-old should be able to attempt to catch a thrown object.

_____

_____

____ 5. A 13- to 18-month-old should be able to speak in short sentences.

_____

_____

____ 5. An infant may be hearing-impaired if he is not startled by loud noises.

_____

_____

____ 7. The hepatitis B vaccine is given at birth.

_____

_____

____ 8. Infants should begin receiving the influenza vaccine at three months of age.

_____

_____

____ 9. The deepening of a boy's voice would be considered a secondary sex characteristic.

_____

_____

____ 10. Measuring the chest circumference is an additional calculation that is used to identify low birth weight in preterm babies.

_____

_____

____ 11. The age range for toddlers is considered to be late in the first year of life to preschool age.

_____

_____

____ 12. A caliper is a device that is used to weigh an infant.

_____

_____

____ 13. Macrocephaly is usually indicated if a child's head measures above the 80th percentile.

_____

_____

____ 14. The brachial and femoral arteries can be used to take an infant's pulse.

_____

_____

____ 15. A pulse rate of 85 BPM would be normal in a child who is five years of age.

_____

_____

____ 16. A startle reflex to noise or other environmental stimuli causing an infant's arms to fling out to the side with the palms up is termed as a rooting reflex.

_____

_____

____ 17. By age 20 months most children should be able to kick a ball.

_____

_____

____ 18. Babies between the age of 10 and 12 months should be able to understand simple words and commands.

_____

_____

Assignment 19-5: Short Answer

1. Explain the importance of correctly plotting height, weight, and head circumference measurements on the pediatric patient.

_____

_____

2. Fill in the normal pulse and respiratory rates for each of the ages listed.

Age	Average Heart Rate	Average Respiratory Rate
Birth	140 BPM	30–60/min.
0–6 months	_____	_____
6–12 months	_____	_____
12–24 months	_____	_____
2–6 years	_____	_____
6–10 years	_____	_____
10–14 years	_____	_____
14 years–adult	_____	_____

3. List and describe six reflexes that are tested in the newborn.

A. _____

B. _____

C. _____

D. _____

E. _____

F. _____

4. Explain how weight is calculated after an infant is weighed in a diaper and a t-shirt.

_____

_____

Assignment 19-6: Certification Practice

Choose the best answer and place the corresponding letter in the blank.

____ 1. Which of the following age classifications would be given to a child who is $2\frac{1}{2}$ years old?

A. Child

B. Infant

C. Preschooler

D. Toddler

____ 2. The main purpose for performing height and weight measurements on pediatric patients is:

A. to provide statistical information.

B. to determine growth trends.

C. to detect potential health problems.

D. to measure rapid growth.

____ 3. At what age can a child be weighed and measured on an upright scale?

A. 2 years

B. 3 years

C. 18 months

D. When the child is able to stand alone

____ 4. Transferring an object from one hand to the other would be considered to be which type of development in an infant?

A. Gross motor

B. Fine motor

C. Sensory

D. None of the above

____ 5. Pediatric visual screenings begin at what age?

A. 18 months

B. 2 years

C. During infancy

D. 3 years

____ 6. Hearing impairment is often mistaken for which of the following conditions?

A. Intellectual delay

B. Speech delay

C. Mental retardation

D. Learning disability

____ 7. Documentation of the immunization may be recorded in all but which of the following records?

A. The immunization log that is provided to the insurance company

B. The parents' personal immunization log for the child

C. The global immunization log for the practice

D. The immunization log within the patient's chart

____ 8. The preferred location for the administration of an intramuscular injection in the young pediatric patient is:

A. dorsogluteal.

B. deltoid.

C. gluteal.

D. vastus lateralis.

____ 9. If cystic fibrosis is suspected in an infant, which of the following tests is usually performed?
   A. PKU
   B. IRT
   C. Ketonuria
   D. Galactosemia

____ 10. All of the following immunizations will be given to a six-month-old *except:*
   A. DTaP.
   B. HepB.
   C. Hib.
   D. MMR.

____ 11. Which of the following signs could be an indication of childhood depression?
   A. Dangerous behavior
   B. Increased physical complaints
   C. Increased boredom
   D. All of the above

____ 12. Which of the following conditions could be present when a teenager seems to eat a large amount of food but never gains weight?
   A. Anorexia nervosa
   B. Metabolisia nervosa
   C. Bulimia nervosa
   D. Heredity

____ 13. Which of the following tests is required for newborns in most states?
   A. IRT
   B. Sickle cell test
   C. PKU
   D. Blood typing

____ 14. Which of the following could contribute to childhood obesity?
   A. Fast food
   B. School nutrition programs
   C. Removal of physical education programs
   D. Genetics
   E. All of the above

____ 15. Common immunizations given at age two months include:
   A. DTaP.
   B. HepB.
   C. Hib.
   D. all of the above.

____ 16. When taking vital signs on a patient that is four months old, you notice that the pulse rate is 128 beats per minute. What action should be taken by the medical assistant?
   A. Record the information in the chart and notify the physician right away.
   B. Record the information in the chart and allow the physician to read it as he reviews the chart before entering the room.
   C. Notify the EMS.
   D. Gather heart monitor, oxygen, and IV equipment.

____ 17. What communication style is best when talking to the parents of a toddler?
   A. Alright, Mrs. Timmons, can you remove Connor's clothes down to his diaper?
   B. Alright, mommy, can you remove Connor's clothes down to his diaper?
   C. Alright, Sharon, can you remove Connor's clothes down to his diaper?
   D. Alright, Connor's mommy, can you remove Connor's clothes down to his diaper?

___ 18. Which of the following abbreviations are connected with a disease that causes infants to stop breathing during periods of sleep?

   A. SADS

   B. SIDS

   C. SIDDS

   D. SADDS

___ 19. Which of the following actions would be *best* when working with a child that does not want to have his blood pressure taken?

   A. Ask the provider to perform the procedure.

   B. Ask the mother to help by holding the child still while you take the blood pressure.

   C. Attempt to reduce the child's fear by allowing him to experiment with the equipment that will be used during the procedure.

   D. Attempt to reduce the child's fear by telling him that he won't feel any pain during the procedure.

___ 20. When sharing information with a mother of a 15-month-old son regarding normal milestones in language development, the mother becomes concerned because her child's development does not match those listed on the chart for her child's age group. Which of the following responses would be *best* for addressing the mother's concerns?

   A. Tell the mother that each child is unique and may not reach projected milestones at the exact age listed on the chart.

   B. Tell mother that each chart is different and you are certain that some charts do match the child's development.

   C. Tell the mother it may be best to have the child's hearing evaluated.

   D. Tell the mother that she should keep a close eye on the child and that if he is not talking by his next appointment, she should share the information with the physician.

SKILL APPLICATION CHALLENGE

Assignment 19-7: Web Assignments

1. Research recent findings on the different forms of autism and present information to the class on your findings. Include an explanation of the different forms along with available treatment options and the prognosis for each.

2. Gather statistics on the occurrence of heart attacks among high-school and college-age athletes. Present facts on possible screenings that could be made mandatory before a student can participate in these activities.

COMPLETING SPECIAL FORMS

Assignment 19-8: Plotting Percentiles on a Growth Chart

Work Form Necessary: FORM 19-1

Directions: Complete the growth chart (Work Form 19-1) using the following information.

The child's name is Ashur Green. His chart number is 125655. His mother's stature is 62 inches and his father's stature is 66 inches. Measurements to be plotted are listed below.

Date	Age	Weight	Length	Head Circumference
10-10-05	Birth	9 pounds	20 inches	12 inches
01-12-06	3 months	12 pounds 3 ounces	21.5 inches	13.5 inches
04-11-06	6 months	15 pounds 6 ounces	24.75 inches	14 inches
07-11-06	9 months	22 pounds	26 inches	15 inches
10-12-06	12 months	26 pounds	28 inches	15.5 inches
04-15-07	18 months	30 pounds	30.5 inches	16 inches

FIELD APPLICATION CHALLENGE
Assignment 19-9

Read the following Field Application Challenge and respond to the questions following the scenario.

You are scheduled to give Mason Pendleton his four-month immunizations today. You give the paperwork and vaccination information statements (VIS) to Mason's mother and ask her to read over VIS forms while you prepare the vaccines. After reading them over, Mrs. Pendleton tells you that she does not want her son to receive the vaccines. When you ask her why, she responds by saying that she just watched a documentary on safety concerns regarding early infant immunizations and she just doesn't feel comfortable with having her son vaccinated.

1. What can you do to help Mason's mother feel reassured that it is in her son's best interest to be vaccinated?

_____

_____

_____

_____

2. Should the medical assistant have drawn up the vaccination medication before the mother signed the release forms?

_____

_____

3. Should the provider be alerted about the mother's hesitancy, even if she ends up allowing the child to be vaccinated?

_____

_____

4. If the child's mother declines the vaccinations, can the same vaccine be used on someone else?

_____

_____

JOURNALING EXERCISE
Assignment 19-10

What content within this chapter was most meaningful to you? Why? List some examples of how you might apply information contained in this chapter, both during your training and after you enter the health care industry.

Work Form 19-1

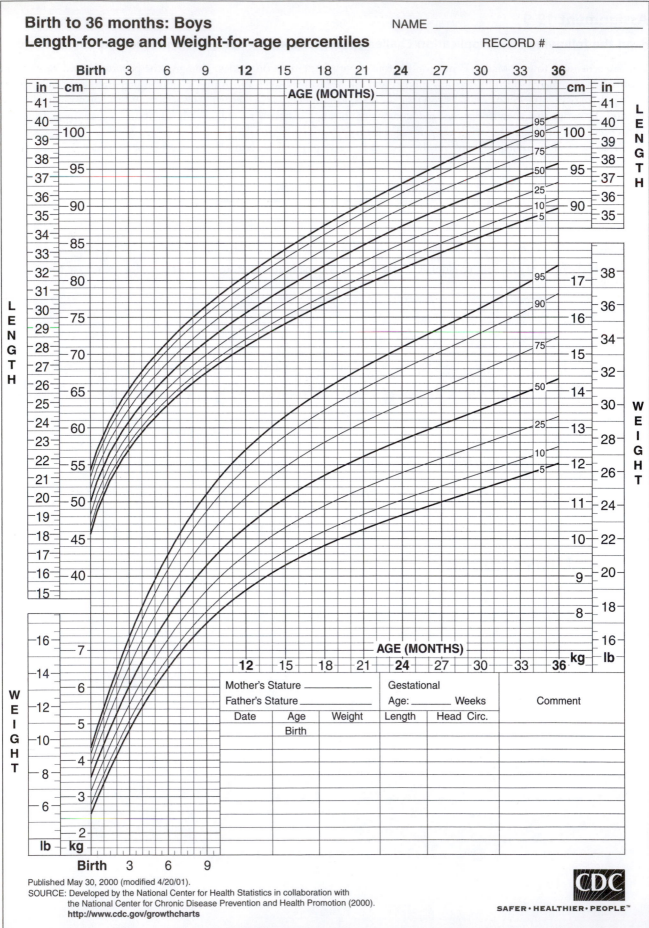

Birth to 36 months: Boys
Length-for-age and Weight-for-age percentiles

NAME _____

RECORD # _____

Published May 30, 2000 (modified 4/20/01).
SOURCE: Developed by the National Center for Health Statistics in collaboration with
the National Center for Chronic Disease Prevention and Health Promotion (2000).
http://www.cdc.gov/growthcharts

CDC

SAFER • HEALTHIER • PEOPLE™

C H A P T E R **20**

Evaluation and Care of the Geriatric Patient

FIELD RELEVANCY AND BENEFITS

Our aging population is changing the overall climate of health care which makes it more important than ever for the medical assistant to have a basic understanding of the social, psychological, and physical changes that occur during a patient's senior years. Learning the information in this chapter will help prepare the medical assistant to work in a vast array of offices including: geriatrics, internal medicine, family practice, and a variety of specialty practices.

NOTE SHEET

The Process of Aging

_____

_____

_____

_____

Cognitive Functioning and Development

_____

_____

_____

Examination/Screening of the Geriatric Patient

_____

_____

_____

Common Diseases of the Geriatric Patient

_____

_____

_____

Societal Issues and Concerns

_____

_____

_____

_____

VOCABULARY REVIEW

Assignment 20-1: Matching

Match the term with its definition and place the corresponding letter in the blank.

____ 1. Ageism

____ 2. Dementia

____ 3. Dowager's hump

____ 4. Frail senior

____ 5. Geriatrician

____ 6. Hospice

____ 7. Osteoporosis

____ 8. Palliative care

____ 9. Parkinson's disease

____ 10. Passive euthanasia

____ 11. Retinopathy

____ 12. Thanatology

A. Care that simply relieves pain and keeps patients who are seriously or terminally ill comfortable

B. Any disorder of the retina

C. Research that studies death

D. Medical specialist who treats diseases and disorders of the aged or the senior adult population

E. Program that provides palliative care for the terminally ill

F. An aged or senior patient who cannot complete three or more activities of daily living (ADLs) independently

G. Chronic neurological disease which inhibits the production of dopamine

H. Care that allows a patient to die with dignity by withholding procedures or drugs that would prolong life

I. False belief or prejudice against the aged

J. Condition in which the bones become brittle and porous

K. An ongoing and irreversible decrease in mental functioning which affects memory, reasoning, and judgment

L. Curvature of the spine due to osteoporosis

CHAPTER REVIEW

Assignment 20-2: Acronym Review

Write what each of the following acronyms stands for.

1. OAA: _____

2. ADLs: _____

3. IADLs: _____

Assignment 20-3: True or False

Fill in the blank with a "T" for true statements and an "F" for false statements. Rewrite the false statements to make them true.

____ 1. Alzheimer's disease and dementia are the same thing.

_____

_____

____ 2. Primary aging involves physical changes which are irreversible.

_____

_____

____ 3. Bathing is considered to be one of the instrumental activities of daily living (IADLs).

_____

_____

____ 4. Osteoarthritis is considered to be an autoimmune disease.

____ 5. Multiple fractures can occur as a result of osteoporosis in the elderly.

____ 6. Parkinson's disease is a disorder in which body movements are altered due to a deficiency of serotonin in the brain.

____ 7. As caloric intake decreases in a geriatric patient, it is important that food selections are high in nutrients to assist in maintaining good health.

____ 8. Hospice is designed to provide a dignified and caring end to life.

Assignment 20-4: Short Answer

1. Describe the categories of aging.

2. Explain the three types of Alzheimer's disease.

3. List three types of stroke or CVA and list their symptoms.

   A. _____

   B. _____

   C. _____

4. List five different types of abuse seen in the elderly population along with clues to look for during patient screening.

   A. _____

   B. _____

C. _____

_____

D. _____

_____

E. _____

_____

Assignment 20-5: Certification Practice

Choose the best answer and place the corresponding letter in the blank.

____ 1. The best definition for the term gerontology is the study of:

A. geriatrics.

B. old age.

C. the elderly.

D. seniors.

____ 2. Which of the following plays a role in secondary aging?

A. Lifestyle

B. Overall health

C. Exercise and nutrition

D. Plastic surgery

____ 3. Loss of height would be an example of:

A. primary aging.

B. secondary aging.

C. ageism.

D. none of the above.

____ 4. Which of the following would be associated with aging of a sense organ?

A. Thinning of the skin

B. Loss of hair

C. Decrease in height

D. Cataracts

____ 5. Which conditions or diseases will usually *not* result in a decrease of cognitive function in the older adult?

A. Cardiovascular disease

B. Osteoporosis

C. Cancer

D. Depression

____ 6. Between the ages of 30 and 90, the brain shrinks by:

A. 15%.

B. 10%.

C. 20%.

D. 25%.

____ 7. Which of the following causes an increase in constipation *due to aging*?

A. Decreased food intake

B. Decreased production of gastric juices

C. Decreased peristalsis

D. Inactivity

___ 8. A term that is synonymous with dementia is:

    A. Alzheimer's disease.

    B. senility.

    C. Parkinson's disease.

    D. cognitive dysfunction.

___ 9. Which of the following neurotransmitters is thought to play a role in Alzheimer's disease?

    A. Serotonin

    B. Dopamine

    C. Acetylcholine

    D. Epinephrine

___ 10. A diagnosis of Alzheimer's disease that occurs after age 65 is known as:

    A. early onset.

    B. familial.

    C. sporadic.

    D. delayed onset.

___ 11. Which of the following would *not* be a correctable cause or form of dementia?

    A. Vitamin deficiency

    B. Hypothyroidism

    C. Hypoglycemia

    D. Multi-infarct dementia

___ 12. Grocery shopping would be considered an:

    A. ADL.

    B. IADL.

    C. EADL.

    D. OT.

___ 13. Which type of arthritis can affect the organs as well as the bones?

    A. Gout

    B. Simple

    C. Osteoarthritis

    D. Rheumatoid

___ 14. Besides genetics and obesity, which of the following may be the cause for type 2 diabetes in the geriatric patient?

    A. Diet

    B. Inactivity

    C. Less tolerance to glucose and an increase in insulin resistance

    D. Metabolism

___ 15. Which of the following types of fractures are common in patients with osteoporosis?

    A. Hip

    B. Leg

    C. Arm

    D. Skull

___ 16. A type of stroke caused by an arterial blood clot in the brain is called:

    A. TIA.

    B. hemorrhagic.

    C. ischemic.

    D. CVA.

___ 17. Hitting, slapping, and restraining are types of:

    A. physical abuse.

    B. neglect.

    C. exploitation.

    D. emotional abuse.

___ 18. Which of the following is accomplished by withholding drugs that would prolong life?

    A. Palliative care

    B. Passive euthanasia

    C. Assisted suicide

    D. None of the above

___ 19. In regard to nutrition, which of the following is *not* suggested for senior adults?

    A. Decrease overall caloric intake.

    B. Drink plenty of liquids.

    C. Increase overall caloric intake.

    D. Select foods that have lots of nutrients.

___ 20. Examples of senior neglect may include all but which of the following?

    A. Bruising

    B. Fecal smell coming from the patient

    C. Malnutrition

    D. Dehydration

SKILL APPLICATION CHALLENGE

Assignment 20-6: Project

Using the following questionnaires, interview one male and one female over the age of 70. Ask them the following questions. (Share and compare findings with your classmates.)

Female over the age of 70

Name (optional):

Birthdate:

Date of interview:

1. Are you married? If so, how old is your husband? How is the health of your husband?
2. Do you have any responsibilities in caring for your husband?
3. What is/was your occupation?
4. Do you have any responsibilities for watching grandchildren or great-grandchildren? If the answer is yes, how many grandchildren do you care for and how often?
5. What is your favorite hobby?
6. Where is your favorite place to travel?
7. Do you still drive? (If yes, do you still enjoy driving?)
8. What are your current chronic or acute health problems?
9. What medications do you currently take?
10. What troubles you most about your health right now?
11. Does the low reimbursement from Medicare ever prevent you from going to the physician or taking your medication?
12. What do you like most about your physician? How do you feel about the staff members who work in your physician's office?
13. What advice can you give to me as I enter the ambulatory health care setting that will assist me in making a positive connection with my senior patients?

Male over the age of 70

Name (optional

Birthdate:

Date of interview

1. Are you married? If so, how old is your wife? How is the health of your wife?
2. Do you have any responsibilities in caring for your wife?
3. What is/was your occupation?
4. Do you have any responsibilities for watching grandchildren or great-grandchildren? If the answer is yes, how many grandchildren do you care for and how often?
5. What is your favorite hobby?
6. Where is your favorite place to travel?
7. Do you still drive? (If yes, do you still enjoy driving?)
8. What are your current chronic or acute health problems?
9. What medications do you currently take?
10. What troubles you most about your health right now?
11. Does the low reimbursement from Medicare ever prevent you from going to the provider or taking your medication?
12. What do you like most about your physician? How do you feel about the staff members who work in your physician's office?
13. What advice can you give to me as I enter the ambulatory health care setting that will assist me in making a positive connection with my senior patients?

FIELD APPLICATION CHALLENGE
Assignment 20-7

Read the following Field Application Challenge and respond to the questions following the scenario.

While escorting 79-year-old Mr. Leonard to the exam room, you notice a slight tremor of his head and a shuffling gait. He has difficulty stepping up on the scale and needs assistance. After obtaining his weight, you allow him to take a seat in a chair in the exam room. While reviewing his history, you notice a slight slurring of his speech and see that he is having trouble answering questions correctly. Normally, Mr. Leonard is bright and energetic and the signs you have observed are of great concern to you. You also notice that he seems quite depressed and when asked he states that he has recently moved into his son's home. While placing the blood pressure cuff on his arm, you notice a large bruise on his upper arm. When asked about the bruise he simply says that he bumped his arm on the bathroom door.

1. What symptoms should you report immediately to the provider?

_____

_____

2. What could the physical symptoms indicate?

_____

3. What could account for his depression and the bruise on his arm?

_____

_____

_____

JOURNALING EXERCISE
Assignment 20-8

What content within this chapter was most meaningful to you? Why? List some examples of how you might apply information contained in this chapter, both during your training and once you enter the health care industry.

C H A P T E R **21**

Orthopedics, Rehabilitation, and Physical Therapy

FIELD RELEVANCY AND BENEFITS

Medical assistants can choose from among a diverse group of specialties when seeking employment. Orthopedics and rehabilitative medicine offer unique challenges not found in other specialties.

In an orthopedics practice, the medical assistant will assist the orthopedist with exams as well as with cast application and removal, and may also be responsible for applying other immobilization devices such as splints and supportive wraps. In some states, the medical assistant may be permitted to take certain x-rays with the proper training and licensing.

Rehabilitative medicine can also be a rewarding specialty. The medical assistant may be able to perform treatments with physical agents help patients recover from injuries and illness, and may play a part in helping them regain their mobility.

NOTE SHEET

Types of Providers Who Specialize in Treating Diseases and Disorders of the Musculoskeletal System

_____

_____

_____

_____

Patient Screening for the Musculoskeletal System

_____

_____

_____

_____

Assisting with the Orthopedic Exam

_____

_____

_____

Common Diagnostic Procedures Performed on Orthopedic Patients

_____

_____

_____

Strains, Sprains, Fractures, and Dislocations

_____

_____

_____

_____

Alternative Treatment Methods

_____

_____

_____

_____

Rehabilitation

_____

_____

_____

_____

Ambulatory Assistive Devices

_____

_____

_____

_____

VOCABULARY REVIEW

Assignment 21-1: Matching

Match the term with its definition and place the corresponding letter in the blank.

____ 1. Ambulation

____ 2. Cartilage

____ 3. Cryotherapy

____ 4. Arthroscopy

____ 5. Modalities

____ 6. Orthopedist

____ 7. Prosthesis

____ 8. Rehabilitation

____ 9. Sprain

____ 10. Strain

____ 11. Thermotherapy

____ 12. Massage

____ 13. Dislocation

____ 14. Physical therapist

____ 15. Ultrasound

A. Sound waves used to generate heat in deep tissues

B. Use of heat to treat an injury or condition of the body

C. An artificial body part

D. Process of treatments designed to return a body part to its full function, following an illness or injury

E. Trauma to a ligament, which may include a tear

F. Physician who specializes in the treatment of diseases and disorders of the bones and muscles

G. Injury to a muscle or tendon caused by overuse

H. Physical agents, such as heat, cold, water, and electricity, used in physical therapy

I. Use of pressure, friction, and kneading to promote muscle relaxation

J. Health care professional who assesses and manages a patient's rehabilitation using different physical agents or modalities

K. Ability to walk or move about freely

L. Visualization of a joint and joint capsule through a a lighted instrument

M. Bones are displaced from their normal position within a joint

N. Connective tissue located between the articular surfaces of bones, joints, and vertebrae that acts as a shock absorber

O. Therapeutic use of cold modalities to treat an injury or other physical condition

CHAPTER REVIEW

Assignment 21-2: Acronym Review

Write what each of the following acronyms stands for.

1. ROM: _____

2. PT: _____

3. RICE: _____

4. OT: _____

Assignment 21-3: True or False

Fill in the blank with a "T" for true statements and an "F" for false statements. Rewrite the false statements to make them true.

_____ 1. A general orthopedist treats only the bones and muscles of the extremities.

_____

_____

_____ 2. A closed reduction procedure is realignment of a bone without penetrating the skin.

_____

_____

_____ 3. Electromyography involves placing needle electrodes into skeletal muscles to record and measure the strength of their contractions.

_____

_____

_____ 4. Occupational therapy involves the use of physical agents such as heat, cold, massage, and exercise to restore function to muscles that have been damaged.

_____

_____

_____ 5. A hot pack would be an example of thermotherapy.

_____

_____

_____ 6. A paraffin bath is considered to be a dry heat modality.

_____

_____

_____ 7. Cryotherapy is most effective if used frequently during the first 48 hours following an injury.

_____

_____

_____ 8. An ice massage is considered to be a wet cold modality.

_____

_____

_____ 9. One example of hydrotherapy is a contrast bath.

_____

_____

_____ 10. When administering a treatment using a hot water bottle, the water temperature should not exceed 120°F (49°C).

_____

_____

_____ 11. An ice pack may be applied to a cast over the area of the break.

_____

_____

_____ 12. It is permissible to insert a soft object inside a cast to scratch the skin.

_____

_____

Assignment 21-4: Short Answer

1. Explain the differences between a sprain and a strain.

_____

_____

2. Describe the following types of fractures.

   A. Complete: _____

   B. Incomplete: _____

   C. Complicated: _____

   D. Greenstick: _____

   E. Compression: _____

   F. Hairline: _____

   G. Impacted: _____

   H. Pathological: _____

   I. Pott's: _____

   J. Spiral: _____

   K. Stress: _____

   L. Colles: _____

   M. Comminuted: _____

   N. Transverse: _____

   O. Oblique: _____

3. Explain how to measure a patient for a cane, walker, and crutches.

   A. Cane: _____

   _____

   B. Walker: _____

   _____

   C. Crutches: _____

   _____

4. Describe the following joint movement terms.

A. Aduction: _____

B. Adduction: _____

C. Circumduction: _____

D. Dorsiflexion: _____

E. Eversion: _____

F. Extension: _____

G. Flexion: _____

H. Hyperextension: _____

I. Inversion: _____

J. Plantar flexion: _____

K. Pronation: _____

L. Rotation: _____

M. Supination: _____

Assignment 21-5: Certification Practice

Choose the best answer and place the corresponding letter in the blank.

____ 1. Which of the following is not a risk factor for developing osteoporosis?

A. Early menopause before age 45

B. Sedentary lifestyle

C. Smoking

D. A diet low in B complex vitamins

____ 2. The correct synonym for an orthopedist is a(n):

A. orthopedic surgeon.

B. orthopedic technician.

C. sports medicine specialist.

D. physiatrist.

____ 3. Which of the following tests visualizes the distribution of an IV-injected radioactive isotope that collects in the bones and joints?

A. CT scan

B. MRI

C. Bone scan

D. Discography

____ 4. Which of the following tests would be performed to detect a bone infection or muscle atrophy?

A. Arthroscopy

B. Bone/muscle biopsy

C. Electromyography

D. Urine and blood tests

____ 5. Following a fracture, the main objective of the orthopedist is to:

A. realign the bones to their original position.

B. surgically insert pins and/or plates to strengthen the fracture.

C. decrease pain.

D. decrease deformity.

____ 6. When an incision is made in the skin for the purpose of realigning a broken bone, it is referred to as a(n):

    A. surgical intervention.

    B. open reduction.

    C. closed reduction.

    D. realignment.

_____7. The name for a fracture that is a crack in the bone with the ends perfectly aligned is:

    A. greenstick.

    B. incomplete.

    C. pathological.

    D. hairline.

____ 8. The cast should extend between which of the following points?

    A. The joints above and below the fracture site

    B. Over the fracture site and the joint above it

    C. Over the fracture site and the joint below it

    D. A half-inch above and below the fracture

____ 9. A fracture may be treated with all but which of the following devices?

    A. Cast

    B. Splint

    C. Sterile gauze

    D. Sling

____ 10. Viscosupplementation is a treatment used for:

    A. osteoarthritis.

    B. bursitis.

    C. tendonitis.

    D. hairline fractures.

____ 11. Which of the following would be a reason for thermotherapy?

    A. To decrease bruising following an injury

    B. To relax muscles that are tight

    C. To reduce swelling immediately following an injury

    D. To relieve pain immediately following an injury

____ 12. Examples of cryotherapy include all of the following *except:*

    A. ice bag.

    B. dry ice.

    C. chemical ice pack.

    D. ice massage.

____ 13. The transducer of the ultrasound is in continuous motion to:

    A. evenly spread the coupling gel.

    B. reduce swelling.

    C. prevent burns and tissue damage.

    D. concentrate the sound waves.

____ 14. The average length of an ultrasound treatment is:

    A. 10 minutes.

    B. 20 minutes.

    C. 25 minutes.

    D. 5 to 15 minutes.

____ 15. Which of the following assistive devices provides the most stability?

  A. Quad cane

  B. Platform crutches

  C. Forearm crutches

  D. Walker

____ 16. Heat should be applied:

  A. when inflammation is present.

  B. immediately following an injury.

  C. when swelling is present.

  D. in order to relax a strained muscle.

____ 17. A type of strengthening exercise in which the physical therapist moves a body part without any assistance from the patient is referred to as:

  A. passive.

  B. active.

  C. assisted.

  D. active resistance.

____ 18. When applying heat or cold packs to a muscle you should:

  A. always apply the packs directly over the skin.

  B. always keep in place for at least 30 to 60 minutes.

  C. always cover the pack so that there is a barrier between the pack and the patient's skin.

  D. always ask the patient to tense their muscle before applying the pack for better absorption.

____ 19. A physician who specializes in diagnosing and treating diseases and disorders of the nervous system, including the brain, spinal cord, and nerves is a(n):

  A. neurologist.

  B. neurosurgeon.

  C. orthopedist.

  D. physiatrist.

____ 20. A nonphysician who helps to restore function, improve mobility and decrease pain to an area that has been damaged by injury or disease using physical agents or modalities is a(n):

  A. occupational therapist.

  B. physical therapist.

  C. occupational therapy assistant.

  D. physical technician.

____ 21. Patients should report all but which of the following symptoms or signs following the application of a cast?

  A. Burning or stinging sensation

  B. Foul odor coming from the cast

  C. Cold fingers or digits in the area the cast was applied

  D. Itching sensation

____ 22. Which of the following would be considered a deep heating treatment?

  A. Application of a hot compress to the skin

  B. Application of a heat pack to the skin

  C. Application of an ultrasound treatment

  D. A whirlpool treatment

____ 23. Turning the palm downward would be referred to as:

  A. adduction.

  B. abduction.

  C. pronation.

  D. supination.

_____ 24. Which of the following gaits provides three points of support at all times?

    A. Two-point

    B. Three-point

    C. Four-point

    D. Swing gait

_____ 25. A practitioner that assists patients in restoring fine motor skills is a(n):

    A. occupational therapist.

    B. physical therapist.

    C. physical therapy assistant.

    D. occupationalist.

SKILL APPLICATION CHALLENGE
Assignment 21-6: Labeling

1. Label the types of fractures illustrated below.

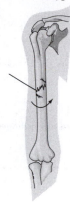
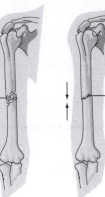
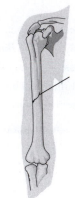
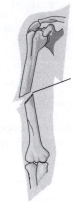

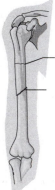
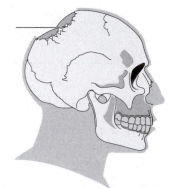
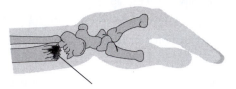

2. Identify the crutch gaits based on the illustrations below.

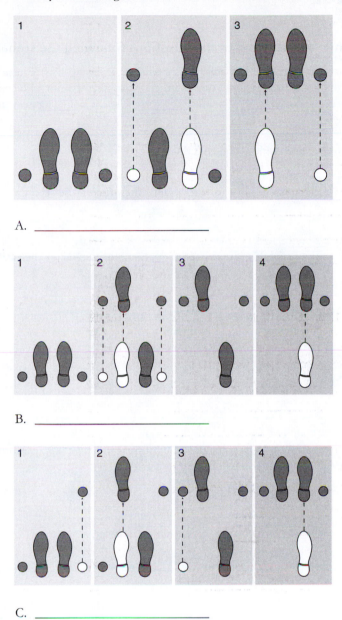

A. _____

B. _____

C. _____

FIELD APPLICATION CHALLENGE
Assignment 21-7

Read the following Field Application Challenge and respond to the questions following the scenario.

A patient calls and states that she fell on her left wrist about an hour ago and that the wrist is really swollen. You schedule the patient for an immediate appointment and give the patient some home care instructions to follow prior to being seen. Following an x-ray examination, the physician diagnoses the patient with a sprain to the wrist. Use the matching items to help you answer the questions below.

A. Rest, ice, compression, and elevation
B. Rest, compression, elevation, movement (alternating periods of heat and cold therapy)
C. Immobilize, elevate, and apply ice

1. Which of the above instructions should be given to the patient prior to coming into the office to be seen by the provider?

    ____

2. Which of the above instructions should be given to the patient for the first 24 to 48 hours or until all of the swelling is gone?

    ____

3. Which of the above instructions may be given to the patient once all of the swelling is diminished?

    ____

JOURNALING EXERCISE
Assignment 21-8

What content within this chapter was most meaningful to you? Why? List some examples of how you might apply information contained in this chapter, both during your training and after you enter the health care industry.

Name _____ Date _____ Score _____

Medical and Surgical Asepsis

FIELD RELEVANCY AND BENEFITS

Ambulatory surgery centers are springing up all over the country. Surgeries that used to be performed only in hospital settings are now being performed in surgical suites located within medical office buildings. Some of these suites are beautiful and quite luxurious.

Urologists, podiatrists, plastic surgeons, proctologists, and dermatologists are just a few of the medical specialists who can perform minor surgeries in ambulatory health centers. Specialized training in minor surgery techniques will assist you in gaining employment in offices that perform these unique procedures.

NOTE SHEET

Asepsis

_____
_____
_____
_____

Care and Maintenance of Surgical Instruments

_____
_____
_____
_____

Sterilization Techniques

_____
_____
_____
_____

VOCABULARY REVIEW

Assignment 22-1: Fill in the Blank

Fill in the blanks below with Essential Terms from this chapter.

1. _____ Free of germs

2. _____ Strips that are used when sterilizing instruments that help to confirm that the necessary environmental conditions needed to achieve complete sterilization in fact met

3. _____ Chemically pure water which helps prevent instruments from rusting

4. _____ Impermeable coating which surrounds the spore protecting it from many environmental factors including: heat, ultraviolet radiation, chemicals, acids, and drying

5. _____ Most common gas used for sterilization because of its ability to kill all forms of microorganisms, including bacterial spores

6. _____ Objects or structures that are nonliving, such as countertop surfaces, flooring, and examination tables

7. _____ The amount of time the disinfecting solution may be used once the bottle has been opened

8. _____ To make sanitary or clean

9. _____ Device that cleans instruments by transmitting sound waves through a cleaning fluid

Assignment 22-2: Matching

Match the term with its definition and place the corresponding letter in the blank.

_____ 1. Wet load

_____ 2. Surgical asepsis

_____ 3. Sterilant

_____ 4. Medical asepsis

_____ 5. Low-level disinfectant

_____ 6. Intermediate-level disinfectant

_____ 7. High-level disinfectant

_____ 8. Disinfection

_____ 9. Biological indicators

_____ 10. Autoclave

_____ 11. Aseptic technique

A. Can kill all forms of microorganisms except large amounts of bacterial spores

B. The process of using special liquids or pasteurization techniques to destroy or inhibit the growth of most microorganisms

C. Inactivates vegetative bacteria, mycobacteria, and most fungi, but does not necessarily kill spores

D. Term that describes what occurs when cold air from the outside rushes into the hot chamber on the inside and causes condensation to form in an autoclave, resulting in wet packs.

E. Used to check that all parameters, including temperature, timing, sterilant, and humidity were reached by the unit's ability to kill endospores

F. The effort that is employed to reduce the spread of microorganisms

G. Sterilizes items by displacing air with steam within a chamber and exposing items to large amounts of heat over a specified time period

H. Procedures that are used to greatly decrease the number of microorganisms and prevent them from being passed from one person to another

I. Kills most types of bacteria and some viruses; does not kill mycobacteria or bacterial spores

J. Term for a high-level chemical disinfectant that has been cleared by the FDA as being capable of destroying all microorganisms, including large amounts of bacterial spores

K. Procedures and practices used to destroy and eliminate all microorganisms from instruments and other objects prior to an invasive procedure

CHAPTER REVIEW

Assignment 22-3: Short Answer

1. Describe the different types of disinfecting solutions and which microorganisms each one is capable of destroying, and explain under which conditions you would use each type.

A. _____

_____

_____

B. _____

_____

_____

C. _____

_____

_____

D. _____

_____

_____

_____

_____

2. List three different types of wrapping materials and unique features of each type.

A. _____

_____

_____

_____

B. _____

_____

_____

_____

C. _____

_____

_____

_____

3. List the chain of events that must occur in order to achieve complete sterilization when using the autoclave as your means of sterilization.

A. _____

B. _____

C. _____

D. _____

E. _____

4. Compare and contrast the differences between and medical and surgical asepsis and list examples of each.

A. _____

_____

_____

_____

_____

B. _____

_____

_____

_____

_____

5. What is a biological indicator and what is the purpose of the indicator? How often should this test be performed?

_____

_____

_____

_____

6. Upon running a spore check on the autoclave, the results come back positive. What would be the next course of action?

_____

_____

Assignment 22-4: True or False

Fill in the blank with a "T" for true statements and an "F" for false statements. Rewrite the false statements to make them true.

____ 1. The only factors which can eliminate endospores altogether is steam under pressure (autoclaving), the proper use of sterilants, certain gases, such as ethyl oxide, and prolonged exposure to radiation.

_____

_____

____ 2. The four methods of sterilization include: dry heat, cool heat, chemicals, and autoclaving.

_____

_____

____ 3. When using sterilizing pouches, you should insert the handle end of the instrument into the bag first.

_____

_____

____ 4. Alcohol will not sterilize the skin.

_____

_____

____ 5. The most dependable form of sterilization is the use of a high-level disinfectant.

_____

_____

____ 6. Instruments that are single-wrapped should be autoclaved for 20 minutes.

_____

_____

____ 7. Disinfecting solutions come in either ready-to-use formulas or as concentrates.

_____

_____

____ 8. The immediate soaking of instruments helps to keep debris from drying on them.

_____

_____

Assignment 22-5: Certification Practice

Choose the best answer and place the corresponding letter in the blank.

_____ 1. Because acidic or alkaline solutions may cause deposits to form resulting in damage to the instrument, surgical soaps used to sanitize instruments should have a pH relatively close to which of the following numbers?

A. 5

B. 6

C. 7

D. 8

_____ 2. The method of sterilization that is ineffective against spores is:

A. dry heat.

B. autoclaving.

C. sterilants.

D. gas.

_____ 3. The method of sterilization that is used in manufacturing plants that package sterile needles, sutures, and catheters is:

A. dry heat.

B. autoclaving.

C. chemical.

D. gas.

_____ 4. What is the shelf life of sterile instruments wrapped with sterilization paper or cloth?

A. 5 days

B. 10 days

C. 20 days

D. 30 days

_____ 5. Before the timing of the autoclave begins, the temperature and pressure should reach:

A. 215°F and 10 pounds.

B. 225°F and 15 pounds.

C. 250°F and 15 pounds.

D. 250°F and 25 pounds.

_____ 6. The least resistant to sterilizing agents of the following microorganisms would be:

A. bacterial spores.

B. mycobacteria.

C. nonlipid or small viruses.

D. fungi.

_____ 7. Instruments that penetrate the skin should be:

A. sanitized.

B. disinfected.

C. dipped in an antiseptic.

D. sterilized.

_____ 8. The method of wrapping used to wrap instruments for autoclaving is:

A. the fanfold method.

B. the circular fold method.

C. the triangular fold method.

D. the square fold method.

____ 9. The exposure time for proper autoclaving begins:

   A. when the temperature and pressure gauges are equal.

   B. when the pressure gauge has reached its desired pressure.

   C. after 20 minutes of preheating.

   D. when the temperature gauge has reached its desired temperature.

   E. when both the temperature and pressure gauges reach desired levels.

____ 10. An object that is free of all living microorganisms is considered to be:

   A. septic.

   B. sanitized.

   C. disinfected.

   D. sterile.

____ 11. The type of asepsis that involves procedures and practices used to *destroy and eliminate all microorganisms* from instruments and other objects prior to an invasive procedure is called:

   A. complete asepsis.

   B. surgical asepsis.

   C. medical asepsis.

   D. microbe asepsis.

____ 12. The most common gas used for sterilization because of its ability to kill all forms of microorganisms including bacterial spores is:

   A. oxygen.

   B. nitrogen.

   C. ethylene oxide.

   D. carbon dioxide.

____ 13. The most dependable method of sterilization is:

   A. autoclaving.

   B. chemical.

   C. dry heat.

   D. gas.

____ 14. Which of the following steps would come last when cleaning and sterilizing an instrument?

   A. Sanitizing

   B. Disinfecting

   C. Soaking

   D. Wiping dry

____ 15. What information is needed on the autoclave tape before the instrument is autoclaved?

   A. Name of instrument, expiration date, date autoclaved

   B. Name of instrument, your initials, expiration date

   C. Expiration date, date autoclaved, your initials

   D. Name of instrument, department, your initials

____ 16. The lowest level of disinfecting solution that may be used on noncritical devices is:

   A. low-level disinfectant.

   B. intermediate-level disinfectant.

   C. high-level disinfectant.

   D. sterilant.

____ 17. Autoclave tape would be an example of a(n):

   A. biological indicator.

   B. internal indicator.

   C. process indicator.

   D. chemical indicator.

____ 18. The amount of time the solution may be stored unopened before losing its potency (the expiration date on the container) is referred to as:

    A. shelf life.

    B. re-use life.

    C. open container life.

    D. potency life.

____ 19. When opening the door to vent on an older, nonautomated autoclave, the door should not be opened more than:

    A. 0.5 to 1 inch.

    B. 1 to 1.5 inches.

    C. 1.5 to 2 inches.

    D. 2.5 to 3 inches.

____ 20. When removing a wrapped pack from the autoclave, you notice that the pack is slightly damp. You should:

    A. place the pack back in the autoclave and allow it to dry for a little while longer.

    B. place the pack on top of the autoclave and allow it to air dry.

    C. place the pack back in the processing pile to be completely reprocessed.

    D. just re-autoclave the instrument.

SKILL APPLICATION CHALLENGE

Assignment 22-6: Ordering Exercise

The following sentences illustrate the steps that are taken to clean and sterilize an instrument. The steps are not in the correct order. In the blanks below, place the letter beside the number that represents the order in which each step is performed.

1. ____

2. ____

3. ____

4. ____

5. ____

6. ____

7. ____

8. ____

9. ____

10. ____

11. ____

12. ____

A. Spray the instrument with lubricant directly to the box locks and dry accordingly.

B. Dry the instrument thoroughly to avoid water spots from drying on it.

C. Soak the instrument in appropriate soaking solution (preferably distilled water).

D. Run the autoclave as directed by the manufacturer. Set a timer if necessary.

E. Thoroughly sanitize the instrument by scrubbing each surface and crevice (using a neutral cleanser is the best).

F. Inspect the instrument for any flaws and make certain it works properly.

G. Label the pack.

H. Rinse the instrument with an appropriate rinsing solution (distilled water is best).

I. Wrap the instrument in the appropriate wrapping material (paper, muslin, or plastic). Place an indicator strip in the pack if necessary before sealing.

J. Correctly load the autoclave.

K. Place the sterilized instrument in the appropriate container, cabinet, etc.

L. Open the autoclave with an oven mitt or allow it to cool completely before removing the sterilized instrument from the autoclave.

Assignment 22-7: Log Practice

Complete the logs below using the information provided.

1. Instrument Disinfecting Log

Date: 02/06/10
Start Time: 12:00 p.m.
End Time: 1:00 p.m.
Items Autoclaved: Laryngoscope
Name of Control: Disnitrol
Results: Solution met MEC requirements
Your initials, followed by SMA

Autoclave Log

Date	Start Time	Finish Time	Items Autoclaved	Name of Control Used to Test Sterility	Strip Met MEC Requirements	Initials

2. Biological Weekly Spore Check

Date Spore Check was Autoclaved: 02/06/10
Date Strip Sent to Virolab: 02/07/10
Date Office Received Report: 02/12/10
Spore Test Results: Negative for Spores
Report Filed in Spore Notebook 02/10/10

Date Spore Check Autoclaved	Date Sent to Lab	Date Office Received Report	Spore Test Results	Report Filed

FIELD APPLICATION CHALLENGE
Assignment 22-8

Read the following Field Application Challenge and respond to the questions following the scenario.

You run a spore check with a load and send it to the lab. You continue to run the autoclave and sterilize six more laceration trays and three incision and drainage (I&D) trays between the time you ran the spore check and the time you receive the results. The report comes back as positive for spores. The chemical indicators in each pack have turned the appropriate color.

1. What will be the plan of action for using the autoclave from this point forward?

_____

_____

_____

_____

2. What should be done with any remaining sterile packs that were autoclaved at the same time the spore check was autoclaved or following the initial spore check?

_____

3. What should be done about the packs that were autoclaved at the time the spore check was performed or following the initial spore check and used on patients?

_____

_____

_____

JOURNALING EXERCISE
Assignment 22-9

What content within this chapter was most meaningful to you? Why? List some examples of how you might apply information contained in this chapter, both during your training and after you enter the health care industry.

C H A P T E R **23**

Instrument Identification and Tray Setups

FIELD RELEVANCY AND BENEFITS

It is important for medical assistants to be familiar with the different types of instruments and trays that are used in ambulatory care settings. Even though instruments will vary from one specialty to another, there are a number instruments that are used regularly regardless of specialty. Medical assistants who are able to identify instruments will be able to retrieve such items much more readily when a provider requests them and will be able to set up trays with more ease because they do not have to constantly refer to pictures for identification. The information in this chapter is applicable to all types of practices, especially family medicine, urgent care, and internal medicine.

NOTE SHEET

Types of Instruments Used in Minor Surgery

_____

_____

_____

_____

Solutions and Supplies Used for Minor Surgery

_____

_____

_____

_____

Types of Procedures Performed in the Medical Office/Tray Setups

_____

_____

_____

_____

VOCABULARY REVIEW

Assignment 23-1: Fill in the Blank

Fill in the blanks below with Essential Terms from this chapter.

1. _____ To cut open or cut apart

2. _____ Material used to tie off tubular structures such as the fallopian tubes or vas deferens

3. _____ Sealants in these products provide the incision site with instant strength usually within a matter of minutes of application

4. _____ Jagged wound or cut that may be the result of a traumatic injury

5. _____ Cyst that occurs as the result of a blocked sebaceous gland

6. _____ Removal of excess fluid which builds up as a result of inflammation

7. _____ Part of the instrument that the surgeon uses to hold the instrument

8. _____ Special hinge found on ring-handled instruments

9. _____ Device used to remove small foreign bodies from the eye, ear, or wound

10. _____ A type of medication that is used to produce a lack of feeling in patients during a surgical procedure

11. _____ Type of strand or fiber that is used to sew

12. _____ infection

13. _____ Instrument that uses a powerful, high-focused beam of light to remove unwanted tissue and to control bleeding in a variety of invasive and noninvasive procedures

14. _____ Procedure in which unwanted tissue such as skin lesions and warts are destroyed by freezing the tissue

Assignment 23-2: Matching I

Match the term with its definition and place the corresponding letter in the blank.

_____ 1. Atraumatic needles

_____ 2. Electrocoagulation

_____ 3. Electrodessication

_____ 4. Electrofulgration

_____ 5. Electrosurgical procedures

_____ 6. Electrosection

_____ 7. Fenestrated

_____ 8. Jaws

_____ 9. Ratchet

_____ 10. Shanks

_____ 11. Serrations

_____ 12. Traumatic needles

A. These are found on the inside tips of some instruments; their purpose is to help improve gripping power when working with tissue that is slippery

B. Electrode is held 1 to 2 mm away from the skin and produces a sparking sensation to remove polyps and cancer cells.

C. The tips of certain instruments that are used to grasp or clamp items

D. The locking mechanism that tightens or locks the tips of an instrument at varying degrees

E. Swaged needles

F. The long straight portion of the instrument that connects the handle with the tip of the instrument

G. Electrical procedures performed to destroy benign and malignant lesions, to cut or excise tissue, and/or to control bleeding

H. Eyed needles

I. A procedure in which an electrode from an electrosurgical unit touches the skin to stimulate tissue destruction; it is frequently performed to treat spider angiomas, warts, and polyps

J. A procedure using an electrosurgical unit that helps to control bleeding during minor office procedures

K. A procedure using the tip of an electrode from an electrosurgery unit; the electrode is shaped like a fine needle, a wire loop, or a triangle, and is used to incise or cut tissue for the removal of a specimen

L. Having one or more openings

CHAPTER REVIEW

Assignment 23-3: Acronym Review

Write what the following acronym stands for.

LASER: _____

Assignment 23-4: Short Answer

1. List and describe four types of anesthesia.

A. _____

_____

_____

B. _____

_____

_____

C. _____

_____

_____

D. _____

_____

_____

2. List six common solutions used in minor surgery and explain their use.

A. _____

_____

B. _____

_____

C. _____

_____

D. _____

_____

E. _____

_____

F. _____

_____

3. Describe the function of a surgical wick.

_____

_____

_____

4. List and explain various ways to close the skin other than the use of sutures and staples.

A. _____

_____

_____

B. _____

_____

_____

Assignment 23-5: True or False

Fill in the blank with a "T" for true statements and an "F" for false statements. Rewrite the false statements to make them true.

____ 1. Epinephrine, which is often combined with a local anesthetic, constricts the blood vessels and reduces bleeding during surgery.

_____

_____

____ 2. After 14 days, sutures may be removed from joint area.

_____

_____

____ 3. Sebaceous glands are responsible for producing sebum or the oil which helps to keep the skin moisturized.

_____

_____

____ 4. A tetanus shot needs to be updated every 5 years.

_____

_____

____ 5. The two most common solutions used during minor office surgeries are iodine and rubbing alcohol.

_____

_____

____ 6. Probes are instruments that are used to explore wounds, body cavities, and/or hidden structures.

_____

_____

____ 7. Needle holders are used to grasp and firmly hold a needle during the suturing process.

_____

_____

____ 8. Hemostats are a type of ratchet.

_____

_____

____ 9. Dressing, tissue, thumb, and splinter are types of forceps.

_____

_____

____ 10. Remove the sutures by pulling toward the incision.

_____

_____

Assignment 23-6: Matching II

Match the instrument to its use.

Answer   Instrument

_____   1. Speculum

_____   2. Surgical knife

_____   3. Needle holder

_____   4. Dressing forceps

_____   5. Hemostats

_____   6. Uterine curette

_____   7. Bandage scissors

_____   8. Operating scissors

_____   9. Dilators

_____   10. Tissue forceps

Use of instrument

A. Grasps suture needle during suturing

B. Grasps tissue

C. Clamps small blood vessels

D. Makes incisions

E. Cuts tissue and sutures

F. Opens structures that are constricted

G. Used to obtain tissue from the endocervical and uterine area

H. Examines body orifices

I. Used to cut bandages

J. Grasps dressings

Assignment 23-7: Certification Practice

Choose the best answer and place the corresponding letter in the blank.

_____ 1. When removing bandages from a wound; the correct method is to:

A. pull away from the wound.

B. pull with the wound.

C. pull toward the wound.

D. pull up and in one quick motion.

_____ 2. When a bandage appears to be stuck to the wound; which of the following methods is the best way to remove it without further injuring the wound?

A. Carefully and slowly continue to pull the bandage off.

B. Saturate the dressing with tap water prior to removal.

C. Apply alcohol around the edges of the bandage to loosen the bandage.

D. Saturate the dressing with sterile saline prior to removal.

_____ 3. The type of electrosurgical procedure that uses a special tip on the electrosurgical unit to touch the skin to stimulate tissue destruction and is frequently used to treat spider angiomas, warts, and polyps is called:

A. electrodesiccation.

B. electrofulguration.

C. electrocoagulation.

D. electrosection.

_____ 4. The tip of the electrode used during which of the following electrosurgical procedures is shaped like a fine needle, a wire loop, or a triangle and is used to incise or cut tissue for the removal of a specimen?

A. Electrodesiccation

B. Electrofulguration

C. Electrocoagulation

D. Electrosection

_____ 5. The type of procedure that uses liquid nitrogen to remove unwanted tissue is called:

A. laser surgery.

B. cryosurgery.

C. electrofulguration.

D. cautery.

____ 6. Which of the following terms is another name for a boil?

    A. Cyst

    B. Abscess

    C. Furuncle

    D. Sebum

____ 7. The type of suture material that is used when suturing deeper layers of the skin or when suturing structures that are difficult to reach is called:

    A. absorbable.

    B. nonabsorbable.

    C. glue.

    D. cold spray.

____ 8. Which of the following suture sizes is the largest?

    A. 2-0

    B. 3-0

    C. 4-0

    D. 5-0

____ 9. Which of the following surgical procedures is used to remove abscesses?

    A. Cyst removal

    B. Aspiration

    C. Incision and drainage

    D. Suture removal

____ 10. Which of the following types of medications is a long-acting anesthetic used for local infiltration or nerve blocks?

    A. Xylocaine®

    B. Carbocaine®

    C. Marcaine®

    D. Novacaine®

____ 11. Lidocaine is the most commonly used:

    A. dressing.

    B. disinfectant.

    C. antiseptic.

    D. anesthetic.

____ 12. Which of the following instruments is used to remove splinters or small objects from skin tissue?

    A. Splinter forceps

    B. Needle holders

    C. Dressing forceps

    D. Sponge forceps

____ 13. The purpose of which of the following instruments is to open or enlarge structures that are constricted such as the urethra or cervix?

    A. Probes

    B. Scopes

    C. Speculums

    D. Dilators

____ 14. Which of the following is a skin antiseptic used to prepare the skin prior to surgery (it also helps reduce bacteria that could potentially cause skin infection)?

    A. Sterile saline

    B. Betadine

    C. Hydrogen peroxide

    D. Tincture of benzoin

____ 15. Which of the following is used to increase the adhesive capabilities of sterile adhesive skin closure strips?

    A. Sterile saline

    B. Betadine

    C. Hydrogen peroxide

    D. Tincture of benzoin

____ 16. Which of the following is used to flush and clean an open wound and to remove foreign particles from a wound?

    A. Sterile saline

    B. Betadine

    C. Hydrogen peroxide

    D. Tincture of benzoin

____ 17. The knee is the most common area of the body where which of the following procedures is performed?

    A. Incision and drainage (I&D)

    B. Joint aspiration

    C. Sutures

    D. Excision of a sebaceous cyst

____ 18. An instrument used to grasp or clamp down objects is a(n):

    A. scalpel.

    B. bandage scissors.

    C. retractor.

    D. forceps.

____ 19. Which of the following is applied as a protective coating over ulcers and abrasions (it can also be placed under adhesive tape to increase holding power and decrease skin sensitivity to tape)?

    A. Hydrogen peroxide

    B. Tincture of benzoin

    C. Povidone-iodine

    D. Iodoform gauze strips

____ 20. Which of the following are used to pack abscesses, to draw out infection, and to act as a local antibacterial?

    A. Saline applicators

    B. Steri-strips

    C. Iodoform gauze strips

    D. Wicks

____ 21. Which of the following is a topical anesthetic of very short duration and its application is sometimes referred to as "freezing"?

    A. Silver nitrate

    B. Ethyl chloride

    C. Iodine

    D. Rubbing alcohol

____ 22. Which of the following is a vasoconstrictor and bronchodilator used to control hemorrhaging and shock, and can also be used to reverse allergic reactions?

    A. Formalin

    B. Silver nitrate

    C. Ether

    D. Epinephrine

____ 23. Which of the following solutions is used to preserve excised tissue?

    A. Hydrogen peroxide

    B. Ether

    C. Formalin 10%

    D. Nitrous oxide

___ 24. All of the following are ways anesthetics may be introduced into the body *except:*

    A. injection.

    B. intravenous.

    C. inhalation.

    D. orally.

    E. topical.

___ 25. Which of the following anesthetics is flammable and should not be used prior to or during electrotherapy or laser procedures?

    A. Epinephrine

    B. Ethyl chloride

    C. Xylocaine

    D. Nitrous oxide

SKILL APPLICATION CHALLENGE
Assignment 23-8: Labeling

  1. Label the parts of the following instrument:

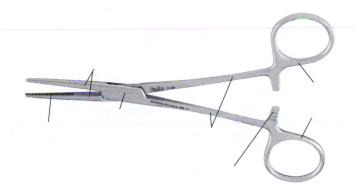

  2. Identify the instruments below and record the name of each instrument in the blank.

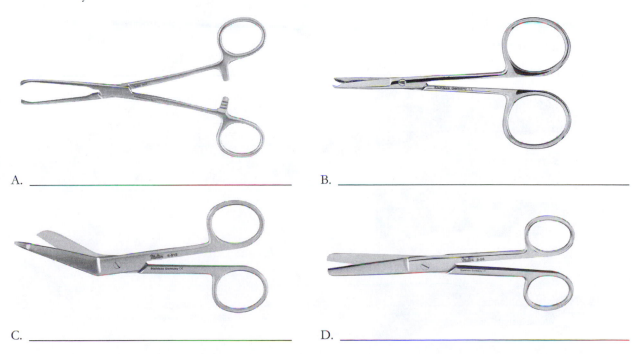

A. _____

B. _____

C. _____

D. _____

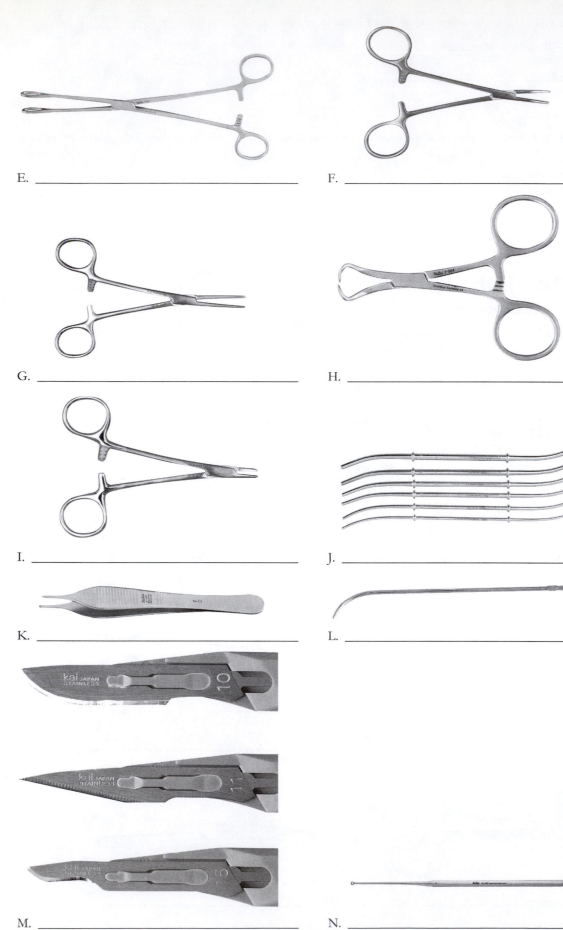

E. _____

F. _____

G. _____

H. _____

I. _____

J. _____

K. _____

L. _____

M. _____

N. _____

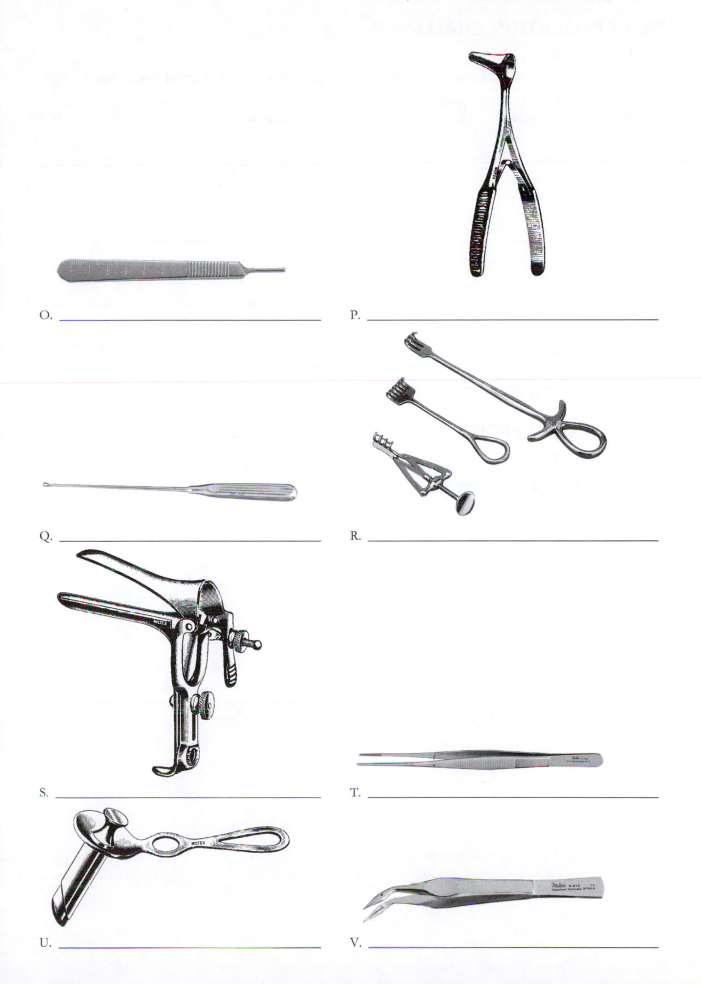

O. _____

P. _____

Q. _____

R. _____

S. _____

T. _____

U. _____

V. _____

FIELD APPLICATION CHALLENGE
Assignment 23-9
Read the following Field Application Challenge and complete the table following the scenario.

Pam is setting up a laceration tray for a patient who cut his right index finger on a meat slicer. Complete the table below by filling in the instruments and supplies that should be directly on the tray and the instruments and supplies that should be off to the side of the tray.

Laceration Tray	
On the Sterile Tray	**Off to the Side**
1.	1.
2.	2.
3.	3.
4.	4.
5.	5.
6.	6.
7.	7.
	8.
	9.

JOURNALING EXERCISE
Assignment 23-10

What content within this chapter was most meaningful to you? Why? List some examples of how you might apply information contained in this chapter, both during your training and after you enter the health care industry.

Name _____   Date _____   Score _____

C H A P T E R **24**

Assisting with Minor Office Surgeries and Wound Care Procedures

FIELD RELEVANCY AND BENEFITS

Assisting with minor office surgery is fairly common in many types of practices. Medical assistants should be familiar with aseptic guidelines so that they can be proactive in preventing postoperative (postop) infections. Instructing the patient on how to prepare for the procedure and how to care for the site following the procedure will result in a positive outcome. The information in this chapter is relevant to many types of practices including: family practice, OB-GYN, urgent care, and dermatology practices.

NOTE SHEET

Developing a Sterile Conscience

_____

_____

_____

_____

Patient Safety Considerations

_____

_____

_____

_____

Preparing for Office Surgeries

_____

_____

_____

_____

Performing a Surgical Handwash and Applying Surgical Attire

_____

_____

_____

_____

Assisting the Provider before and during the Procedure

Wound Care

_____

_____

_____

_____

_____

_____

_____

_____

VOCABULARY REVIEW

Assignment 24-1: Misspelled Words

Underline the correctly spelled term.

2. Purulint   Purelent   Purulent

3. Exedate   Exodate   Exudate

4. Debribdement   Debridement   Debribment

5. Bandge   Bandage   Bandege

6. Serosangunious   Serosanguineous   Seronsangious

7. Sterile consceince   Sterile conscience   Stirele conscious

8. Sanguineous   Sangunious   Sangious

Assignment 24-2: Definitions

Define the following terms.

1. Closed wound: _____

   _____

2. Concentric circle: _____

   _____

3. Dressing: _____

   _____

4. Open wound: _____

   _____

5. Primary dressing: _____

   _____

6. Secondary dressing: _____

   _____

7. Subatmospheric pressure device: _____

   _____

CHAPTER REVIEW

Assignment 24-3: Acronym Review

Write what each of the following acronyms stands for.

1. HBO_2: _____

2. JC: _____

Assignment 24-4: Short Answer

1. Describe two different types of alternative treatments used to treat chronic wounds that will not heal.

    A. _____

    _____

    _____

    _____

    _____

    _____

    _____

    B. _____

    _____

    _____

    _____

    _____

    _____

    _____

2. List the proper technique for preparing a Mayo stand for a surgical procedure.

    _____

    _____

    _____

    _____

    _____

3. Describe the three stages of healing.

    A. _____

    _____

    _____

    B. _____

    _____

    _____

    _____

C. _____

_____

_____

_____

4. Describe how a sterile conscience will help to reduce the patient's risk of developing a postop infection.

_____

_____

_____

_____

_____

_____

Assignment 24-4: True or False

Fill in the blank with a "T" for true statements and an "F" for false statements. Rewrite the false statements to make them true.

____ 1. Statistics show it is best not to shave the skin prior to surgery unless absolutely necessary.

_____

_____

____ 2. The skin can be sterilized.

_____

_____

____ 3. The provider is responsible for explaining the necessity for the procedure, what the procedure entails, the risks associated with the procedure, and alternatives in place of the procedure.

_____

_____

____ 4. The two most common prescriptions given to patients following a surgical procedure are antidotes and analgesics.

_____

_____

____ 5. The circulator is considered sterile and she must be careful not to contaminate herself during the procedure.

_____

_____

____ 6. When bandaging, always wrap distal to proximal.

_____

_____

____ 7. The surgery tray should be cleaned with a disinfectant starting from the center and working toward the periphery.

_____

_____

____ 8. Cleaning the wound with anything other than sterile saline could actually inhibit the healing process.

_____

_____

____ 9. Cool moist dressings help to speed up the healing process by stimulating the re-epithelialization rate, increasing collagen synthesis, and increasing the amount of fluid gained from the wound.

_____

_____

____ 10. Dead skin can improve the healing process.

_____

_____

____ 11. Always approach a sterile tray or a scrubbed person head on.

_____

_____

____ 12. It is all right to leave a sterile tray unattended as long as it has a sterile drape over it.

_____

_____

____ 13. When setting up a sterile tray, it should be positioned at the level of your hip.

_____

_____

____ 14. The outer $1/2$ inch of a sterile drape is considered nonsterile.

_____

_____

____ 15. Electrocautery equipment should be kept at a minimum of 12 to 24 inches away from the sterile field.

_____

_____

____ 16. The latest recommendations from the Association of periOperative Registered Nurses (AORN) states that moving drapes or applying new drapes over a sterile field could set the field up to become contaminated.

_____

_____

Assignment 24-5: Certification Practice

Choose the best answer and place the corresponding letter in the blank.

____ 1. Which of the following types of drape should be placed under the patient before cleansing the skin?
   A. Fenestrated drape
   B. Waterproof drape
   C. Sterile barrier
   D. Surgical towel

____ 2. When setting up the surgical tray, it should be positioned so that the top of the tray is:
   A. 12 inches from the knees.
   B. even with the waist of the provider.
   C. countertop height.
   D. even with the waist of the preparer.

____ 3. The two most common solutions used in minor office surgeries are:

     A. iodine and hydrogen peroxide.

     B. iodine and Hibiclens.

     C. sterile saline and sterile iodine.

     D. sterile saline and hydrogen peroxide.

____ 4. When bandaging, one needs to check for signs of poor circulation. All of the following are signs *except:*

     A. blueness around the nail beds.

     B. pallor.

     C. tingling sensation.

     D. numbness.

     E. itching.

____ 5. Which of the following exudates contains serum only?

     A. Serous

     B. Sanguineous

     C. Serosanguineous

     D. Purulent

____ 6. Which of the following exudates contains both serum and blood?

     A. Serous

     B. Sanguineous

     C. Serosanguineous

     D. Purulent

____ 7. Which of the following exudates contains pus?

     A. Serous

     B. Sanguineous

     C. Serosanguineous

     D. Purulent

____ 8. Which of the following exudates contains blood only?

     A. Serous

     B. Sanguineous

     C. Serosanguineous

     D. Purulent

____ 9. If using an antibacterial ointment over an open wound, it should be applied using a:

     A. tongue depressor.

     B. Q-tip.

     C. cotton ball.

     D. sterile cotton tip applicator.

____ 10. Which of the following types of bandage is used when wrapping body parts that are uniform in size?

     A. Circular turn

     B. Spiral turn

     C. Reverse spiral turn

     D. Figure-eight bandage

____ 11. Which of the following types of bandage is used to immobilize a joint?

     A. Circular turn

     B. Spiral turn

     C. Reverse spiral turn

     D. Figure-eight bandage

____ 12. Which of the following bandaging techniques is used to anchor a bandage at the beginning of most bandaging applications?

    A. Circular turn

    B. Spiral turn

    C. Reverse spiral turn

    D. Figure-eight bandage

____ 13. A card that lists all of the specifics regarding surgical procedures performed in the provider's office is referred to as a:

    A. tickler card file.

    B. surgical card file.

    C. surgery consent form.

    D. none of the above.

____ 14. Which of the following items is considered at least partially sterile?

    A. Shoe covers

    B. Mask

    C. Gown

    D. Cap

____ 15. Which of the following handwashes is much more thorough and is designed to eliminate large numbers of microorganisms on the skin by removing dirt, oils, and dead skin cells?

    A. Medical aseptic handwash

    B. Surgical handwash

____ 16. The medical assistant's role at the conclusion of the surgery includes:

    A. assisting the provider with removal of surgical attire.

    B. applying sterile dressing and bandage over the surgical wound.

    C. cleaning the patient's skin.

    D. all of the above.

____ 17. The stage of wound healing in which scar tissue forms is the called the:

    A. inflammatory stage.

    B. proliferative stage.

    C. maturation and remolding stage.

    D. granulation.

____ 18. Angiogenesis is defined as:

    A. the formation of blood vessels.

    B. the regeneration of heart vessels.

    C. the formation of a bloody discharge.

    D. a blood condition.

____ 19. The three main goals for the treatment of wounds include all of the following *except* to:

    A. increase moisture.

    B. control bacteria.

    C. increase temperature

    D. absorb exudates.

____ 20. You just finished setting up a sterile tray for an incision and drainage procedure. You are considered nonsterile during the procedure and will be assisting the physician as she needs items. The physician sticks her head in the room and tells you that she will be in just as soon as she performs a surgical scrub. You realize that you forgot to obtain the suture material, but the physician is almost scrubbed in and is ready for you to help her apply her PPE. You can't leave the room because you can't leave the tray unattended. What action would be best based on this scenario?

     A. Inform the physician that you are going to have to set up the tray again because you forgot an important item.

     B. Remain facing the tray, but work your way toward the door and yell down the hall for someone to bring the suture material to you.

     C. Once the physician has started the procedure and has taken ownership of the tray, inform the physician that you need to slip out to get the suture material.

     D. Ask the physician when she enters the room if she will get the suture material and just perform a new scrub.

Assignment 24-6: Matching

Match the dressing to its use.

Answer	Type of Dressing		When to Use
_____	1.	Alginates	A. Absorb exudates; provide a moist environment
_____	2.	Collagens	B. Used on wounds with light to heavy drainage or on wounds that are granulating
_____	3.	Foams	C. Used as a secondary dressing; can also be used to secure IVs
_____	4.	Gauze	D. Good for clean exudating wounds; aid in debridement
_____	5.	Hydrocolloids	E. Good for wounds with large amounts of drainage
_____	6.	Hydrogels	F. Should only be used on minor wounds or as a secondary dressing
_____	7.	Transparent films	G. Very useful on burns

SKILL APPLICATION CHALLENGE
Assignment 24-7: Preparing for Surgical Procedures

Fill in the table below with: (1) common patient instructions, (2) surgery room responsibilities, and (3) insurance responsibilities that are performed prior to, during, and following the surgical procedure.

(1) Provide the patient with the following instructions:	(2) Surgery room responsibilities:	(3) Insurance responsibilities:

FIELD APPLICATION CHALLENGE
Assignment 24-8
Read the following Field Application Challenge and respond to the questions following the scenario.

This is your first day working with Dr. Janelle Speelman and you are assisting with a mole removal. You gather the supplies and set up a sterile tray for the procedure. The physician asks for 1% Lidocaine and you hold the vial so that the physician can draw up the medication. The physician anesthetizes the patient and goes out of the room for a few minutes to allow time for the medication to take effect. While the physician is out of the room, you pick up the Lidocaine bottle to return it to its proper storage and notice that the label on the bottle reads 2% Lidocaine with epinephrine.

1. What should be your first course of action?

   A. Leave the surgery room and tell the physician about the mixup.

   B. Leave the surgery room for just long enough to alert someone to ask the physician to return ASAP.

   C. Tell the patient what happened.

   D. Privately tell the physician what happened upon her return to the surgery room.

2. Why did you choose this as your first course of action?

   _____

   _____

   _____

   _____

3. If after returning, the physician states that there is no problem and that she wants to go forward with the procedure, what will need to be done?

   A. Continue where you left off.

   B. Send someone new in to take your place.

   C. Set up an entirely new sterile tray and reprep the patient.

4. Why did you choose this response?

   _____

   _____

5. How can you make certain that nothing like this will ever happen again?

   _____

   _____

JOURNALING EXERCISE
Assignment 24-9

What content within this chapter was most meaningful to you? Why? List some examples of how you might apply information contained in this chapter, both during your training and after you enter the health care industry.

C H A P T E R **25**

Fundamentals of the Medical Laboratory

FIELD RELEVANCY AND BENEFITS

The medical lab can be an exciting place to work. Obtaining lab specimens, preparing them for transportation, and even conducting particular lab tests are all skills performed by medical assistants. In order to do well in this area, you must be familiar with laws that govern the laboratory, have thorough knowledge on how to properly collect and store specimens, and also know how to perform CLIA waived testing. You must also have a basic understanding of the variables that can affect each test.

The information in this chapter will be beneficial for anyone working in a laboratory setting or working in offices where laboratory tests are performed.

NOTE SHEET

Rationale for Laboratory Tests

_____

_____

_____

Laboratory Regulations

_____

_____

_____

Implications of CLIA '88 for the Medical Assistant

_____

_____

_____

Other Accreditation Options for POLs

_____

_____

_____

Classifications of Laboratories

_____

_____

_____

_____

Laboratory Personnel

_____

_____

_____

_____

Quality Assurance

_____

_____

_____

_____

Safety in the Laboratory

_____

_____

_____

_____

Processing Requests for Laboratory Tests

_____

_____

_____

_____

General Guidelines for Specimen Collection, Handling, and Transport

_____

_____

_____

_____

Laboratory Departments

_____

_____

_____

_____

Quality Control

_____

_____

_____

_____

Proficiency Testing

_____

_____

_____

_____

Hazards

_____

_____

_____

_____

Preparing the Patient for Laboratory Testing

_____

_____

_____

_____

The Microscope

_____

_____

_____

_____

The Centrifuge

_____

_____

_____

_____

VOCABULARY REVIEW
Assignment 25-1: Definitions
Define the following terms.

1. Assay: _____

_____

2. Baseline value: _____

_____

3. Centrifuge: _____

_____

4. Clinical diagnosis: _____

_____

5. Condenser: _____

_____

6. Cytology: _____

_____

7. Differential diagnosis: _____

_____

8. Histology: _____

_____

9. Panic value: _____

_____

10. Profile: _____

_____

11. Reference value: _____

_____

Assignment 25-2: Sentence Completion
Fill in the blanks below with Essential Terms from this chapter.

1. A _____ is a request form that accompanies each specimen sent to the lab.

2. A _____ is a large independently owned regional laboratory that performs complex or specialty tests.

3. Satellite locations where samples are collected are known as _____.

4. The _____ is the eyepiece of the microscope.

5. The part of the microscope that opens and closes to control the amount of light directed on the specimen is the _____.

6. _____ is the study of the structures of the immune system and their functions.

7. _____ is the study of blood and blood-forming tissues.

8. _____ is the laboratory department that grows and identifies microorganisms.

9. The part of the microscope that contains a magnifying lens for viewing specimens is the _____.

10. A patient who is without symptoms is _____.

CHAPTER REVIEW

Assignment 25-3: Acronym Review

Write what each of the following acronyms stands for.

1. ASCP: _____

2. AMT: _____

3. CLIA '88: _____

4. CLS: _____

5. COLA: _____

6. DHHS: _____

7. MLT: _____

8. MSDS: _____

9. MT: _____

10. PBT (ASCP): _____

11. POCT: _____

12. POL: _____

13. PPM: _____

14. QA: _____

15. QC: _____

16. STAT: _____

Assignment 25-4: True or False

Fill in the blank with a "T" for true statements and an "F" for false statements. Rewrite the false statements to make them true.

____ 1. Point-of-care testing can be performed in the exam room.

   _____

   _____

____ 2. A procurement station is the same thing as a satellite lab.

   _____

   _____

___ 3. COLA is an accrediting agency for pharmaceutical laboratories.

___ 4. Proficiency testing is a program that ensures the results of laboratory testing.

___ 5. Different laboratories may have different reference values.

___ 6. The proper way to carry the microscope is by the arm while supporting the base with the other hand.

___ 7. The objectives of the microscope should be cleaned once every day.

___ 8. The process of centrifugation is designed to separate components in a specimen.

___ 9. The total magnification of an object that is viewed under the 10x objective is 10.

___ 10. A microscopic examination of urine sediment would fall under waived testing.

Assignment 25-5: Short Answer

1. List at least four reasons for performing laboratory tests.

2. Explain why different laboratories have different normal values or reference ranges.

3. Explain the purpose of CLIA '88.

4. Describe the following laboratory classifications.

   A. Reference or independent: _____

   _____

   B. Hospital: _____

   _____

   C. Physician's office laboratory (POL): _____

   _____

   D. Point-of-care testing: _____

   _____

   E. Procurement station: _____

   _____

5. Describe the terms quality control and quality assurance.

   A. _____

   _____

   B. _____

   _____

6. Hazards in the lab are divided into what three categories?

   _____

7. List eight general specimen collection guidelines.

   A. _____

   B. _____

   C. _____

   D. _____

   E. _____

   F. _____

   G. _____

   H. _____

Assignment 25-6: Certification Practice

Choose the best answer and place the corresponding letter in the blank.

_____ 1. A POL is required to obtain which of the following before performing any low complexity tests?
   A. Approval by DHHS
   B. CLIA approval
   C. Certificate of waiver
   D. Pass proficiency tests

_____ 2. A waived test must meet all *but which* of the following criteria?
   A. Has been cleared for home use by the FDA
   B. Test method is simple and accurate
   C. Is unlikely to produce erroneous results
   D. Should not need to have controls performed to check the accuracy of the test

____ 3. All of the following are CLIA waived tests, *except:*

    A. Hgb A1c.

    B. differential count.

    C. hematocrit.

    D. ESR.

____ 4. Into which of the following categories does PPM fall?

    A. Low complexity

    B. Waived

    C. Moderately complex

    D. High complexity

____ 5. Which of the following tests is classified as PPM?

    A. Hemoglobin

    B. Urine sediment examination

    C. Occult blood testing

    D. Hematocrit

____ 6. The provider requests some coagulation studies on a patient who is scheduled for surgery. Which of the following departments of the laboratory will conduct the testing?

    A. Blood bank

    B. Clinical chemistry

    C. Serology

    D. Hematology

____ 7. A patient is suspected of having rheumatoid arthritis. Which of the following departments in the laboratory will perform the test to confirm the diagnosis?

    A. Serology

    B. Hematology

    C. Immunology

    D. Histology

____ 8. Medical assistants are permitted to perform which of the following job responsibilities in the POL?

    A. Phlebotomy

    B. Differential counts

    C. Wet mounts

    D. Microscopic urinalysis

____ 9. Procedures that are designed to ensure the accuracy and precision of laboratory tests are known as:

    A. proficiency testing.

    B. quality assurance.

    C. quality control.

    D. CEUs.

____ 10. You are preparing to test some patient samples on a handheld cholesterol instrument. You run a low-normal control and a high control. The result for the low-normal control is 85 mg/dl and the result for the high control is 350 mg/dl. The acceptable reference range for the low-normal control is 60-90 mg/dl and 190-280 mg/dl for the high control. Which of the following should you do before performing testing on the patient samples?

    A. Repeat the controls before running the patient samples. If they still are not accurate, go ahead and perform the patient samples; however, set up a maintenance call for the unit.

    B. Go ahead and run the patient samples anyway.

    C. Inform the provider.

    D. Repeat the controls one more time; if still not accurate, do not run patient samples until the problem is corrected.

___ 11. You are reading the temperature on the refrigerator where patient samples and test kits are stored. The acceptable range is 36–38°F, but the thermometer reads 42°F. Which of the following statements is true regarding the impact storing samples and test kits in this refrigerator would have on test results?

    A. None, since there really isn't that much of a difference.

    B. Test kits could be altered and may not produce accurate results.

    C. There may be a bit of an odor, but this shouldn't affect the overall results.

    D. It will vary depending on the tests that are to be performed.

___ 12. The Occupational Exposure to Hazardous Chemicals in the Laboratory Standard law was designed to:

    A. inform employees of the risks involved while working with particular chemicals in the laboratory.

    B. set the standards for the types of chemicals used in a laboratory setting.

    C. establish protocol for documenting test methods.

    D. educate lab personnel regarding the molecular structure of each chemical.

___ 13. Which of the following activities would *not* fall under chemical hazards cautions?

    A. Proper storage of chemicals

    B. Labeling of reagents

    C. Instructions of what to do in the event of accidental exposure

    D. A listing of all the uses for each chemical

___ 14. All of the following items are required information on a laboratory requisition form *except:*

    A. clinical diagnosis.

    B. specimen source.

    C. date and time of collection.

    D. an explanation of how the specimen was stored.

___ 15. *All* specimens sent to an outside laboratory should be:

    A. kept at room temperature.

    B. frozen.

    C. documented in an outside lab log.

    D. refrigerated.

___ 16. A patient calls the office demanding to know the results of her laboratory tests that were drawn over a week ago. You notice that they have not been reviewed by the physician. Which of the following statements is correct about what you should tell the patient?

    A. If results are normal, inform the patient of the results.

    B. Tell the patient that results seem to be normal but that they will have to talk to the physician for confirmation.

    C. Read the report to the patient, but inform her that you cannot interpret the results.

    D. Inform the patient that the physician has not had an opportunity to review the results but that you will get back in touch with her just as soon as the physician does.

SKILL APPLICATION CHALLENGE

Assignment 25-7: Labeling

Label the parts of the microscope and describe their use in the table below.

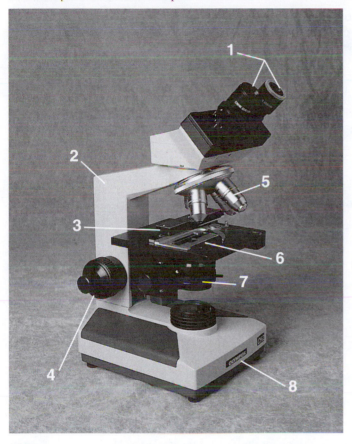

Name of Part	Use
1.	
2.	
3.	
4.	
5.	
6.	
7.	
8.	

COMPLETING SPECIAL FORMS

Assignment 25-8: Completing a Lab Requisition

Work Form Necessary: FORM 25-1

Directions: Complete the laboratory requisition form (Work Form 25-1) using the following information. The bill is to be sent directly to the provider so no insurance information is listed for the patient. (Hint: You will not use all of the information that is listed.)

Provider information: Robert Aniso, MD, Welleville Family Physicians, 1010 Carter Drive, Welleville, OH 12345-0987, Dr ID 20A

Patient information: Jane Karnes, 18168 August Avenue, Hometown, OH, 12345-7780, 50 years old, DOB: 05-11-60

Specimen source: Whole blood and serum

Date and time of collection: 05-12-10, 14:00, patient is fasting

Tests requested: Hemoglobin A_{1c}, and cholesterol

Medications: Lisinopril, Glucophage, Lipitor

Clinical diagnosis: 250.02; 272.0

FIELD APPLICATION CHALLENGE

Assignment 25-9

Read the following Field Application Challenge and respond to the questions following the scenario.

The provider has requested that you obtain a blood sample to be sent to the lab for a blood glucose, cholesterol, and PT/INR. After consulting the lab catalog, you notice that the patient must be fasting for the glucose and cholesterol levels and that serum is the specimen requirement. The PT does not require fasting but the specimen requirement is plasma. You obtain one SST tube and one light-blue top tube. After centrifugation, you pour off the serum and the plasma into tubes that will be sent to the lab. You forgot to label the tubes before pouring off the samples so you do not know which one is serum and which one is plasma.

1. How can you rectify the problem?

   _____

   _____

2. What could happen if you send the specimens to the lab anyway?

   _____

3. How could you prevent this kind of mistake from happening again?

   _____

JOURNALING EXERCISE

Assignment 25-10

What content within this chapter was most meaningful to you? Why? List some examples of how you might apply information contained in this chapter, both during your training and after you enter the health care industry.

Work Form 25-1

BILL	PLEASE LEAVE BLANK	C-3 REQUEST FORM	
☐ ACCOUNT	AREA _____	INSTRUCTIONS ① FOR PATIENT BILLING, COMPLETE BOX A.	**USA Biomedical Labs**
☐ PATIENT SEE ①	DEPT. _____	② FOR 3RD PARTY BILLING, COMPLETE BOX A	**957 Central Avenue**
☐ 3RD PARTY SEE ②	BILL CD _____	AND FILL IN DIAGNOSIS, THEN EITHER B, C, or D.	**Heartland, NY 11112**

N7708

PATIENT NAME (LAST)   (FIRST)   SPECIES SEX   AGE YRS. MOS.   DATE COLLECTED MO. DAY YR.   TIME COLLECTED

PATIENT ADDRESS   STREET   MISC. INFORMATION   DR. I.D.   MEDICARE: #

CITY   STATE   ZIP   DIAGNOSIS

PHYSICIAN   WELFARE: #   CASE NAME:

PROGRAM: PATIENT 1ST NAME: DATE OF BIRTH ALL CLAIMS   MO. DAY YR.

INSURANCE GR. #   I.D.   SERVICE CODE:

SUBSCRIBER NAME: RELATION: PHONE

STANDARD PROFILES

2987	( )	Diagnostic (Multi-Chem) Profile
2804	( )	Health Survey (SMA-12)
2824	( )	Executive Profile A
2825	( )	Executive Profile B
2826	( )	Executive Profile C
2858	( )	Amenorrhea Profile
7330	( )	Anticonvulsant Group
2927	( )	Autoimmune Profile
2801	( )	Calcium Metabolism Profile
2859	( )	Diabetes Management Profile
7701	( )	Drug Abuse Screen
	( )	Drug Analysis Comprehensive (S & U or G)
	( )	Drug Analysis, Qual (U/G)
7340	( )	Drug Analysis, Quant. (S)
2022	( )	Electrolyte Profile
	( )	Exanthem Group
	( )	Glucose/Insulin Response
2871	( )	Hepatitis Profile I
2872	( )	Hepatitis Profile II
2873	( )	Hepatitis Profile III
2874	( )	Hepatitis Profile IV
2875	( )	Hepatitis Profile V
2876	( )	Hepatitis Profile VI
2879	( )	Hepatitis Profile VII
2864	( )	Hirsutism Profile
2865	( )	Hypertension Screen

8350	( )	Immunologic Evaluation*
2814	( )	Lipid Profile A
2817	( )	Lipid Profile B
2003	( )	Lipid Profile C
2805	( )	Liver Profile A
2867	( )	Liver Profile B
2868	( )	MMR Immunity Panel
2869	( )	Myocardial Infarction Profile
2585	( )	Parathyroid Panel A (Mid-Molecule)
2586	( )	Parathyroid Panel B (Dialysis)
2587	( )	Parathyroid Panel C (Adenoma)
2818	( )	Prenatal Profile A
2819	( )	Prenatal Profile B
2820	( )	Prenatal Profile C
2877	( )	Prenatal Profile D
	( )	Respiratory Infection Profile A
	( )	Respiratory Infection Profile B
	( )	Respiratory Infection Profile C
	( )	Respiratory Infection Profile D
2821	( )	Rheumatoid Profile A
2878	( )	Rheumatoid Profile B
2882	( )	T & B Lymphocyte Differential Panel
2883	( )	Testicular Function Profile
2832	( )	Thyroid Panel A
2032	( )	Thyroid Panel B
2833	( )	Thyroid Panel C

SINGLE TESTS

5165	( )	ABO and Rho (B) (G)
6555	( )	Alpha-Fetoprotein RIA (S)
3015	( )	Alk. Phosphatase (S)
3041	( )	Amylase (S)
5163	( )	Antibody Screen ( ) If pos. ID & Titer (S) (B)
5166	( )	Antibody ID (B&S)
5104	( )	Antibody Titer (B&S) (Previous Pat. # _____)
5208	( )	ANA. Fluorescent (S)
5169	( )	ASO Titer (B) (S)
3147	( )	Bilirubin, Direct (S)
3010	( )	BUN (S)
3018	( )	Calcium (S)
6472	( )	CEA (RIA) (Plasma Only)
2995	( )	CBC with Automated Diff. (Abnormal Follow-Up Studies) (B) (SL)
2996	( )	CBC less Diff. (B)
3022	( )	Cholesterol (S)
3042	( )	CPK (S)
6500	( )	Digoxin (S)
6501	( )	Digitoxin (S)
3606	( )	GGT (S)
3006	( )	Glucose (S) Fasting
3009	( )	Glucose (P) Fasting
3023	( )	Glucose P.P. (P) Hrs. _____
3650	( )	HDL Cholesterol (S)
5180	( )	Heterophile Screen (Mono) (S)
5179	( )	Heterophile Absorption (S)
3342	( )	Hemoglobin A1C (B)
6416	( )	IgE (S)
3078	( )	Iron and T.I.B.C. (S)

6526	( )	Neonatal T_4 (S)
6525	( )	Neonatal TSH (S)
7941	( )	Neonatal T_4 Blood Spot
3019	( )	Phosphorus (S)
4132	( )	Platelet Count (B) (S)
3026	( )	Potassium (S)
	( )	Pregnancy Test, (S or U)
5167	( )	Premarital RPR (S)
6505	( )	Prostatic Acid Phosphatase (RIA) (S)*
2992	( )	Protein Electrophoresis (S) IEP if Abnormal ( ) 9085
4149	( )	Prothrombin Time (P)*
4144	( )	Reticulocyte Count (B)
5207	( )	RA Latex Fixation (S)
5194	( )	RPR
5195	( )	Rubella H.I. (S)
3016	( )	SGOT (S)
3045	( )	SGPT (S)
3031	( )	T-3 Uptake (S)
3032	( )	T-4 (S)
2832	( )	Thyroxine Index, Free (T_7) (S)
3036	( )	Triglycerides (S)
4111	( )	Urinalysis (U)
5277	( )	Urogenital GC Assay

UNLISTED TESTS OR PROFILES

_____
_____
_____
_____
_____
_____

★ FROZEN • (B) BLOOD • (P) PLASMA • (U) URINE • (S) SERUM • (SL) SLIDES   (Rev. 1-84)

FOLD THIS FORM IN HALF SO TEST(S) ORDERED IS CLEARLY VISIBLE

C H A P T E R **26**

Collecting the Blood Sample

FIELD RELEVANCY AND BENEFITS

Proper collection and preservation of laboratory specimens are critical to the diagnosis and treatment of patient conditions. The medical assistant must become proficient in collection techniques and specimen handling to preserve the integrity of the specimen and to ensure that the provider will receive the most accurate results possible.

NOTE SHEET

Why Do We Collect Blood?

_____

_____

_____

_____

Venipuncture

_____

_____

_____

_____

Vacuum Tube System

_____

_____

_____

_____

Winged Infusion (Butterfly) System

_____

_____

_____

_____

Blood Collection Tray

_____

_____

_____

_____

Specimen Collection by the Syringe Method

_____

_____

_____

_____

Specimen Collection by the Butterfly Method

_____

_____

_____

_____

The Failed Venipuncture

_____

_____

_____

_____

The Capillary Puncture

_____

_____

_____

_____

Performing the Venipuncture

_____

_____

_____

_____

Specimen Collection by the Vacuum Tube Method

_____

_____

_____

_____

Patient Response and Complications

_____

_____

_____

_____

Criteria for Specimen Rejection

_____

_____

_____

_____

General Guidelines for Specimen Handling

_____

_____

_____

_____

VOCABULARY REVIEW

Assignment 26-1: Matching

Match the term with its definition and place the corresponding letter in the blank.

____ 1. Aliquot

____ 2. Constrict

____ 3. Lipemia

____ 4. Evacuated tube

____ 5. Hematoma

____ 6. Lancet

____ 7. Gauge

____ 8. Phlebotomy

____ 9. Serum

____ 10. Tourniquet

____ 11. Primary container

____ 12. Venipuncture

____ 13. Plasma

____ 14. Butterfly

____ 15. Integrity

A. Device used to distend veins to assist with venipuncture

B. Liquid portion of the blood that remains after the blood has clotted

C. Piercing a vein with a needle to obtain a blood specimen

D. Small winged needle used for venipuncture

E. Narrowing of a blood vessel

F. Portion of a specimen that is used for testing

G. Sterile disposable sharp-pointed blade used to puncture the skin to collect a blood sample

H. Diameter of the lumen of a needle

I. Guarantees the purity or quality of the specimen

J. Swelling or accumulation of blood due to leakage from a blood vessel during or after venipuncture

K. Abnormal amount of fat in the blood causing the serum or plasma to appear cloudy or milky

L. Collection tube which contains a vacuum that facilitates the collection of blood during venipuncture

M. Original container in which the specimen is collected

N. Puncture of a vein to collect a blood sample

O. Liquid portion of whole blood which comes from a sample which contains an anticoagulant

Assignment 26-2: Sentence Completion

Fill in the blanks below with Essential Terms from this chapter.

1. A gel contained in some separator tubes which forms a barrier between the cellular portion of the specimen and the serum or plasma after centrifugation is _____.

2. _____ is a pooling of blood at the venipuncture site that is caused by leaving the tourniquet in place too long.

3. The medical assistant will _____ the vein to determine its location.

4. A rupturing of the red blood cells during venipuncture is known as _____.

5. The veins used for venipuncture are located in the _____.

6. A _____ is a skin puncture method used to obtain small amounts of blood for testing.

7. An _____ in the vacuum tube can help to preserve the integrity of the specimen.

CHAPTER REVIEW

Assignment 26-3: Acronym Review

Write what each of the following acronyms stands for.

1. QNS: _____

2. EDTA: _____

3. CLSI: _____

Assignment 26-4: Fill in the Blank

Fill in the blanks below with the appropriate word or phrase.

1. To ensure patient _____ with fasting instructions, the patient should be questioned to determine if fasting instructions were followed.

2. Venipuncture requires special equipment, _____, and _____.

3. _____ should be used for patients with a latex allergy.

4. Color-coding of needles is not _____ and may vary by manufacturer.

5. The range of syringe volumes most commonly used for blood collection is _____.

6. It is best to have patients _____ if they have a history of fainting during a venipuncture.

7. When palpating for a vein, _____ are often mistaken for a vein.

8. A _____ is one of the most common complications resulting from a venipuncture.

9. A _____ is the preferred method for blood collection for infants and children under the age of two and for patients with extremely small, fragile veins.

10. When performing a capillary puncture, the _____ should be collected last.

Assignment 26-5: Short Answer

1. List all the equipment needed to perform a venipuncture (evacuated tube method).

   _____

   _____

2. List the additive in each of the following tubes:

   A. Lavender: _____

   B. Red (plain): _____

   C. Red/gray: _____

   D. Gray: _____

   E. Light blue: _____

   F. Green: _____

3. Explain the purpose of following the correct order of draw.

   _____

   _____

4. In the table below, list causes for failed venipuncture attempts and provide possible remedies for each cause.

Causes of Failed Attempt	Possible Remedy

5. Explain the importance of mixing the blood sample in a tube that contains an additive.

_____

_____

_____

_____

6. List five hematoma prevention tips.

A. _____

B. _____

C. _____

D. _____

E. _____

7. List and describe four criteria for specimen rejection.

A. _____

B. _____

C. _____

D. _____

Assignment 26-6: Certification Practice

Choose the best answer and place the corresponding letter in the blank.

____ 1. You have collected several tubes of blood to be sent to the lab for testing. Which of the following methods applies to the transportation of all of the tubes?

A. Protected from light

B. Placed on ice

C. Placed in a bag, lying down

D. Kept in an upright position

____ 2. All of the following are reasons for a failed venipuncture *except:*

A. the needle inserted bevel down.

B. a collapsed vein.

C. the needle bevel is against the wall of the vein.

D. the needle was inserted bevel up.

____ 3. Leaving a tourniquet on the patient's arm for more than one minute can result in:

A. hematoma.

B. reflux.

C. hemoconcentration.

D. reduced specimen volume.

____ 4. Which of the following is the correct level of placement for the tourniquet on the arm?

A. One inch above the puncture site

B. Three to four inches above the puncture site

C. Anywhere on the arm as long as it is above the puncture site

D. As close to the axilla as possible

____ 5. After cleansing the venipuncture site, the medical assistant cannot remember where the vein is located and palpates the site again. Which of the following actions should be the next step in performing the venipuncture?

A. Clean the site again following palpation

B. Collect the sample

C. Remove the tourniquet

D. Start over

____ 6. Generally the gauge of needles used to perform venipunctures is:

A. 16G to 18G.

B. 19G to 20G.

C. 21G to 23G.

D. 23G to 25G .

____ 7. The size of syringe used for collection of a blood sample is determined by:

A. the amount of blood needed.

B. provider preference.

C. medical assistant preference.

D. no need to determine since the same size is used for all collections.

____ 8. Which of the following is *not* an advantage of the vacuum tube system?

A. Collection of numerous tubes with one stick

B. Specimen is immediately mixed with additive

C. Closed system

D. Reusable needle holders

____ 9. In 2002, OSHA released new regulations regarding the removal of contaminated needles from used blood tube holders. Which of the following was not included in the guidelines?

A. Reuse is prohibited because 50% to 80% of the adapters are contaminated after a single use.

B. Multisample needles are double-ended which increases the risk of accidental needlesticks.

C. Holders can be reused if they are first disinfected.

D. The tube holder or needle must have a safety device.

____ 10. An under-filled vacuum tube can result in a(n):

A. dilution of the sample.

B. incorrect ratio of blood to additive.

C. inaccurate test result.

D. all of the above.

____ 11. When placing a tourniquet on the patient's arm, all of the following statements are correct *except:*

A. Apply tourniquet 3 to 4 inches above the draw site.

B. Apply the tourniquet firmly.

C. If the tourniquet falls on the floor after releasing, immediately pick it up off the floor so it doesn't get dirty.

D. Do not leave the tourniquet in place more than one minute.

____ 12. Which of the following is the first step following a skin puncture?

A. Wipe away the first drop of blood.

B. Squeeze the finger firmly.

C. Collect the specimen immediately.

D. Cleanse the area again before collecting the specimen.

____ 13. Approximately how long should it take for blood that was collected in a nonadditive tube to clot?

A. 20 minutes

B. 2 hours

C. 60 minutes

D. 45 minutes

____ 14. After inspecting both of the patient's arms and applying the tourniquet, you realize that the veins are very small and fragile and very hard to palpate. Which of the following should be your next step?

A. Inspect the veins of the hand.

B. Inspect the veins of the wrist.

C. Ask for help.

D. Inform the provider that the patient has no veins.

____ 15. Which of the following is an OSHA requirement regarding a blood collection tray?

A. Should be well-stocked

B. Should be black in color

C. Should be red in color or have the biohazard symbol prominently displayed

D. Should have an ammonia capsule taped on the tray in the event the patient faints

____ 16. You are asked to collect a blood sample from a new patient. All of the following questions should be asked of the patient, *except:*

A. Have you ever had a reaction to an adhesive bandage?

B. Are you on aspirin therapy or blood thinners?

C. Is there any reason that you should not have a tourniquet on your arm (for example, patient has had a mastectomy, has a port, etc.)?

D. Are you afraid of needles?

____ 17. Which of the following techniques would you *not* use when selecting a vein for venipuncture?

A. Always inspect both arms.

B. Always select veins in the antecubital regions first, before looking at other sites.

C. Always select veins in the forearm region first, before looking at other sites.

D. Always palpate the vein so that you get a grasp of the direction the vein is running.

____ 18. When performing a venipuncture, all of the following procedures are correct *except:*

    A. the tourniquet is applied 3 to 4 inches above site.

    B. the needle is inserted at a 30° angle.

    C. the patient's arm is in a downward position.

    D. the tourniquet is in place less than one minute.

____ 19. Which of the following is a disadvantage of the syringe method for collecting blood?

    A. Pulling on the plunger can result in the needle being pulled out of the vein.

    B. The amount of blood collected is limited by the volume of the syringe.

    C. Blood must be transferred to a collection tube immediately.

    D. All of the above

____ 20. Each blood specimen must have a label which contains all of the following information *except* the:

    A. patient's full name or ID number.

    B. date and time of collection.

    C. patient's birth date.

    D. initials of person collecting the specimen.

____ 21. Which of the following vacuum tubes is unaffected by a short draw?

    A. Light blue

    B. Lavender

    C. Plain red top

    D. Gray

____ 22. Which of the following is the rationale for wiping away the first drop of blood following a capillary puncture?

    A. Contains electrolytes

    B. Contains skin cells

    C. Diluted with tissue fluid

    D. None of the above

SKILL APPLICATION CHALLENGES

Assignment 26-7: Tube Label Exercise

Complete the tube label below using the following information:

Patient: Carter Leonard
Time collected: 9:30 a.m.
Date collected: 10-10-2012
Tests ordered: CBC and ESR
You are the phlebotomist

ASSIGNMENT 26-8: Order of Draw

Fill in the following table with the appropriate information concerning the order of draw established by the CLSI.

Order of Draw	Tube Color
1.	
2.	
3.	
4.	
5.	
6.	

Assignment 26-9: Selecting the Proper Color Tube

Choose the appropriate tube top color that should be collected for the following laboratory tests.

1. CBC _____

2. Blood glucose _____

3. Cholesterol level _____

4. PT/INR _____

5. HIV testing _____

6. Medication level _____

7. Differential _____

8. Alcohol level _____

9. STAT chemistry test _____

10. ESR _____

Assignment 26-10: Documentation Exercise

Correctly document the following information in charting format in the progress note below.

Dr. Julieanne Young has ordered the following laboratory tests for patient Julie Vance: CBC, PT, and Chem Profile. You collect a lavender top tube, a light blue top tube, and a SST tube from the patient's left antecubital space using the vacuum tube method. The tests are sent to ABC Laboratories. The patient complains of pain following the venipuncture. There is no swelling, numbness, or tingling in the area. Dr. Young advises you to tell the patient to put some ice over the site upon returning home. The patient is to call if there are any complications.

COMPLETING SPECIAL FORMS

Assignment 26-11: Outside Specimen Tracking Log

Work Form Necessary: FORM 26-1

Directions: Complete the outside specimen tracking form (Work Form 26-1) using the following information.

10-10-2012, Dr. Young orders a CBC, PT, and Chem profile on Carter Leonard. Enter the correct tube types, your initials, and ABC Laboratories.

FIELD APPLICATION CHALLENGE

Assignment 26-12

Read the following Field Application Challenge and respond to the questions following the scenario.

After processing specimens collected for a CBC and potassium level, you notice that the serum in the red top tube is hemolyzed. The provider needs the results STAT so you send the specimen to the lab for testing. Will the results be accurate? What could have been done to prevent the hemolysis?

_____

_____

_____

_____

_____

JOURNALING EXERCISE

Assignment 26-13

What content within this chapter was most meaningful to you? Why? List some examples of how you might apply information contained in this chapter, both during your training and after you enter the health care industry.

Work Form 26-1

DOUGLASVILLE MEDICINE ASSOCIATES
5076 BRAND BLVD
DOUGLASVILLE, NY 01234
(123) 456-7890

OUTSIDE LAB SPECIMEN TRACKING LOG								
Date Sent	Patient Name/ID	Ordering Provider	Tests Ordered	Number and Type of Specimens Sent to Laboratory (Include Tube Colors)	Prepared By	Laboratory	Date Results Received	Results Received By

C H A P T E R **27**

Urinalysis

FIELD RELEVANCY AND BENEFITS

Urinalysis testing can provide practitioners with a vast amount of information regarding a patient's state of health. It is quick and easy to perform, but requires careful attention to detail from the medical assistant and a thorough knowledge and understanding of testing procedures. The medical assistant must become proficient at specimen handling and preservation, performing both physical and chemical urinalysis, and spinning down and setting up the specimen for microscopic evaluation. By being proficient at all these skills, the medical assistant will be prepared to work in a physician's office lab or in any practice that performs urinalysis testing.

NOTE SHEET

Composition of Urine

_____

_____

_____

_____

Specimen Collection

_____

_____

_____

_____

Quality Control

_____

_____

_____

Routine Urinalysis

_____

_____

_____

Physical Examination

_____

_____

_____

_____

Chemical Examination

_____

_____

_____

_____

Confirmatory Tests

_____

_____

_____

_____

Microscopic Examination

_____

_____

_____

_____

VOCABULARY REVIEW

Assignment 27-1: Matching

Match the term with its definition and place the corresponding letter in the blank.

____ 1. Turbid

____ 2. Urochrome

____ 3. pH

____ 4. Hemoglobinuria

____ 5. Bilirubin

____ 6. Cast

____ 7. Refractometer

____ 8. Renal threshold

____ 9. Sediment

A. Point at which a substance reaches a concentration high enough for it to spill over into the urine

B. Opaque appearance of urine

C. Structures sometimes found in urine caused by the accumulation of protein in the renal tubule

D. Orange-yellow pigment found in bile which is formed when RBCs are broken down

E. Blood found in urine without the presence of intact red blood cells

F. Instrument used to measure the specific gravity of urine

G. Pigment that gives urine its color

H. Solid material found in urine, after centrifugation, that is examined microscopically

I. Acidity or alkalinity of a urine specimen

Assignment 27-2: Sentence Completion

Fill in the blanks below with Essential Terms from this chapter.

1. A _____ is used to perform a chemical urinalysis.

2. A _____ urine specimen is collected with no special preparation.

3. The _____ is the clear liquid portion of urine that is discarded after centrifugation.

4. The amount of dissolved substances found in the urine is measured as its _____.

5. _____ is the presence of blood in the urine with the presence of intact red cells upon microscopic examination.

CHAPTER REVIEW

Assignment 27-3: True or False

Fill in the blank with a "T" for true statements and an "F" for false statements. Rewrite the false statements to make them true.

____ 1. A urobilinogen of 2.0 in the urine may indicate a liver dysfunction.

_____

_____

____ 2. 1+ protein in the urine could be the result of a gastrointestinal disorder.

_____

_____

____ 3. A specific gravity of 1.035 would indicate a concentrated urine specimen.

_____

_____

____ 4. Along with a positive glucose result, you may also expect to have a positive protein.

_____

_____

____ 5. Red blood cells should be seen during the microscopic exam when there is a positive result for hemoglobin on the reagent strip.

_____

_____

____ 6. The pH is important when determining the type of amorphous crystals present in urine.

_____

_____

____ 7. If urobilinogen is positive on the reagent test strip, you may also expect to see a positive bilirubin result.

_____

_____

____ 8. It is only necessary to test a control sample when a new bottle of reagent strips is used for the first time.

_____

_____

____ 9. Specific gravity of urine provides information on the kidney's ability to concentrate and dilute substances.

_____

_____

____ 10. Presence of bacteria is one cause of urine cloudiness.

_____

_____

Assignment 27-4: Short Answer

1. List changes that will occur in a urine specimen left standing at room temperature for more than one hour.

   Clarity: _____

   Odor: _____

   pH: _____

   Glucose: _____

   Ketones: _____

   Bilirubin: _____

   Urobilinogen: _____

   Nitrites: _____

   RBCs and WBCs: _____

   Casts: _____

   Bacteria: _____

2. Describe the different collection methods for urine specimens.

   Random: _____

   _____

   First-morning: _____

   _____

   Fasting/timed: _____

   _____

   Clean-catch midstream: _____

   _____

   Catheterization: _____

   _____

   24-hour collection: _____

   _____

   _____

   _____

3. List and describe the three parts of a complete urinalysis, including test methods used in each.

   A. _____

   _____

   B. _____

   _____

   C. _____

   _____

4. List and describe three confirmatory tests performed for glucose, bilirubin, and ketones.

   A. _____

   _____

B. _____

_____

C. _____

_____

5. Describe the proper procedure for preparing a slide for a microscopic urinalysis.

_____

_____

_____

_____

6. Fill in the missing information in the following urine color chart.

Color	Potential Cause
Colorless	
	Normal color
Dark yellow/amber	
	Hematuria; intact red cells present in the urine; menstrual contamination
Clear pink, red, or reddish/brown	
	Bilirubin present; bilirubin converted to biliverdin
	UTI caused by Pseudomonas bacteria; antidepressants such as Amitriptiline; Clorets®
Brown	
Black	

Assignment 27-5: Certification Practice

Choose the best answer and place the corresponding letter in the blank.

____ 1. Approximately which of the following percentages of urine is water?
   A. 50%
   B. 75%
   C. 95%
   D. 80%

____ 2. If a patient with diabetes has a positive glucose in their urine, which of the following has occurred?
   A. Patient is not following diet.
   B. Renal threshold has been reached.
   C. Patient is not taking medication properly.
   D. Patient is in acidosis.

____ 3. All of the following pieces of information may be requested to appear on a urine specimen container *except* the:

    A. patient's name.

    B. date of collection.

    C. diagnosis.

    D. patient's gender.

____ 4. Which of the following specimen types would be the most concentrated?

    A. Clean-catch

    B. Random

    C. Catheterization

    D. First-morning

____ 5. What is the purpose of a clean-catch midstream urine specimen?

    A. It is the most concentrated.

    B. It removes normal flora that may be present in the distal urethra and urinary meatus and extraneous epithelial cells from the vagina in females.

    C. It is the most sterile.

    D. It is the most accurate.

____ 6. A urine specimen collected by catheterization should be placed into which of the following containers?

    A. Sterile container

    B. Urine specimen cup

    C. Any type of container as long as it has been thoroughly cleaned

    D. Centrifuge tube

____ 7. If the provider orders a quantitative test for urine creatinine, which of the following types of specimen should be collected?

    A. First-morning

    B. Clean-catch midstream

    C. 24-hour

    D. Random

____ 8. Which of the following findings would be abnormal for a urine microscopic?

    A. 8–10 WBCs/hpf

    B. Few calcium oxalate crystals

    C. 0–1 hyaline cast

    D. Few mucus threads

____ 9. Which of the following amounts of urine is necessary for testing?

    A. 5 mL

    B. 8 mL

    C. 10–12 mL

    D. 15 mL

____ 10. Which of the following might a sweet fruity odor in a urine specimen indicate?

    A. Ingestion of fruit

    B. Contamination

    C. Ketoacidosis

    D. Presence of glucose

____ 11. If a control test does not fall within the acceptable range, which of the following steps should be taken?

    A. Repeat the test.

    B. Check the expiration date of the strips.

    C. Check the expiration date of the control sample.

    D. All of the above

____ 12. Which of the following is a confirmatory test for ketones?

    A. SSA

    B. Ictotest

    C. Acetest

    D. Clinitest

____ 13. Which of the following findings would be abnormal on a urine microscopic exam?

    A. 1–2 renal epithelial cells

    B. Few squamous epithelial cells

    C. Few bacteria

    D. 0–3 WBCs

____ 14. Which of the following cells could be present in an incorrectly collected clean-catch midstream specimen?

    A. White blood cells

    B. Yeast cells

    C. Red blood cells

    D. Bacteria

____ 15. Which of the following crystals would be clinically significant if found in the urine?

    A. Amorphous

    B. Calcium oxalate

    C. Triple phosphate

    D. Tyrosine

SKILL APPLICATION CHALLENGE

Assignment 27-7: Application Activity

Using the two urinalysis reports on the following pages, identify the abnormal results in the blanks below and state the clinical significance of each abnormal result.

Example A

1. _____

2. _____

3. _____

4. _____

5. _____

6. _____

7. _____

8. _____

9. _____

_____

_____

Example B

1. _____

2. _____

3. _____

4. _____

Example A

URINALYSIS REPORT FORM

PHYSICIAN INFORMATION		PATIENT INFORMATION
DOUGLASVILLE MEDICINE ASSOCIATES **5076 BRAND BLVD.** **DOUGLASVILLE, NY 01234** **(123) 456-7890** Ordering Physician: Dr. C. Leonard Physician ID #345679234		Name: Mr. Joshua Leonard Address: 1234 Main Street City / State / Zip: Mytown, OH 23333 Phone #: 216-888-8888 ID #: 12345678
Date and Time of Collection		**Date Results Received**
02-24-10 9:00 a.m.		02-25-10
Test Ordered	**Results**	**Reference Range**
Complete Urinalysis (UA):		
Physical UA:		
Color	Reddish/brown	Straw to Dark Yellow
Clarity/Transparency	Turbid	Clear to Hazy
Chemical UA/Reagent Strip:		
Specific Gravity	1.0430	1.005-1.030
pH	8.0	5.0-9.0
Protein	3+ (300)	Negative/trace
Glucose	Negative	Negative
Ketones	Negative	Negative
Blood	2+ (moderate)	Negative
Bilirubin	2+ (moderate)	Negative
Urobilinogen	1	0.1-1.0
Nitrite	Positive	Negative
Leukocytes	2+ (moderate)	Negative
Microscopic UA:		
Hyaline Casts		0-2/LPF
Granular Casts		0/LPF
Cellular Casts	4-6 WBC casts/lpf	0/LPF
WBCs	5-10/hpf	0-5/HPF
RBCs	TNTC	0-2/HPF
Squamous epithelial cells	Few	Few
Transitional epithelial cells		Rare
Bacteria	moderate	Rare to few
Yeast		Small amount
Crystals:		
Artifacts:		

Example B

URINALYSIS REPORT FORM

PHYSICIAN INFORMATION		PATIENT INFORMATION	
DOUGLASVILLE MEDICINE ASSOCIATES **5076 BRAND BLVD.** **DOUGLASVILLE, NY 01234** **(123) 456-7890** Ordering Physician: Dr. Alan Manning Physician ID #345679234		Name: Ms. Kelly Lynn ID #: 456-88-6523 **Date Results Received**	
Date and Time of Collection			
02-15-10 2:00 p.m.		02-19-10	
Test Ordered	**Results**	**Reference Range**	
Complete Urinalysis (UA):			
Physical UA:			
Color	Dark yellow	Straw to Dark Yellow	
Clarity/Transparency	Hazy	Clear to Hazy	
Chemical UA/Reagent Strip:			
Specific Gravity	1.025	1.005-1.030	
pH	6.0	5.0-9.0	
Protein	Trace	Negative/trace	
Glucose	1/4 (250)	Negative	
Ketones	Moderate	Negative	
Blood	Negative	Negative	
Bilirubin	Negative	Negative	
Urobilinogen	Negative	0.1-1.0	
Nitrite	Negative	Negative	
Leukocytes	Negative	Negative	
Microscopic UA:			
Hyaline Casts	0-1/lpf	0-2/LPF	
Granular Casts		0/LPF	
Cellular Casts		0/LPF	
WBCs	None seen	0-5/HPF	
RBCs	None seen	0-2/HPF	
Squamous epithelial cells	Moderate	Few	
Transitional epithelial cells		Rare	
Bacteria		Rare to few	
Yeast		Small amount	
	Few mucus threads		
Crystals:			
Artifacts:			

Assignment 27-8: Documentation Exercise

Document the physical and chemical lab results from Assignment 27-7, Example B, as though you performed the urinalysis, using in correct charting format. Use 02/19/10 as the date and 9:30 a.m. as the time you performed the testing. (The order from Dr. Manning is for a Physical and Chemical UA.)

COMPLETING SPECIAL FORMS

Assignment 27-8: Lab Requisition Form

Work Form Necessary: FORM 27-1

Directions: Complete the lab requisition (Work Form 27-1) with the scenario information given below.

Today's date: 02/15/2010 Time: 2:00 p.m. Patient name: Kelly J. Lynn, Address: 725 Mapleview Ave, Polaris, NY 01658, Telephone number: (123)888-8888, Patient ID # 4523, DOB: 08-12-1984, Age: 25, Sex: female, Fasting: no, Tests ordered: complete UA, Urine Culture, Sample: Urine specimen, and UA Culture Tube, Referring provider: Dr. Alan Manning, Address: Douglasville Medicine Associates, 5076 Brand Blvd., Douglasville, NY 01234, Telephone number: (123) 456-7890, Provider ID#: 345679234. Bill to patient. Patient is a self-pay with no insurance.

Assignment 27-9: Outside Specimen Tracking Log

Work Form Necessary: FORM 27-2

Directions: Enter the following information regarding Kelly Lynn's urine sample and requested tests into the outside lab specimen tracking log (Work Form 27-2). Additional information that you will need is listed below.

Name of lab: ABC Lab
Initials of employee who prepared the specimen: LMV
Initials of employee who received the results: MEH
Date results received: 02/19/2010

FIELD APPLICATION CHALLENGE
Assignment 27-10

Read the following Field Application Challenge and respond to the questions following the scenario.

A patient being treated for the past 10 days for a UTI has dropped off a urine sample at the office for a recheck. You obtain the sample from the front desk and take it to the lab for a complete urinalysis. You place the sample on the counter and prepare to complete the physical and chemical urinalysis. Another medical assistant calls for your help with obtaining a blood sample from the patient in exam room two. You are then called to the front desk to speak with a patient who has a question about his medication. You room three more patients and return to the lab and realize that it has been over two hours since the patient dropped off the urine specimen. The specimen is quite cloudy and has an abnormal odor. You perform the reagent strip testing. Some tests are abnormal. You prepare the slide for the microscopic exam and notify the provider that it is ready for viewing.

1. Should the results you received be reported as accurate? Why or why not?

_____

_____

2. What should you have done with the urine specimen when you received it?

_____

_____

3. What implication could your actions have on the treatment of this patient?

_____

_____

JOURNALING EXERCISE
Assignment 27-11

What content within this chapter was most meaningful to you? Why? List some examples of how you might apply information contained in this chapter, both during your training and after you enter the health care industry.

Work Form 27-1

LABORATORY REQUISITION

PATIENT LAST NAME	FIRST	M.I.	REFERRING PROVIDER

PROVIDER ID #	PATIENT ID #	BILL: ☐ PHYSICIAN	☐ MEDICAL ☐ HMO ☐ CHDP	D.O.B	AGE	SEX
			☐ MEDICARE ☐ INSURANCE ☐ PATIENT			

PLEASE COMPLETE INSURANCE BILLING INFORMATION AT BOTTOM

PROVIDER NAME, ADDRESS, AND PHONE NUMBER	PATIENT ADDRESS	PATIENT PHONE NUMBER ( )	DATE COLLECTED	TIME COLLECTED
	CITY	STATE	ZIPCODE	FASTING YES | NO	STAT	CALL RESULT
	PATIENT MEDICARE #	PATIENT MEDICAID #	INFO. BELOW WILL APPEAR ON REPORT

CUSTOM PROFILES & ADDITIONAL TESTS

173 [ ] CHEMISTRY PANEL, COMPLETE BLOOD COUNT (ZPP), LIPID PROFILE, T4

05050 [ ] CHOL, TRIG, HDL CHOL, VLDL CHOL, LDL CHOL, RISK FACTOR

PROFILES

00011	☐ SPECIAL COMPREHENSIVE	2 SS,L	03536	☐ HYPERTHYROID PROFILE		SS
00001	☐ COMPREHENSIVE HEALTH SURVEY	SS,L	05037	☐ HYPOTHYROID PROFILE		SS
00002	☐ GENERAL SURVEY	SS,L	05051	☐ LIPID PROFILE		SS
00003	☐ CHEMISTRY PANEL	SS,L	05021	☐ LIVER PROFILE		SS
CH7	☐ CHEM 7 PANEL	SS	03359	☐ LUPUS PROFILE		SS
03280	☐ ANEMIA PROFILE	SS,L	03959	☐ MENOPAUSAL PROFILE SS /03960 ☐ POST MENOPAUSAL		SS
06016	☐ ARTHRITIS PROFILE	SS,L	02280	☐ OVARIAN FUNCTION PROFILE SS /02281 ☐ TESTICULAR FUNC. PROF.		SS
05725	☐ COMPREHENSIVE THYROID SURVEY	SS	02808	☐ PRENATAL PROFILE		L,R
02691	☐ EPSTEIN BARR PROFILE	SS	05006	☐ THYROID PROFILE		SS
05010	☐ ELECTROLYTES	SS	03191	☐ TORCH PANEL		SS
06826	☐ HEPATITIS PROFILE	SS	5756	☐ URINE DRUG SCREEN U / ☐ VENIPUNCTURE		

TESTS

0361	☐ ABO & Rh TYPE	R,L	0141	☐ C-REACTIVE PROTEIN	SS	0673	☐ HEPATITIS B SURFACE ANTIGEN	SS	0237	☐ PTT	B
0302	☐ ALKALINE PHOSPHATASE	SS	1341	☐ DHEA-S	SS	0245	☐ HEPATITIS C ANTIBODY	SS	0317	☐ RA FACTOR	SS
0109	☐ AMYLASE	SS	0119	☐ DIGOXIN	SS	0257	☐ IRON	SS	0321	☐ RUBELLA	SS
0613	☐ ANA	SS	0224	☐ DILANTIN	LDL-A	☐ LDL CHOLESTEROL	SS	0331	☐ RPR	SS
0366	☐ ANTIBODY SCREEN	R	0835	☐ ESTRADIOL	SS	0283	☐ LEAD BLOOD	RB	0335	☐ SEMEN ANALYSIS	SEMEN
0110	☐ ASO (STREPTOZYME)	SS	0833	☐ FERRITIN	SS	0281	☐ LIPASE	SS	0328	☐ SEDIMENTATION RATE (ESR)	L
0126	☐ BILIRUBIN TOTAL	SS	0003	☐ FOLIC ACID & VITAMIN B12	SS	8225	☐ LH	SS	0349	☐ SGOT (AST)	SS
0132	☐ BUN	SS	0651	☐ FSH	SS	0247	☐ MONONUCLEOSIS	SS	0348	☐ SGPT (ALT)	SS
8726	☐ CA125	SS	0140	☐ FTA-ABS	SS	0778	☐ PHENOBARBITAL	SS	0330	☐ SICKLE CELL SCREEN	L
0142	☐ CALCIUM	SS	0210	☐ GGTP	SS	0307	☐ POTASSIUM	SS	0354	☐ T4 (THYROXINE)	SS
0130	☐ CBC	L	0536	☐ GLUCOSE, FASTING	GY	0557	☐ PREGNANCY (SERUM)	SS	1358	☐ T4 FREE	SS
0388	☐ CEA-ROCHE	SS		☐ GLUCOSE, ____ HR PP	GY	0308	☐ PREGNANCY (URINE)	U	8456	☐ TESTOSTERONE	SS
0152	☐ CHOLESTEROL	SS	0771	☐ GLYCOHEMOGLOBIN	L	0359	☐ PROGESTERONE	SS	0824	☐ THEOPHYLLINE	SS
0788	☐ CORTISOL	SS	0534	☐ H. PYLORI	SS	8041	☐ PROLACTIN	SS	0360	☐ TRIGLYCERIDE	SS
0162	☐ CPK	SS	0823	☐ HGG QUANTITATIVE	SS	0103	☐ PROTEIN, TOTAL	SS	0672	☐ TSH	SS
0445	☐ CKMB ISOENZYME	SS	1856	☐ HIV (ANTIBODY)	SS	2000	☐ PROSTATE SPECIFIC ANTIGEN (PSA)	SS	0373	☐ URIC ACID	SS
0161	☐ CREATININE	SS	0558	☐ HDL CHOLESTEROL	SS	0310	☐ PT (PROTHROMBIN TIME)	B	0219	☐ URINALYSIS	U

CYTOPATHOLOGY

☐ PREGNANT ☐ ABORTION ☐ POST-PARTUM ☐ POST-MENOPAUSE

HISTORY _____

PREV. ABNORMAL CYTOL FINDINGS _____

☐ CONTRACEPTIVES DATE _____
☐ HYSTERECTOMY ☐ HORMONES ☐ IUD
☐ COPHORECTOMY ☐ TOTAL ☐ SUPRA CX
☐ RADIATION Rx DATE _____
☐ OTHER _____ ☐ HORMONES Rx ☐ CHEMO Rx

LMP _____ DATE COLLECTED _____
SOURCE ☐ CERVIX ☐ ENDOCERVIX ☐ VAGINA
☐ CYTOBRUSH ☐ OTHER SITE _____

MICROBIOLOGY

THCUL ☐ THROAT	URTHC ☐ URETHRAL	9391 ☐ CHLAMYDIA DNA
EACUL ☐ EAR	VACUL ☐ VAGINAL	9390 ☐ GONORRHEA DNA
EYCUL ☐ EYE	WOCUL ☐ WOUND	9391 ☐ OCCULT BLOOD
GOCUL ☐ GC	ROCUL ☐ CULTURE (Routine)	0293 ☐ OVA & PARASITE
SPCUL ☐ SPUTUM	URCUL ☐ URINE	WTM ☐ WET MOUNT
STCUL ☐ STOOL	GSP ☐ GRAM STAIN	
SOURCE _____	OTHER _____	

DIAGNOSIS OR COMMENTS

LAB USE ONLY (DO NOT WRITE BELOW THIS SPACE)

DATE RECEIVED | DATE REPORTED

STATEMENT OF SPECIMEN ADEQUACY

GENERAL CATEGORIZATION

DESCRIPTIVE DIAGNOSIS

HORMONAL EVALUATION

ADDITIONAL COMMENT

CYTOTECHNOLOGIST | PATHOLOGIST

INSURANCE BILLING INFORMATION

PRIMARY INSURED | INSURANCE COMPANY

ADDRESS

POLICY NO. & I.D. NO. | ICD9 CODE

LEGEND

SS	Serum Separator	GY	Grey	B	Blue	U	Urine
R	Red	L	Lavender	RB	Royal Blue	G	Green

Work Form 27-2

DOUGLASVILLE MEDICINE ASSOCIATES
5076 BRAND BLVD
DOUGLASVILLE, NY 01234
(123) 456-7890

OUTSIDE LAB SPECIMEN TRACKING LOG								
Date Sent	Patient Name/ ID	Ordering Provider	Tests Ordered	Number and Type of Specimens Sent to Laboratory (Include Tube Colors)	Prepared By	Laboratory	Date Results Received	Results Received By

C H A P T E R **28**

Hematology and Coagulation Studies

FIELD RELEVANCY AND BENEFITS

A small sample of blood can yield a great deal of information about the well being of a patient as well as any disease states that may be present in the body. The medical assistant should possess a basic knowledge of normal values for common hematology tests, the function of the various types of blood cells, and the rationale for performing standard tests. Alerting the provider to abnormal lab results is often the medical assistant's duty. Understanding the significance of those results is part of being a competent member of the health care team.

NOTE SHEET

Hemopoesis

_____

_____

_____

_____

Blood Components

_____

_____

_____

_____

Basic Hematology Studies

_____

_____

_____

_____

The Complete Blood Count (CBC)

_____

_____

_____

_____

Erythrocyte Sedimentation Rate (ESR)

_____

_____

_____

_____

Automated Hematology Analyzers

_____

_____

_____

Coagulation Tests

_____

_____

_____

_____

VOCABULARY REVIEW

Assignment 28-1: Matching

Match the term with its definition and place the corresponding letter in the blank.

____ 1. Differential count

____ 2. Complete blood count

____ 3. Erythrocyte sedimentation rate

____ 4. Thrombocyte

____ 5. Normocyte

____ 6. Serum

____ 7. Lymphocyte

____ 8. Hematocrit

____ 9. Monocyte

____ 10. Macrocyte

____ 11. Hemoglobin

____ 12. Microcyte

____ 14. Leukocyte

A. Term used to describe a larger than normal red blood cell

B. Percentage of packed red blood cells in the total volume of blood

C. The largest of all white blood cells; contains no granules in cytoplasm; has a large, irregularly shaped nucleus; may contain holes in the cytoplasm because it is active in phagocytosis

D. Term used to describe a normal sized cell

E. Platelet

F. Liquid portion of the blood after the blood has been allowed to clot; contains no coagulation factors

G. Group of blood tests that includes a hemoglobin, hematocrit, red and white blood counts, differential count, platelet count or estimate, and red blood cell indicies

H. Measurement of how far red cells fall in a given amount of blood in a one-hour time frame

I. Count of 100 white blood cells on a stained blood smear for the purpose of determining the approximate percentage of each type of white blood cell

J. The smallest of all white blood cells; contains no granules in cytoplasm; elevated in viral infections

K. Iron pigment on the red blood cells that carries oxygen

L. Term used to describe a smaller than normal red blood cell

M. Another name for white blood cell; its main function is to fight infection

Assignment 28-2: Misspelled Words

Underline the correctly spelled term.

1. <u>morphology</u>   mourphology   morphologie

2. eaosenophil   <u>eosinophil</u>   eosenophil

3. poickilocytosis   poicilocitosis   <u>poikilocytosis</u>

4. newtrofil   <u>neutrophil</u>   neutraphil

5. <u>erythrocyte</u>   erythracyte   erythrocite

6. <u>hemostasis</u>   homeostasis   hemeostasis

7. anisocitosis   anisositosis   <u>anisocytosis</u>

8. bascophil   <u>basophil</u>   bazophil

CHAPTER REVIEW

Assignment 28-3: Acronym Review

Write what each of the following acronyms stands for.

1. CBC: _____

2. WBC: _____

3. RBC: _____

4. ESR: _____

5. MCV: _____

6. MCH: _____

7. MCHC: _____

8. PT: _____

9. INR: _____

Assignment 28-4: Fill in the Blank

Fill in the blanks below with the correct word or phrase.

1. One function of hemoglobin is to _____ to the cells throughout the body.

2. While ESR is not a specific test for any one disease, it is used as an indicator for _____.

3. Glass capillary tubes are being replaced with _____ or tubes with a special mylar coating to decrease the possibility of accidental _____ due to broken tubes during the sealing process.

4. A patient's hemoglobin level would be _____ in a condition such as COPD.

5. A heparinized capillary tube is coated with the anticoagulant _____.

6. A microhematocrit tube fills by _____ action.

7. The most common method for preparing a blood smear is the _____ or _____ method.

8. The two most common types of stains used to stain a blood smear are _____ and _____.

9. The differential count is performed using the _____ on the microscope.

10. A U-shaped nucleus in a neutrophil would indicate that the cell is a(n) _____ or _____.

ASSIGNMENT 28-5: SHORT ANSWER

1. Describe the process of hemopoesis and state the different parts of the body in which hemopoesis takes place throughout a person's life.

   _____

   _____

   _____

   _____

   _____

   _____

2. Describe the function of each of the following cellular components.

Cellular Components	*Function*

   Erythrocytes (RBCs)   _____

   _____

   _____

   _____

   Leukocytes (WBCs)   _____

   _____

   _____

   _____

   Thrombocytes (Platelets)   _____

   _____

   _____

   _____

3. List the normal values for components of the CBC.

Component	*Normal Value*

   Red blood cell count   Males: _____

   Females: _____

   Neonates: _____

   White blood cell count   Adults: _____

   Neonates: _____

   Platelet count or estimate   _____

   Hemoglobin   Males: _____

   Females: _____

   Neonates: _____

   Hematocrit   Males: _____

   Females: _____

   Neonates: _____

Differential   Neutrophils: _____

                      Bands: _____

                      Eosinophils: _____

                      Basophils: _____

                      Lymphocytes: _____

                      Monocytes: _____

4. Give an explanation of why the hematocrit would be increased in a patient with dehydration.

   _____

   _____

5. Explain the importance of the information obtained from the red cell indicies.

   _____

   _____

   _____

   _____

6. List the different types of white blood cells found on a differential and reasons for an increase and decrease of each type.

Name of Cell	Increase	Decrease
_____	_____	_____
	_____	_____
	_____	_____
_____	_____	_____
	_____	_____
	_____	_____
_____	_____	_____
	_____	_____
	_____	_____
_____	_____	_____
	_____	_____
	_____	_____
_____	_____	_____
	_____	_____
	_____	_____
_____	_____	_____
	_____	_____

7. Fill in the blanks listing possible sources of error when preparing a blood smear.

Error   *Possible Cause*

Too long or too thin

_____

_____

_____

Too short or too thick

_____

_____

_____

Waves or ridges

_____

_____

Abnormal cell morphology/artifacts

_____

_____

_____

Holes in the smear

_____

_____

Uneven cell distribution

_____

_____

_____

_____

Assignment 28-6: Certification Practice

Choose the best answer and place the corresponding letter in the blank.

____ 1. The following laboratory results have been received on a 79-year-old female. Which of the following results is abnormal?

A. WBC: 11,500/cumm

B. RBC: 3.5 million/cumm

C. Hgb: 10 gm/dL

D. Hct: 33%

E. All of the above

____ 2. Which of the following is a component of red blood cells that allows for easy movement through small blood vessels?

A. Their small diameter

B. The viscosity of the hemoglobin found on the RBC

C. Their biconcave shape

D. Their cellular coating

____ 3. A mature erythrocyte remains functional in the blood stream for approximately:

    A. 21 days.

    B. 120 days.

    C. 30 days.

    D. 180 days.

____ 4. A leukocyte in which holes are commonly found in the cytoplasm because of its function in phagocytosis is:

    A. neutrophil.

    B. monocyte.

    C. eosinophil.

    D. basophil.

____ 5. If anisocytosis is reported on a differential count, this means that there are variations in the:

    A. hemoglobin content of the red blood cells.

    B. size of the red blood cells.

    C. shape of the red blood cells.

    D. color of the red blood cells.

____ 6. Which of the following types of anemia is characterized by a decrease in red blood cell production due to a bone marrow disorder?

    A. Hemolytic anemia

    B. Pernicious anemia

    C. Sickle-cell anemia

    D. Aplastic anemia

____ 7. A decrease in all blood cell types is known as:

    A. poikilocytosis.

    B. pancytopenia.

    C. polycythemia.

    D. leukocytopenia.

____ 8. Which of the following is an inherited disorder caused by Hemoglobin S?

    A. Shistocytosis

    B. Spherocytosis

    C. Sickle-cell anemia

    D. Shigellocytosis

____ 9. Which of the following counts within a CBC would help with the differentiation of particular types of anemias?

    A. RBC count

    B. Hemoglobin

    C. Hematocrit

    D. RBC indicies

____ 10. The readings of both tubes for a hematocrit determination must be:

    A. within ± 2%.

    B. within ± 1%.

    C. within ± 3%.

    D. exactly the same.

____ 11. When performing a hematocrit determination, the sealed end of the capillary tube should be placed:

    A. pointing inward.

    B. against the outside rim of the centrifuge or toward the gasket.

    C. pointing in opposite directions.

    D. none of the above.

____ 12. Depending on the unit used, the microhematocrit is spun for:

    A. 1–2 minutes.

    B. 2–3 minutes.

    C. 1–4 minute.

    D. 2–5 minutes.

____ 13. Medical assistants are generally permitted to perform which of the following hematology tests?

    A. Hemoglobin

    B. Hematocrit

    C. Differential

    D. Only A and B are correct

____ 14. If the neutrophil count on a differential is reported as 75%, which of the following conditions would likely be responsible?

    A. Bacterial infection

    B. Viral infection

    C. Leukemia

    D. Polycythemia

____ 15. If a WBC count is reported as 2,000/cumm, which of the following may apply?

    A. The patient has a bacterial infection.

    B. The patient has leukemia.

    C. The patient is taking chemotherapy.

    D. The patient has a parasitic infection.

____ 16. All of the following are true of the ESR *except* the:

    A. test must be timed precisely for one hour.

    B. tube must remain in a vertical position for one hour.

    C. tube rack should be placed on a surface free from vibrations.

    D. tube should be placed in a cool, dark place.

____ 17. In which of the following conditions would you expect to see an increased ESR?

    A. Inflammatory conditions

    B. Polycythemia

    C. Sickle cell anemia

    D. None of the above

____ 18. Which of the following rationales would apply for performing a PT/INR?

    A. Patient has diabetes

    B. Patient is on anticoagulant therapy

    C. Patient has a decreased platelet count

    D. Patient has arthritis

____ 19. When preparing a slide for a differential, the slide should go under which of the following objectives?

    A. Oil immersion (100x)

    B. High power (40x)

    C. Low power (10x)

    D. None of the above

SKILL APPLICATION CHALLENGES

Assignment 28-7: Normal and Abnormal Results

1. Read and record the following ESR result and state whether it is normal or abnormal. The patient is male.

A. The result is: _____.

B. This result is normal/abnormal. (Circle one.)

2. Identify the abnormal results from the following lab report and explain their clinical significance in the blanks on the next page.

ABC LABORATORY HEMATOLOGY REPORT FORM

PHYSICIAN INFORMATION		PATIENT INFORMATION
DOUGLASVILLE MEDICINE ASSOCIATES **5076 BRAND BLVD.** **DOUGLASVILLE, NY 01234** **(123) 456-7890** Ordering Physician: Dr. Carl Veach Physician ID #23658A		Name: Kathleen Beavers ID #: 25698

Date and Time of Collection		Date Results Received
10-29-11 8:30 a.m.		10-30-11

Test Ordered	Results	Reference Range
Complete blood count (CBC):		
White Blood Cell Count	15,000/cu mm	4,500–11,000/cu mm
Red Blood Cell Count	5.0 million/cu mm	M: 4.5–6.0 million/cu mm F: 4.0–5.5/cu mm
Hemoglobin	10 gm/dL	M: 13–18 gm/dL F: 12–16 gm/dL
Hematocrit	32%	M: 42–52% F: 36–45%
MCV	96 fL	82–98 fL
MCH	30 pG	26–34 pG
MCHC	34 g/dL	32–36 g/dL
Platelet Count	300,000/cu mm	150,000–400,000/ cu mm
Differential white blood cell count:		
Neutrophilic Bands	6%	0–2%
Neutrophils	75%	40–65%
Eosinophils	1%	1–3%
Basophils	0	0–1%
Lymphocytes	10%	25–40%
Monocytes	9%	3–9%
RBC Morphology:	Hypochromic	Normochromic
	Microcytic	Normocytic
Coagulation Studies:		11–13 seconds
PT		Will vary by laboratory
INR		

COMPLETING SPECIAL FORMS

Assignment 28-8: Lab Requisition Form

Work Form Necessary: FORM 28-1

Directions: Complete the lab requisition form (Work Form 28-1) with the scenario information given below.

Today's date 10-29-11, 8:30 a.m., Patient name: Kathleen L. Beavers, Address: 8900 Gracie Blvd., Westerville, NY 01563, Telephone number: 123-469-7449, DOB: 10-29-47 Age: 64, Sex: female, Billing information: The patient should be billed for the lab work (patient does not have any health insurance), Fasting: no, Tests ordered: CBC, Referring provider information: Dr. Carl Veach, Address: Douglasville Medicine Associates, 5076 Brand Blvd., Douglasville, NY 01234, Telephone number: 123-456-7890, Provider ID#: 23658A, Billing information: Dr. Veach, Diagnosis: ICD-9 Code: V78.0

Assignment 28-9: Outside Specimen Tracking Log

Work Form Necessary: FORM 28-2

Directions: Enter the specimen from the lab requisition in Work Form 28-1 into the lab log (Work Form 28-2). Additional information is included below.

- Type of specimen: One lavender-top tube

- Prepared by: LMV

- Date received: 10-30-11

- Received by: MEH

- Lab name: ABC Laboratory

FIELD APPLICATION CHALLENGE

Assignment 28-10

Read the following Field Application Challenge and respond to the questions following the scenario.

You are asked to run a hemoglobin and hematocrit on a female patient who suffers from anemia. The hematocrit results are 46% and the hemoglobin is 11 gm/dL.

1. Are the test results normal?

2. Do the results correlate with one another? Why or why not?

3. Could there be a correlation? If so, what?

_____

_____

JOURNALING EXERCISE
Assignment 28-11

What content within this chapter was most meaningful to you? Why? List some examples of how you might apply information contained in this chapter, both during your training and after you enter the health care industry.

Work Form 28-1

LABORATORY REQUISITION

PATIENT LAST NAME	FIRST		M.I.	REFERRING PROVIDER

PROVIDER ID #	PATIENT ID #	BILL: ☐ PHYSICIAN ☐ MEDICAL ☐ HMO ☐ CHDP ☐ MEDICARE ☐ INSURANCE ☐ PATIENT	D.O.B	AGE	SEX

PLEASE COMPLETE INSURANCE BILLING INFORMATION AT BOTTOM

PROVIDER NAME, ADDRESS, AND PHONE NUMBER	PATIENT ADDRESS	PATIENT PHONE NUMBER ( )	DATE COLLECTED	TIME COLLECTED
	CITY	STATE	ZIP CODE	FASTING YES NO	STAT	CALL RESULT
	PATIENT MEDICARE #	PATIENT MEDICAID #	INFO. BELOW WILL APPEAR ON REPORT	

CUSTOM PROFILES & ADDITIONAL TESTS

```
173   [ ] CHEMISTRY PANEL, COMPLETE BLOOD COUNT (ZPP), LIPID PROFILE, T4
05050 [ ] CHOL, TRIG, HDL CHOL, VLDL CHOL, LDL CHOL, RISK FACTOR
```

PROFILES

00011 ☐	SPECIAL COMPREHENSIVE	2 SS,L	03536 ☐	HYPERTHYROID PROFILE	SS
00001 ☐	COMPREHENSIVE HEALTH SURVEY	SS,L	05037 ☐	HYPOTHYROID PROFILE	SS
00002 ☐	GENERAL SURVEY	SS,L	05051 ☐	LIPID PROFILE	SS
00003 ☐	CHEMISTRY PANEL	SS,L	05021 ☐	LIVER PROFILE	SS
CH7 ☐	CHEM 7 PANEL	SS	03359 ☐	LUPUS PROFILE	SS
03280 ☐	ANEMIA PROFILE	SS,L	03959 ☐	MENOPAUSAL PROFILE SS /03960 ☐ POST MENOPAUSAL	SS
06016 ☐	ARTHRITIS PROFILE	SS,L	02280 ☐	OVARIAN FUNCTION PROFILE SS /02281 ☐ TESTICULAR FUNC. PROF.	SS
05725 ☐	COMPREHENSIVE THYROID SURVEY	SS	02808 ☐	PRENATAL PROFILE	L,R
02691 ☐	EPSTEIN BARR PROFILE	SS	05006 ☐	THYROID PROFILE	SS
05010 ☐	ELECTROLYTES	SS	03191 ☐	TORCH PANEL	SS
06826 ☐	HEPATITIS PROFILE	SS	5756 ☐	URINE DRUG SCREEN U / ☐ VENIPUNCTURE	

TESTS

0361 ☐ ABO & Rh TYPE	R,L	0141 ☐ C-REACTIVE PROTEIN	SS	0673 ☐ HEPATITIS B SURFACE ANTIGEN	SS	0237 ☐ PTT	B
0302 ☐ ALKALINE PHOSPHATASE	SS	1341 ☐ DHEA-S	SS	0245 ☐ HEPATITIS C ANTIBODY	SS	0317 ☐ RA FACTOR	SS
0109 ☐ AMYLASE	SS	0119 ☐ DIGOXIN	SS	0257 ☐ IRON	SS	0321 ☐ RUBELLA	SS
0613 ☐ ANA	SS	0224 ☐ DILANTIN	SS	LDL-A ☐ LDL CHOLESTEROL	SS	0331 ☐ RPR	SS
0366 ☐ ANTIBODY SCREEN	R	0835 ☐ ESTRADIOL	SS	0283 ☐ LEAD BLOOD	RB	0335 ☐ SEMEN ANALYSIS	SEMEN
0110 ☐ ASO (STREPTOZYME)	SS	0833 ☐ FERRITIN	SS	0281 ☐ LIPASE	SS	0328 ☐ SEDIMENTATION RATE (ESR)	L
0126 ☐ BILIRUBIN TOTAL	SS	0003 ☐ FOLIC ACID & VITAMIN B12	SS	8225 ☐ LH	SS	0349 ☐ SGOT (AST)	SS
0132 ☐ BUN	SS	0651 ☐ FSH	SS	0247 ☐ MONONUCLEOSIS	SS	0348 ☐ SGPT (ALT)	SS
8726 ☐ CA125	SS	0140 ☐ FTA-ABS	SS	0778 ☐ PHENOBARBITAL	SS	0330 ☐ SICKLE CELL SCREEN	L
0142 ☐ CALCIUM	SS	0210 ☐ GGTP	SS	0307 ☐ POTASSIUM	SS	0354 ☐ T4 (THYROXINE)	SS
0130 ☐ CBC	L	0536 ☐ GLUCOSE, FASTING	GY	0557 ☐ PREGNANCY (SERUM)	SS	1358 ☐ T4 FREE	SS
0388 ☐ CEA-ROCHE	SS	☐ GLUCOSE, _____ HR PP	GY	0308 ☐ PREGNANCY (URINE)	U	8456 ☐ TESTOSTERONE	SS
0152 ☐ CHOLESTEROL	SS	0771 ☐ GLYCOHEMOGLOBIN	L	0359 ☐ PROGESTERONE	SS	0824 ☐ THEOPHYLLINE	SS
0788 ☐ CORTISOL	SS	0534 ☐ H. PYLORI	SS	8041 ☐ PROLACTIN	SS	0360 ☐ TRIGLYCERIDE	SS
0162 ☐ CPK	SS	0823 ☐ HGG QUANTITATIVE	SS	0103 ☐ PROTEIN, TOTAL	SS	0672 ☐ TSH	SS
0445 ☐ CKMB ISOENZYME	SS	1856 ☐ HIV (ANTIBODY)	SS	2000 ☐ PROSTATE SPECIFIC ANTIGEN (PSA)	SS	0373 ☐ URIC ACID	SS
0161 ☐ CREATININE	SS	0558 ☐ HDL CHOLESTEROL	SS	0310 ☐ PT (PROTHROMBIN TIME)	B	0219 ☐ URINALYSIS	U

CYTOPATHOLOGY

☐ PREGNANT ☐ ABORTION ☐ POST-PARTUM ☐ POST-MENOPAUSE

HISTORY _____

PREV. ABNORMAL CYTOL FINDINGS _____

☐ CONTRACEPTIVES   DATE _____
☐ HYSTERECTOMY   ☐ HORMONES   ☐ IUD
☐ COPHORECTOMY   ☐ TOTAL   ☐ SUPRA CX
☐ RADIATION Rx   DATE _____
☐ OTHER _____   ☐ HORMONES Rx   ☐ CHEMO Rx

LMP _____   DATE COLLECTED _____
SOURCE ☐ CERVIX   ☐ ENDOCERVIX   ☐ VAGINA
☐ CYTOBRUSH   ☐ OTHER SITE _____

MICROBIOLOGY

THCUL ☐ THROAT	URTHC ☐ URETHRAL	9391 ☐ CHLAMYDIA DNA
EACUL ☐ EAR	VACUL ☐ VAGINAL	9390 ☐ GONORRHEA DNA
EYCUL ☐ EYE	WOCUL ☐ WOUND	9391 ☐ OCCULT BLOOD
GOCUL ☐ GC	ROCUL ☐ CULTURE (Routine)	0293 ☐ OVA & PARASITE
SPCUL ☐ SPUTUM	URCUL ☐ URINE	WTM ☐ WET MOUNT
STCUL ☐ STOOL	GSP ☐ GRAM STAIN	

SOURCE _____   OTHER _____

DIAGNOSIS OR COMMENTS

LAB USE ONLY (DO NOT WRITE BELOW THIS SPACE)

DATE RECEIVED	DATE REPORTED

STATEMENT OF SPECIMEN ADEQUACY

GENERAL CATEGORIZATION

DESCRIPTIVE DIAGNOSIS

HORMONAL EVALUATION

ADDITIONAL COMMENT

CYTOTECHNOLOGIST	PATHOLOGIST

INSURANCE BILLING INFORMATION

PRIMARY INSURED	INSURANCE COMPANY

ADDRESS

POLICY NO. & I.D. NO.	IOD9 CODE

LEGEND

SS	Serum Separator	GY	Grey	B	Blue	U	Urine
R	Red	L	Lavender	RB	Royal Blue	G	Green

Work Form 28-2

DOUGLASVILLE MEDICINE ASSOCIATES
5076 BRAND BLVD
DOUGLASVILLE, NY 01234
(123) 456-7890

				OUTSIDE LAB SPECIMEN TRACKING LOG				
Date Sent	Patient Name/ID	Ordering Provider	Tests Ordered	Number of and Type of Specimens Sent to Laboratory (Include Tube Colors)	Prepared By	Laboratory	Date Results Received	Results Received By

C H A P T E R **29**

Microbiology

FIELD RELEVANCY AND BENEFITS

Microbiology is one branch of science that is constantly changing with the discovery of new diseases and the organisms that cause them. While the medical assistant cannot be expected to have knowledge of all pathogenic microorganisms, he should be familiar with the more common ones that cause diseases such as strep throat, infectious mononucleosis, hepatitis, tuberculosis, staph infections, etc. The medical assistant will often be the first one to process lab results and may need to educate patients about certain tests.

While the medical assistant will perform tests such as a rapid strep test in the POL, his primary role will be proper specimen collection and processing to ensure that accurate results are obtained from the laboratory. The specimen must be collected from the appropriate site using sterile supplies to avoid contamination of the specimen. Precise and accurate specimen collection by the medical assistant will benefit both the provider and the patient. Quick turn-around of test results will allow the provider to begin treatment much sooner.

NOTE SHEET

Classification of Microorganisms

_____

_____

_____

_____

Blood Components

_____

_____

_____

_____

Binomial Nomenclature System for Bacteria

_____

_____

_____

_____

Characteristics of Bacteria

_____

_____

_____

_____

Specimen Collection and Safe Handling Requirements

_____

_____

_____

_____

Sensitivity Testing

_____

_____

_____

_____

Virology

_____

_____

_____

_____

Mycology

_____

_____

_____

_____

Identification of Bacteria

_____

_____

_____

_____

Special Microscopic Techniques

_____

_____

_____

_____

Parasitology

_____

_____

_____

_____

Quality Control

_____

_____

_____

_____

VOCABULARY REVIEW
Assignment 29-1: Matching
Match the term with its definition and place the corresponding letter in the blank.

_____ 1. Culture

_____ 2. Agar

_____ 3. Aerobic

_____ 4. Inoculation

_____ 5. Opportunistic infection

_____ 6. Fastidious

_____ 7. Pathogen

_____ 8. Pure culture

_____ 9. Sensitivity testing

_____ 10. Taxonomy

_____ 11. Bacilli

_____ 12. Cocci

_____ 13. Culture medium

_____ 14. Normal flora

_____ 15. Microbiology

_____ 16. Incubate

_____ 17. Fungi

_____ 18. Parasite

_____ 19. Gram positive

_____ 20. Anaerobic

_____ 21. Bacteria

_____ 22. Colony

A. Liquid or solid material in which bacteria are grown

B. Class of bacteria that do not require oxygen to grow

C. Microorganisms grown in a laboratory from a patient sample

D. Infection that develops in patients with depressed immune systems

E. Group of microorganisms that includes yeasts and molds

F. Applying a microorganism onto a culture medium

G. Study of microorganisms, especially as they relate to diseases

H. Place a culture in an apparatus that provides optimum conditions for growth and multiplication of microorganisms

I. Bacteria that have special growth requirements; difficult to culture

J. Single-celled microbes that lack a nucleus (the most prevalent of all microorganisms)

K. Disease-causing microorganism

L. Culture that contains only one pathogen

M. Technique that evaluates which antibiotics will destroy a particular pathogen

N. Classification of living organisms into the proper category using a specific set of laws and principles

O. Microorganisms normally present in different parts of the human body which pose no health threat under ordinary circumstances

P. Organism that lives within, upon, or at the expense of the host

Q. Round or spherical shaped bacteria

R. Rod-shaped bacteria; may contain spores

S. Class of bacteria that requires oxygen to grow

T. Gelatin-like substance that may contain added nutrients, used to support the growth of particular microorganisms

U. Visible growth of microorganisms that appear on a culture medium

V. Term used to describe bacteria that stain purple during the Gram staining process

CHAPTER REVIEW

Assignment 29-2: Acronym Review

Write what each of the following acronyms stands for.

1. DNA: _____

2. CSF: _____

3. C&S: _____

4. BA: _____

5. SBA: _____

6. TM: _____

7. EMB: _____

8. HE: _____

9. EBV: _____

10. RSV: _____

11. KOH: _____

12. ELISA: _____

Assignment 29-3: True or False

Fill in the blank with a "T" for true statements and an "F" for false statements. Rewrite the false statements to make them true.

____ 1. Virology is a branch of microbiology dedicated strictly to the study of viruses.

_____

_____

____ 2. Normal flora are designed to help protect the body and are never the cause for infection in particular parts of the body.

_____

_____

____ 3. A sensitivity test helps to identify the antibiotic(s) that will have the greatest effect on a specific pathogenic microorganism.

_____

_____

____ 4. The wet mount is used to determine the cause of vaginosis; it is very useful for diagnosing trichomonas vaginalis.

_____

_____

____ 5. A *Salmonella* infection must be reported to the Public Health Department.

_____

_____

____ 6. Bacteria are named with two names based on the person who discovered them.

_____

_____

____ 7. Bacteria are identified by their structure, morphology, and staining characteristics.

_____

_____

____ 8. Intestinal flora can be the cause of a UTI.

_____

_____

____ 9. The name for bacteria appearing in clusters would include the prefix strepo.

_____

_____

____ 10. Colonies of some bacteria have a characteristic appearance which can be seen on the culture.

_____

_____

Assignment 29-4: Short Answer

1. Draw examples of each of the following.

Cocci	Bacilli	Spirilla
Diplococci	Bacilli (flagellated)	Spirilla
Streptococci	Diplobacilli	Spirochete
Staphylococci	Streptobacilli	

2. List the different reagents used in the Gram staining process and explain the purpose of each.

_____

_____

_____

_____

_____

3. Describe the three methods used to identify viruses.

   A. _____

   _____

   B. _____

   _____

   C. _____

   _____

4. Explain the purpose of a safety hood when working with molds.

   _____

   _____

   _____

5. List precautions that should be observed to ensure safe handling of microbiology specimens.

   A. _____

   _____

   B. _____

   _____

   C. _____

   _____

   D. _____

   _____

   E. _____

   _____

   F. _____

   _____

6. For the following specimen types, state whether or not normal flora could be present and list two possible pathogens that might be found in each.

Type of Specimen	Normal Flora Present	Two Types of Pathogens
Urine	_____	_____
Blood	_____	_____
Cerebrospinal Fluid	_____	_____
Sputum	_____	_____
Stool	_____	_____
Wound	_____	_____
Genital	_____	_____
Nasal	_____	_____
Throat	_____	_____
Eyes	_____	_____
Ears	_____	_____

7. Name and describe the three general classifications of growth media contained in culture plates.

A. _____

_____

B. _____

_____

C. _____

_____

8. List common diseases caused by the following types of bacteria.

A. Escherichia coli: _____

B. Salmonella species: _____

C. Citrobacter: _____

D. Bacillus species: _____

E. Psuedomonas species: _____

_____

F. Listeria species: _____

G. Helicobacter pylori: _____

H. Bordetella pertussis: _____

9. List pathogenic conditions caused by the following common viruses.

A. Rhinovirus: _____

B. Epstein-Barr virus: _____

C. Respiratory syncytial virus: _____

D. Rotavirus: _____

E. Varicella-zoster virus: _____

F. Human papilloma virus: _____

Assignment 29-5: Certification Practice

Choose the best answer and place the corresponding letter in the blank.

____ 1. Microorganisms are usually classified using a set of laws and principles known as:

A. binomial standards.

B. taxonomy.

C. microbe classification standards.

D. prokaryote standards.

____ 2. Which of the following is reportable to the Public Health Department?

A. Salmonella

B. Shigella

C. Gonorrhea

D. Chlamydia

E. All of the above

____ 3. Bacteria have two names the first being the genus, the second being the:

A. species.

B. class.

C. family.

D. group.

____ 4. Which of the following is a common type of bacilli?

   A. *Spirilla*

   B. *Vibrio*

   C. *E. coli*

   D. *Clostridium*

____ 5. Which of the following is an example of an acid-fast stain?

   A. Gram

   B. MacConkey

   C. Ziehl-Neelsen

   D. Methylene blue

____ 6. When collecting a microbiology specimen, the medical assistant should do all of the following *except:*

   A. collect the specimen from the site of infection, not surrounding areas.

   B. immediately place the specimen in the refrigerator.

   C. immediately place the specimen in the appropriate transport media.

   D. collect a sufficient amount of the specimen.

____ 7. When separating organisms from the primary culture and then replating them on the appropriate media, the new growth is known as the:

   A. subculture.

   B. secondary culture.

   C. mixed culture.

   D. pure culture.

____ 8. If the provider asks you to prepare the culture media for a suspected case of gonorrhea, which type of media would you select?

   A. Sheep's blood agar

   B. Thayer-Martin

   C. Hektoen-Enteric

   D. MacConkey

____ 9. A common method of streaking the plate for colony growth and isolation is called:

   A. lawn streak.

   B. full-plate streak.

   C. four-quadrant streak.

   D. two-division streak.

____ 10. All of the following are correct procedures regarding the four-quadrant method except to:

   A. allow plate to come to room temperature before inoculation.

   B. replace the lid immediately after streaking.

   C. not use a plate that has reached its expiration date.

   D. label the bottom of the plate and place in the incubator with the lid facing upward.

____ 11. A wide clear zone around the colonies on a sheep's blood agar plate indicates which of the following?

   A. Alpha hemolysis

   B. Gamma hemolysis

   C. Beta hemolysis

   D. Epi hemolysis

____ 12. Which of the following antibiotics is impregnated on the "A" disc used to determine the presence of group A beta strep?

   A. Methicillin

   B. Bacitracin

   C. Optichin

   D. Zithrocin

____ 13. Which of the following methods is used to determine the sensitivity of a microorganism to an antibiotic?

    A. Ziehl-Neelsen method

    B. Leonard-Gram method

    C. Kirby-Bauer method

    D. Kelso method

____ 14. Which of the following classifications would indicate the antibiotic of choice?

    A. (I)

    B. (S)

    C. (R)

    D. (V)

____ 15. A wet mount is valuable when trying to diagnose the cause of which of the following?

    A. STDs

    B. Vaginosis

    C. UTI

    D. URI

____ 16. The hanging drop method is used to ascertain:

    A. flagella.

    B. fluorescence.

    C. trichomonas motility (trichmonas infection).

    D. spores.

____17. Which of the following organisms would be suspect in a case of necrotizing fasciitis?

    A. *Streptococcus pneumoniae*

    B. *Streptococcus agalactiae*

    C. *Streptococcus pyogenes*

    D. *beta hemolytic group A strep*

____ 18. Which of the following organisms is known to cause skin and wound infections?

    A. *Staphylococcus epidermidis*

    B. *Staphylococcus aureus*

    C. *Proteus* species

    D. *Pseudomonas* species

____ 19. *Salmonella* species can cause all of the following illnesses *except:*

    A. typhoid fever.

    B. urethritis.

    C. food poisoning.

    D. bacteremia.

____ 20. A parasite can be identified by detecting which of the following in a stool specimen?

    A. Ova

    B. Larvae

    C. Trophozoite

    D. All of the above

____ 21. Which of the following parasites can enter the body by the larvae in soil penetrating the bare skin of the foot?

    A. *Giardia lamblia*

    B. *Necator americanus*

    C. *Entamoeba histolytica*

    D. *Cryptosporidium parvum*

_____ 22. Which of the following pathogenic fungi is responsible for vaginal yeast infections?

    A. *Candida* species

    B. *Coccidioides immitus*

    C. *Aspergillus*

    D. *Histoplasma capsulatum*

_____ 23. Which of the following tests is used to identify certain fungi?

    A. Wet mount

    B. Biochemical

    C. KOH prep

    D. Stained prep

SKILL APPLICATION CHALLENGES

Assignment 29-6: Application Activity

The lab report is back on Maryn Leonard. Read the findings and state whether or not treatment will be necessary and why you feel that treatment is or is not necessary.

_____

ABC LABORATORY
MISCELLANEOUS LABORATORY TEST REPORT FORM

PHYSICIAN INFORMATION	PATIENT INFORMATION
DOUGLASVILLE MEDICINE ASSOCIATES **5076 BRAND BLVD.** **DOUGLASVILLE, NY 01234** **(123) 456-7890** **Ordering Physician:** Dr. Carl Daniels **Physician ID #** 23658B	**Name:** Maryn Leonard **Address:** 6789 Avery Lane **City/State/Zip:** Blondeville, NY 12345 **Phone #:** 123-891-5030 **ID #:** 87652364546

Date and Time of Collection		Reporting Date	
07/24/11	9:00 a.m.	07/26/11	

Test Ordered	Results	Reference Range	Abnormal Results
Pregnancy Test			
Rapid Strep Test		Negative	
Mono Test		Negative	
Influenza Test		Negative	
H. Pylori		Negative	
Culture Results	**No Growth**	No Growth	
Serology Tests:			
VDRL/RPR		Nonreactive	
HIV		Negative	
CRP		Less than 6 mg/L	
Rheumatoid Factor		Negative	
ASO titer		Negative	

Assignment 29-7: Web Assignments

1. Research MRSA (methicillin-resistant *Staphylococcus aureus*) infections and design an informational pamphlet to distribute to patients who might be at-risk for developing this type of infection, such as those using gyms or workout facilities, students using equipment in school gymnasiums, and hospital patients.
2. Search the Internet and obtain information on diseases that were once thought to be eradicated in the United States, such as tuberculosis and whooping cough, but are now making a comeback.

COMPLETING SPECIAL FORMS

Assignment 29-8: Lab Requisition Form

Work Form Necessary: FORM 29-1

Directions: Complete the lab requisition (Work Form 29-1) with the scenario information given below.

Patient name: Maryn L. Leonard, Address: 6789 Avery Lane, Blondeville, NY 12345, Telephone number: (123) 891-5030, DOB: 05/09/90, Age: 21, Date of collection: 07/24/2011, Time of collection: 9:00 a.m., Bill the provider for the lab services, Sex: female, Fasting: no, Tests ordered: Throat culture, ICD9 code: 462.0, Referring provider: Dr. Carl Daniels, Douglasville Medicine Associates, 5076 Brand Blvd., Douglasville, NY 01234, (123) 456-7890, ID#: 23658B

Assignment 29-9: Outside Specimen Tracking Log

Work Form Necessary: FORM 29-2

Directions: Enter the following information regarding outside specimen tracking into the log (Work Form 29-2). Additional information is included below.

- Type of specimen: Throat swab

- Prepared by: LMV

- Date received: 07/26/2011

- Received by: MEH

- Lab name: ABC Laboratory

FIELD APPLICATION CHALLENGE

Assignment 29-10

Read the following Field Application Challenge and respond to the questions following the scenario.

When collecting a wound specimen from a patient, you accidentally touch the swab to the skin at the edge of the wound. The area appears to be infected and the patient appears to be in a lot of pain and asks you to stop swabbing the wound. You don't want to upset the patient any further, so you place the swab in the appropriate transport media to be sent to the lab.

1. What type of transport media should be used for a wound specimen?

_____

_____

2. Should you have collected another sample? Why or why not?

_____

_____

_____

_____

3. What impact could your actions have on this patient's treatment?

_____

_____

JOURNALING EXERCISE
Assignment 29-11

What content within this chapter was most meaningful to you? Why? List some examples of how you might apply information contained in this chapter, both during your training and after you enter the health care industry.

Work Form 29-1

LABORATORY REQUISITION

PATIENT LAST NAME		FIRST	M.I.	REFERRING PROVIDER

PROVIDER ID #	PATIENT ID #	BILL: ☐ PHYSICIAN ☐ MEDICAL ☐ HMO ☐ CHDP ☐ MEDICARE ☐ INSURANCE ☐ PATIENT	D.O.B	AGE	SEX

PLEASE COMPLETE INSURANCE BILLING INFORMATION AT BOTTOM

PROVIDER NAME, ADDRESS, AND PHONE NUMBER	PATIENT ADDRESS	PATIENT PHONE NUMBER ( )	DATE COLLECTED	TIME COLLECTED
	CITY	STATE	ZIP CODE	FASTING YES | NO	STAT	CALL RESULT
	PATIENT MEDICARE #	PATIENT MEDICAID #	INFO. BELOW WILL APPEAR ON REPORT	

CUSTOM PROFILES & ADDITIONAL TESTS

```
173    [ ] CHEMISTRY PANEL, COMPLETE BLOOD COUNT (ZPP), LIPID PROFILE, T4
05050 [ ] CHOL, TRIG, HDL CHOL, VLDL CHOL, LDL CHOL, RISK FACTOR
```

PROFILES

00011 ☐	SPECIAL COMPREHENSIVE	2 SS,L	03536 ☐	HYPERTHYROID PROFILE	SS
00001 ☐	COMPREHENSIVE HEALTH SURVEY	SS,L	05037 ☐	HYPOTHYROID PROFILE	SS
00002 ☐	GENERAL SURVEY	SS,L	05051 ☐	LIPID PROFILE	SS
00003 ☐	CHEMISTRY PANEL	SS,L	05021 ☐	LIVER PROFILE	SS
CH7 ☐	CHEM 7 PANEL	SS	03359 ☐	LUPUS PROFILE	SS
03280 ☐	ANEMIA PROFILE	SS,L	03959 ☐	MENOPAUSAL PROFILE SS /03960 ☐ POST MENOPAUSAL	SS
06016 ☐	ARTHRITIS PROFILE	SS,L	02280 ☐	OVARIAN FUNCTION PROFILE SS /02281 ☐ TESTICULAR FUNC. PROF.	SS
05725 ☐	COMPREHENSIVE THYROID SURVEY	SS	02808 ☐	PRENATAL PROFILE	L,R
02691 ☐	EPSTEIN BARR PROFILE	SS	05006 ☐	THYROID PROFILE	SS
05010 ☐	ELECTROLYTES	SS	03191 ☐	TORCH PANEL	SS
06826 ☐	HEPATITIS PROFILE	SS	5756 ☐	URINE DRUG SCREEN U / ☐ VENIPUNCTURE	

TESTS

0361 ☐	ABO & Rh TYPE	R,L	0141 ☐	C-REACTIVE PROTEIN	SS	0673 ☐	HEPATITIS B SURFACE ANTIGEN	SS	0237 ☐	PTT	B
0302 ☐	ALKALINE PHOSPHATASE	SS	1341 ☐	DHEA-S	SS	0245 ☐	HEPATITIS C ANTIBODY	SS	0317 ☐	RA FACTOR	SS
0109 ☐	AMYLASE	SS	0119 ☐	DIGOXIN	SS	0257 ☐	IRON	SS	0321 ☐	RUBELLA	SS
0613 ☐	ANA	SS	0224 ☐	DILANTIN	SS	LDL-A ☐	LDL CHOLESTEROL	SS	0331 ☐	RPR	SS
0366 ☐	ANTIBODY SCREEN	R	0835 ☐	ESTRADIOL	SS	0283 ☐	LEAD BLOOD	RB	0335 ☐	SEMEN ANALYSIS	SEMEN
0110 ☐	ASO (STREPTOZYME)	SS	0833 ☐	FERRITIN	SS	0281 ☐	LIPASE	SS	0328 ☐	SEDIMENTATION RATE (ESR)	L
0126 ☐	BILIRUBIN TOTAL	SS	0003 ☐	FOLIC ACID & VITAMIN B12	SS	8225 ☐	LH	SS	0349 ☐	SGOT (AST)	SS
0132 ☐	BUN	SS	0651 ☐	FSH	SS	0247 ☐	MONONUCLEOSIS	SS	0348 ☐	SGPT (ALT)	SS
8726 ☐	CA125	SS	0140 ☐	FTA-ABS	SS	0778 ☐	PHENOBARBITAL	SS	0330 ☐	SICKLE CELL SCREEN	L
0142 ☐	CALCIUM	SS	0210 ☐	GGTP	SS	0307 ☐	POTASSIUM	SS	0354 ☐	T4 (THYROXINE)	SS
0130 ☐	CBC	L	0536 ☐	GLUCOSE, FASTING	GY	0557 ☐	PREGNANCY (SERUM)	SS	1358 ☐	T4 FREE	SS
0388 ☐	CEA-ROCHE	SS	☐	GLUCOSE, ___ HR PP	GY	0308 ☐	PREGNANCY (URINE)	U	8456 ☐	TESTOSTERONE	SS
0152 ☐	CHOLESTEROL	SS	0771 ☐	GLYCOHEMOGLOBIN	L	0359 ☐	PROGESTERONE	SS	0824 ☐	THEOPHYLLINE	SS
0788 ☐	CORTISOL	SS	0534 ☐	H. PYLORI	SS	8041 ☐	PROLACTIN	SS	0360 ☐	TRIGLYCERIDE	SS
0162 ☐	CPK	SS	0823 ☐	HGG QUANTITATIVE	SS	0103 ☐	PROTEIN, TOTAL	SS	0672 ☐	TSH	SS
0445 ☐	CKMB ISOENZYME	SS	1856 ☐	HIV (ANTIBODY)	SS	2000 ☐	PROSTATE SPECIFIC ANTIGEN (PSA)	SS	0373 ☐	URIC ACID	SS
0161 ☐	CREATININE	SS	0558 ☐	HDL CHOLESTEROL	SS	0310 ☐	PT (PROTHROMBIN TIME)	B	0219 ☐	URINALYSIS	U

CYTOPATHOLOGY

☐ PREGNANT   ☐ ABORTION   ☐ POST-PARTUM   ☐ POST-MENOPAUSE
HISTORY _____

PREV. ABNORMAL CYTOL FINDINGS _____
☐ CONTRACEPTIVES   DATE _____
☐ HYSTERECTOMY   ☐ HORMONES   ☐ IUD
☐ COPHORECTOMY   ☐ TOTAL   ☐ SUPRA CX
☐ RADIATION Rx   DATE _____
☐ OTHER _____   ☐ HORMONES Rx ☐ CHEMO Rx

LMP _____ DATE COLLECTED _____
SOURCE ☐ CERVIX   ☐ ENDOCERVIX   ☐ VAGINA
       ☐ CYTOBRUSH   ☐ OTHER SITE _____

MICROBIOLOGY

THCUL ☐ THROAT	URTHC ☐ URETHRAL	9391 ☐ CHLAMYDIA DNA
EACUL ☐ EAR	VACUL ☐ VAGINAL	9390 ☐ GONORRHEA DNA
EYCUL ☐ EYE	WOCUL ☐ WOUND	9391 ☐ OCCULT BLOOD
GOCUL ☐ GC	ROCUL ☐ CULTURE (Routine)	0293 ☐ OVA & PARASITE
SPCUL ☐ SPUTUM	URCUL ☐ URINE	WTM ☐ WET MOUNT
STCUL ☐ STOOL	GSP ☐ GRAM STAIN	

SOURCE _____   OTHER _____

DIAGNOSIS OR COMMENTS

LAB USE ONLY (DO NOT WRITE BELOW THIS SPACE)

DATE RECEIVED	DATE REPORTED

STATEMENT OF SPECIMEN ADEQUACY

GENERAL CATEGORIZATION

DESCRIPTIVE DIAGNOSIS

HORMONAL EVALUATION

ADDITIONAL COMMENT

CYTOTECHNOLOGIST	PATHOLOGIST

INSURANCE BILLING INFORMATION

PRIMARY INSURED	INSURANCE COMPANY
ADDRESS	
POLICY NO. & I.D. NO.	ICD9 CODE

LEGEND

SS	Serum Separator	GY	Grey	B	Blue	U	Urine
R	Red	L	Lavender	RB	Royal Blue	G	Green

Work Form 29-2

DOUGLASVILLE MEDICINE ASSOCIATES
5076 BRAND BLVD
DOUGLASVILLE, NY 01234
(123) 456-7890

OUTSIDE LAB SPECIMEN TRACKING LOG								
Date Sent	Patient Name/ID	Ordering Provider	Tests Ordered	Number of and Type of Specimens Sent to Laboratory (Include Tube Colors)	Prepared By	Laboratory	Date Results Received	Results Received By

C H A P T E R **30**

Clinical Chemistry and CLIA Waived Rapid Tests

FIELD RELEVANCY AND BENEFITS

While medical assistants may not perform some of the common lab tests discussed in this chapter, they will be responsible for collecting and correctly processing the specimens for most of them. The medical assistant should possess a basic knowledge of the testing process itself, the normal/reference values, and any pathologic conditions related to increased or decreased levels of a substance in the body.

The medical assistant is often the first member of the health care team to receive both normal and abnormal laboratory test results and is responsible for alerting the provider to any potential problems immediately. The importance of the lab test and the result received from it becomes more relevant when the medical assistant has a clear understanding of the results as well as the ramifications of not acting accordingly when a result is abnormal.

NOTE SHEET

Clinical Chemistry Tests

_____

_____

_____

_____

Specimen Requirements

_____

_____

_____

_____

Appearance of Serum and Plasma

_____

_____

_____

_____

Profiles and Panels

_____

_____

_____

_____

Glucose Testing

_____

_____

_____

_____

Additional Chemistry Tests

_____

_____

_____

_____

Serology/Immunology Tests

_____

_____

_____

_____

Blood Typing

_____

_____

_____

_____

Drug Testing

_____

_____

_____

_____

VOCABULARY REVIEW

Assignment 30-1: Matching

Match the term with its definition and place the corresponding letter in the blank.

_____ 1. Antiserum

_____ 2. Agglutination

_____ 3. Blood urea nitrogen

_____ 4. Analyte

_____ 5. Homeostasis

_____ 6. Lipoprotein

_____ 7. Triglycerides

_____ 8. Antibody

A. Fat found in the blood stream that is often stored as adipose tissue

B. Simple protein, bound to fat, that transports lipids in the blood

C. Serum that contains antibodies to a specific antigen used to perform blood typing

D. Antigen-antibody reaction which involves clumping of cells due to the antibody attaching itself to the antigen

E. Any substance that is being chemically analyzed

F. Kidney function indicator test which measures the amount of nitrogen in the blood

G. Particle produced in response to an antigen for the purpose of neutralizing or destroying that antigen

H. State of equilibrium within the body when body systems are functioning normally

Assignment 30-2: Sentence Completion

Fill in the blanks below with Essential Terms from this chapter.

1. _____ is an orange-yellow pigment produced from the breakdown of red blood cells that is excreted in bile.

2. Made in the liver, _____ is the major component of bile.

3. A(n) _____ is a substance that stimulates antibody production within the body.

4. The term for an increase in blood glucose levels is _____ and the term for a decrease in blood glucose levels is _____.

5. _____ is the fraction of cholesterol that carries and deposits lipids in the arteries and other body tissues.

6. "Good cholesterol" is known as _____.

7. A hormone produced by the placenta in pregnant females is _____ _____.

CHAPTER REVIEW

Assignment 30-3: Acronym Review

Write what each of the following acronyms stands for.

1. HDL: _____
2. LDL: _____
3. BUN: _____
4. hCG: _____
5. GTT: _____
6. ALT: _____
7. AST: _____
8. LDH: _____
9. GGT: _____
10. ALP: _____
11. CPK: _____
12. SGOT: _____
13. TSH: _____
14. HbA1c: _____
15. CRP: _____
16. ALB: _____
17. CEA: _____
18. PSA: _____
19. TP: _____
20. UA: _____

Assignment 30-4: Short Answer

1. List the clinical significance for performing the following tests, along with the normal values for the tests.

Test	Normal Value	Clinical Significance
FBS	_____	_____
BUN	_____	_____
HbA1c	_____	_____
Creatinine	_____	_____
Total cholesterol	_____	_____
HDL	Males: _____	_____
	Females: _____	_____
LDL	_____	_____
Triglycerides	_____	_____

2. Explain the purpose of a laboratory profile.

   _____

   _____

3. Explain the importance of proper specimen collection and handling.

   _____

   _____

4. Explain the purpose of the two-hour postprandial blood sugar test.

   _____

   _____

   _____

   _____

5. List the electrolytes and explain their function in the body.

   A. _____

   _____

   _____

   B. _____

   _____

   _____

   C. _____

   _____

   _____

6. List the three tests commonly included in a thyroid panel and provide the clinical significance of each.

   A. _____

   B. _____

   C. _____

7. Discuss the role of HbA1c in the management of diabetes.

   _____

   _____

8. Explain the differences between Type 1, Type 2, and gestational diabetes.

   A. _____

   _____

   _____

   B. _____

   _____

   _____

   C. _____

   _____

   _____

9. Describe the appearance and causes of icteric, lipemic, and hemolyzed serum.

   A. _____

   B. _____

   C. _____

10. Explain the difference between serum and plasma.

   _____

   _____

   _____

11. Explain the purpose of the chain of custody.

   _____

   _____

   _____

Assignment 30-5: Certification Practice

Choose the best answer and place the corresponding letter in the blank.

____ 1. Which of the following is a screening test for syphilis?

   A. HEC

   B. SYP

   C. STD

   D. VDRL

____ 2. If a patient's blood demonstrates a positive reaction when tested with Anti-B serum, it indicates which of the following blood types?

   A. AB

   B. B

   C. A

   D. O

____ 3. A blood glucose result of 140 mg/dL would indicate which of the following?

    A. Hypoglycemia

    B. Glycogenemia

    C. Hyperglycemia

    D. Glycemia

____ 4. Patients on anticoagulant therapy must have which of the following tests regularly?

    A. APT

    B. PT/INR

    C. Bleeding time

    D. ALP

____ 5. When homeostasis is disrupted, the body responds by doing which of the following?

    A. It shuts down altogether.

    B. It interrupts blood flow.

    C. It increases or decreases related chemicals or hormones.

    D. It retains water.

____ 6. Which of the following must be a part of any laboratory test method?

    A. Record keeping

    B. Quality control

    C. Quality assurance

    D. All of the above

____ 7. Which of the following special procedures must be followed regarding a blood specimen for arterial blood gases?

    A. Protect from light

    B. Refrigerate

    C. Place on ice

    D. Wrap in aluminum foil

____ 8. All of the following tests would be included in a hepatic profile, *except:*

    A. total and direct bilirubin.

    B. ALT.

    C. AST.

    D. CO_2.

____ 9. A patient presents with symptoms of a MI, with an increased CPK. Which of the following tests should be performed to indicate the extent of damage to the heart muscle?

    A. SGOT

    B. CPK-MB

    C. LDH

    D. CCB

____ 10. Before collecting a specimen for an FBS, the patient is required to:

    A. fast for 8–12 hours.

    B. fast for 6 hours.

    C. eat a high carbohydrate meal.

    D. none of the above.

____ 11. Before beginning a GTT, the patient is required to do all of the following *except:*

    A. fast.

    B. perform daily glucose monitoring during the week prior to testing.

    C. eat a diet high in carbohydrates for three days prior to testing.

    D. refrain from smoking after midnight prior to testing.

____ 12. All of the following are true regarding the administration of a glucose supplement during a GTT *except:*

    A. fasting specimen should be tested before administering the glucose supplement.

    B. chill the glucose supplement before administering.

    C. determine if patient has a preference of flavors.

    D. check with provider prior to administering if patient's blood glucose is normal—you may not need to perform the testing.

____ 13. Which of the following symptoms could indicate hypoglycemia during GTT testing?

    A. Headache

    B. Senseless speech

    C. Perspiration

    D. Irrational behavior

    E. All of the above

____ 14. Which of the following could be the result of decreased amylase levels?

    A. Cirrhosis

    B. Pancreatitis

    C. Bile stones

    D. Bile duct obstruction

____ 15. Which of the following is a tumor marker for colorectal cancer?

    A. PSA

    B. CEA

    C. SST

    D. ALP

____ 16. Which of the following is the most common cause of a peptic ulcer?

    A. Diet

    B. Alcohol consumption

    C. Smoking

    D. *Helicobacter pylori*

____ 17. Which of the following determines a person's blood type?

    A. Antibodies

    B. Antigens

    C. T-cells

    D. B-cells

____ 18. When performing an ABO blood typing, the antigen on the red cells combines with the antibody in the test serum causing which of the following reactions?

    A. Neutralization

    B. Specificity

    C. Agglutination

    D. Autoagglutination

____ 19. A positive test for drugs must be:

    A. reported to the Department of Public Health.

    B. confirmed with more precise tests.

    C. quantified.

    D. repeated.

____ 20. Which of the following insures the validity of a specimen for drug testing?

    A. Quality assurance

    B. Proper preservation

    C. Quality control

    D. Chain of custody

SKILL APPLICATION CHALLENGES
Assignment 30-6: ABO Blood Chart
Fill in the following ABO blood group chart.

ABO Blood Type	*Antigen Present on the Red Cells*	*Antibody Present on the Red Cells*
Type A	_____	_____
Type B	_____	_____
Type AB	_____	_____
Type O	_____	_____

Assignment 30-7: Normal and Abnormal Results

The lab results are back for April Lindsey. Medical assistants cannot diagnose or prescribe; however, knowing the significance of lab results and possible contributing factors for abnormal results will assist you when educating patients in person or over the phone. Record the abnormal results on the lines below, then write an analogy as to why particular results may be abnormal and state what may be a likely course of action based on the findings from the provider.

Abnormal Results	*Analogy*
_____	_____
_____	_____
_____	_____
_____	_____
_____	_____
_____	_____
_____	_____
_____	_____
_____	_____
_____	_____
_____	_____
_____	_____
_____	_____

CLINICAL CHEMISTRY REPORT FORM

PHYSICIAN INFORMATION	PATIENT INFORMATION
DOUGLASVILLE MEDICINE ASSOCIATES **5076 BRAND BLVD.** **DOUGLASVILLE, NY 01234** **(123) 456-7890** **Physician Name:** Dr. J. Leonard **Physician ID #:** 298739750023	**Name:** April Lindsey **Address:** 1234 Lark Lane **City/State/Zip:** Douglasville, NY 01234 **Phone #:** 123-456-9087 **ID #:** 877387477

Date and Time of Collection		Date Results Received
10/12/XX	9:00 a.m.	10/15/XX

Fasting Sample	Random Sample
Yes ___X___	Yes_____

Test Ordered	Results	Reference Range
Profiles/Panels:		
Liver/Hepatic Panel		
Direct Bilirubin	1.0 mg/dL	0.0–0.2 mg/dL
Total Bilirubin	1.4 mg/dL	0.2–1.0 mg/dL
Total Protein	7.8 mg/dL	6.0–8.0 mg/dL
ALT	54 U/L	7–56 U/L
AST	42 U/L	5–40 U/L
LDH	147 mg/dL	less than 130 mg/dL
GGT	42	M: 9–70 U/L F: 5–45 U/L
ALP	116	30–130 mU/L
Renal Panel		
Sodium (Na)		136–145 mEq/L
Potassium (K)		3.5–5.0 mEq/L
Chloride (Cl)		96–110 mEq/L
BUN/Blood Urea Nitrogen		8–25 mg/dL
Creatinine		0.4–1.5 mg/dL
Uric Acid		M: 3.5–7.2 mg/dL F: 2.6–6.0 mg/dL
Carbon Dioxide/CO_2		22–32 mmol/L
Glucose		70–110 mg/dL
Lipid Panel		
Total Cholesterol	256 mg/dL	less than 200 mg/dL
HDL	75 mg/dL	M: 37–70 mg/dL F: 40–85 mg/dL
LDL	150 mg/dL	less than 130 mg/dL
Triglycerides	140 mg/dL	20–180 mg/dL
Thyroid Panel		
	3.0 mU/mL	4.5–13.0 mU/mL
	2.5 mcg/dL	4–11.5 mcg/dL
	6.0 mU/mL	0.3–4.5 mU/mL

Continued

Test Ordered	Results	Reference Range
Cardiac Panel		
LDH		100–225 U/L
CPK		M: 12-70 mcg/L F: 10-55 mcg/L
SGOT		5–40 U/L
Miscellaneous Tests		
Glucose Tests:		
FBS		70–110 mg/dL
2-hr. PP		less than 140 mg/dL
GTT:		
1/2 hr.		110–170 mg/dL
1 hr.		120–170 mg/dL
2 hr.		70–120 mg/dL
3 hr.		60–120 mg/dL
HgbA1c		4.5–6.5
Albumin		3.0–5.0 gm/dL
Globulin		2.3–3.5 mg/dL
Calcium		8.5–10.5 mg/dL
CEA		Nonsmoker: less than 2.5 ng/mL Smoker: less than 5 ng/mL
PSA		
Amylase		Adults: 25–125 IU/L Adults over 70: 21–160 IU/L
Lipase		Adults: 0–1.5 U/mL
Magnesium (Mg)		1.2–2.4 mEq/L
Phosphorous (P)		2.5–4.5 mg/dL

COMPLETING SPECIAL FORMS

Assignment 30-8: Lab Requisition Form

Work Form Necessary: FORM 30-1

Directions: Complete the lab requisition (Work Form 30-1) with the scenario information given below. (Hint: You may not use all of the information listed.)

Complete the lab requisition with the following information: Patient name: April R. Lindsey, Address: 1234 Lark Lane, Douglasville, NY 01234, Telephone number: 123-456-9087, DOB: 10-12-76, Age: 35, Sex: female, Fasting: yes, Date of visit: 06/26/12, Time of collection: 8:00 a.m., Tests ordered: Liver and lipid profile. Primary insurance through husband, Dennis Lindsey, Address: Same as patient: ID #: 56987, Payer: Meditel, 9000 Green Ave., Anytown, OH 45229, ICD9 code: 414.0, Referring provider: Dr. Miguel Gonzales, Address: Douglasville Medicine Associates, 5076 Brand Blvd., Douglasville, NY 01234, Telephone number: 123-456-7890, ID# 298739750023.

ASSIGNMENT 30-9: OUTSIDE SPECIMEN TRACKING LOG

Work Form Necessary: FORM 30-2

Directions: Enter the information from Assignment 30-8 into the log (Work Form 30-2).

FIELD APPLICATION CHALLENGE

Assignment 30-10

Read the following Field Application Challenge and respond to the questions following the scenario.

You have been asked to perform a rapid test for infectious mononucleosis on a patient specimen. You obtain the proper specimen and perform the test according to manufacturer's directions. You obtain a negative result and report your result to the provider.

1. What important step was left out?

   _____

2. Can the results be considered accurate? Why or why not?

   _____

   _____

   _____

3. What impact could this have on the patient?

   _____

JOURNALING EXERCISE

Assignment 30-11

What content within this chapter was most meaningful to you? Why? List some examples of how you might apply information contained in this chapter, both during your training and after you enter the health care industry.

Work Form 30-1

LABORATORY REQUISITION

PATIENT LAST NAME		FIRST		M.I.	REFERRING PROVIDER

PROVIDER ID #	PATIENT ID #	BILL: ☐ PHYSICIAN	☐ MEDICAL ☐ HMO ☐ CHDP ☐ MEDICARE ☐ INSURANCE ☐ PATIENT PLEASE COMPLETE INSURANCE BILLING INFORMATION AT BOTTOM	D.O.B	AGE	SEX

PROVIDER NAME, ADDRESS, AND PHONE NUMBER	PATIENT ADDRESS		PATIENT PHONE NUMBER ( )	DATE COLLECTED	TIME COLLECTED

CITY	STATE	ZIP CODE	FASTING YES | NO	STAT	CALL RESULT

PATIENT MEDICARE #	PATIENT MEDICAID #	INFO. BELOW WILL APPEAR ON REPORT

CUSTOM PROFILES & ADDITIONAL TESTS

```
173    [ ] CHEMISTRY PANEL, COMPLETE BLOOD COUNT (ZPP), LIPID PROFILE, T4
05050 [ ] CHOL, TRIG, HDL CHOL, VLDL CHOL, LDL CHOL, RISK FACTOR
```

PROFILES

00011 ☐ SPECIAL COMPREHENSIVE	2 SS,L	03536 ☐ HYPERTHYROID PROFILE		SS
00001 ☐ COMPREHENSIVE HEALTH SURVEY	SS,L	05037 ☐ HYPOTHYROID PROFILE		SS
00002 ☐ GENERAL SURVEY	SS,L	05051 ☐ LIPID PROFILE		SS
00003 ☐ CHEMISTRY PANEL	SS,L	05021 ☐ LIVER PROFILE		SS
CH7 ☐ CHEM 7 PANEL	SS	03359 ☐ LUPUS PROFILE		SS
03280 ☐ ANEMIA PROFILE	SS,L	03959 ☐ MENOPAUSAL PROFILE SS /03960 ☐ POST MENOPAUSAL		SS
06016 ☐ ARTHRITIS PROFILE	SS,L	02280 ☐ OVARIAN FUNCTION PROFILE SS /02281 ☐ TESTICULAR FUNC. PROF.		SS
05725 ☐ COMPREHENSIVE THYROID SURVEY	SS	02808 ☐ PRENATAL PROFILE		L,R
02691 ☐ EPSTEIN BARR PROFILE	SS	05006 ☐ THYROID PROFILE		SS
05010 ☐ ELECTROLYTES	SS	03191 ☐ TORCH PANEL		SS
06826 ☐ HEPATITIS PROFILE	SS	5756 ☐ URINE DRUG SCREEN	U / ☐ VENIPUNCTURE	

TESTS

0361 ☐ ABO & Rh TYPE	R,L	0141 ☐ C-REACTIVE PROTEIN	SS	0673 ☐ HEPATITIS B SURFACE ANTIGEN	SS	0237 ☐ PTT	B
0302 ☐ ALKALINE PHOSPHATASE	SS	1341 ☐ DHEA-S	SS	0245 ☐ HEPATITIS C ANTIBODY	SS	0317 ☐ RA FACTOR	SS
0109 ☐ AMYLASE	SS	0119 ☐ DIGOXIN	SS	0257 ☐ IRON	SS	0321 ☐ RUBELLA	SS
0613 ☐ ANA	SS	0224 ☐ DILANTIN	SS	LDL-A ☐ LDL CHOLESTEROL	SS	0331 ☐ RPR	SS
0366 ☐ ANTIBODY SCREEN	R	0835 ☐ ESTRADIOL	SS	0283 ☐ LEAD BLOOD	RB	0335 ☐ SEMEN ANALYSIS	SEMEN
0110 ☐ ASO (STREPTOZYME)	SS	0833 ☐ FERRITIN	SS	0281 ☐ LIPASE	SS	0328 ☐ SEDIMENTATION RATE (ESR)	L
0126 ☐ BILIRUBIN TOTAL	SS	0003 ☐ FOLIC ACID & VITAMIN B12	SS	8225 ☐ LH	SS	0349 ☐ SGOT (AST)	SS
0132 ☐ BUN	SS	0651 ☐ FSH	SS	0247 ☐ MONONUCLEOSIS	SS	0348 ☐ SGPT (ALT)	SS
8726 ☐ CA125	SS	0140 ☐ FTA-ABS	SS	0778 ☐ PHENOBARBITAL	SS	0330 ☐ SICKLE CELL SCREEN	L
0142 ☐ CALCIUM	SS	0210 ☐ GGTP	SS	0307 ☐ POTASSIUM	SS	0354 ☐ T4 (THYROXINE)	SS
0130 ☐ CBC	L	0536 ☐ GLUCOSE, FASTING	GY	0557 ☐ PREGNANCY (SERUM)	SS	1358 ☐ T4 FREE	SS
0388 ☐ CEA-ROCHE	SS	☐ GLUCOSE, _____ HR PP	GY	0308 ☐ PREGNANCY (URINE)	U	8456 ☐ TESTOSTERONE	SS
0152 ☐ CHOLESTEROL	SS	0771 ☐ GLYCOHEMOGLOBIN	L	0359 ☐ PROGESTERONE	SS	0824 ☐ THEOPHYLLINE	SS
0788 ☐ CORTISOL	SS	0534 ☐ H. PYLORI	SS	8041 ☐ PROLACTIN	SS	0360 ☐ TRIGLYCERIDE	SS
0162 ☐ CPK	SS	0823 ☐ HGG QUANTITATIVE	SS	0103 ☐ PROTEIN, TOTAL	SS	0672 ☐ TSH	SS
0445 ☐ CKMB ISOENZYME	SS	1856 ☐ HIV (ANTIBODY)	SS	2000 ☐ PROSTATE SPECIFIC ANTIGEN (PSA)	SS	0373 ☐ URIC ACID	SS
0161 ☐ CREATININE	SS	0558 ☐ HDL CHOLESTEROL	SS	0310 ☐ PT (PROTHROMBIN TIME)	B	0219 ☐ URINALYSIS	U

CYTOPATHOLOGY

☐ PREGNANT ☐ ABORTION ☐ POST-PARTUM ☐ POST-MENOPAUSE
HISTORY _____

PREV. ABNORMAL CYTOL FINDINGS _____
☐ CONTRACEPTIVES DATE _____
☐ HYSTERECTOMY ☐ HORMONES ☐ IUD
☐ COPHORECTOMY ☐ TOTAL ☐ SUPRA CX
☐ RADIATION Rx DATE _____
☐ OTHER _____ ☐ HORMONES Rx ☐ CHEMO Rx

LMP _____ DATE COLLECTED _____
SOURCE ☐ CERVIX ☐ ENDOCERVIX ☐ VAGINA
☐ CYTOBRUSH ☐ OTHER SITE _____

MICROBIOLOGY

THCUL ☐ THROAT	URTHC ☐ URETHRAL	9391 ☐ CHLAMYDIA DNA
EACUL EAR	VACUL ☐ VAGINAL	9390 ☐ GONORRHEA DNA
EYCUL ☐ EYE	WOCUL ☐ WOUND	9391 ☐ OCCULT BLOOD
GOCUL ☐ GC	ROCUL ☐ CULTURE (Routine)	0293 ☐ OVA & PARASITE
SPCUL ☐ SPUTUM	URCUL ☐ URINE	WTM ☐ WET MOUNT
STCUL ☐ STOOL	GSP ☐ GRAM STAIN	
SOURCE _____	OTHER _____	

DIAGNOSIS OR COMMENTS

LAB USE ONLY (DO NOT WRITE BELOW THIS SPACE)

DATE RECEIVED	DATE REPORTED

STATEMENT OF SPECIMEN ADEQUACY

GENERAL CATEGORIZATION

DESCRIPTIVE DIAGNOSIS

HORMONAL EVALUATION

ADDITIONAL COMMENT

CYTOTECHNOLOGIST	PATHOLOGIST

INSURANCE BILLING INFORMATION

PRIMARY INSURED	INSURANCE COMPANY
ADDRESS	
POLICY NO. & I.D. NO.	ICD9 CODE

LEGEND

SS	Serum Separator	GY	Grey	B	Blue	U	Urine
R	Red	L	Lavender	RB	Royal Blue	G	Green

Work Form 30-2

DOUGLASVILLE MEDICINE ASSOCIATES
5076 BRAND BLVD
DOUGLASVILLE, NY 01234
(123) 456-7890

OUTSIDE LAB SPECIMEN TRACKING LOG								
Date Sent	Patient Name/ID	Ordering Provider	Tests Ordered	Number of and Type of Specimens Sent to Laboratory (Include Tube Colors)	Prepared By	Laboratory	Date Results Received	Results Received By

C H A P T E R **31**

Diagnostic Imaging

FIELD RELEVANCY AND BENEFITS

There are times when the office examination does not provide all of the necessary information to make a precise diagnosis. Further evaluations may involve the use of radiographic equipment. These evaluations may be performed within the office setting, but, more likely, will be obtained at an alternate facility. To ensure the highest level of patient compliance, the medical assistant must be familiar with procedures in order to provide satisfactory instruction to the patient. The medical assistant may also be the staff member responsible for scheduling these radiographic exams at another facility. In some states, medical assistants who earn a GXMO/general x-ray machine operator's license are permitted to perform flat-plate x-rays. If this is an option in your state, consider getting your license. A medical assistant who can perform general x-ray procedures in the office is a valuable asset to the practice.

NOTE SHEET

Radiology Overview

_____

_____

_____

_____

Legal Considerations for Taking X-Rays

_____

_____

_____

_____

X-Ray Equipment

_____

_____

_____

_____

The Medical Assistant's Role in Radiographic Procedures

_____

_____

_____

_____

Common Types of X-Rays Performed in the Office

_____

_____

_____

_____

Storing and Disposing of X-Ray Films

_____

_____

_____

_____

Scheduling Radiological Procedures Outside the Office

_____

_____

_____

_____

Other Diagnostic Imaging Procedures

_____

_____

_____

_____

Radiation Therapy

_____

_____

_____

_____

Processing and Displaying X-Ray Films

_____

_____

_____

_____

Safety Precautions

_____

_____

_____

_____

Radiological Procedures Commonly Performed Outside the Office

_____

_____

_____

_____

Nuclear Medicine

_____

_____

_____

_____

VOCABULARY REVIEW

Assignment 31-1: Matching

Match the term with its definition and place the corresponding letter in the blank.

____ 1. Fluoroscopy

____ 2. Collimator

____ 3. Angiography

____ 4. Contrast medium

____ 5. Radiolucent

____ 6. Magnetic resonance

____ 7. Cholangiography

____ 8. Bucky

____ 9. Nuclear medicine

____ 10. Ultrasound

____ 11. Rad

____ 12. Radiopaque

A. Diagnostic imaging procedure that uses a magnetic field to produce clear images of the body

B. X-ray procedure that allows visualization of the blood vessels after a radiopaque contrast medium has been injected

C. Substance that is either injected or ingested which enhances the visibility of structures during diagnostic imaging procedures

D. Special film holder that contains a moveable grid to help reduce the scatter of secondary radiation during an x-ray

E. Allows the x-ray beam to pass through, making structures difficult to visualize

F. Diagnostic procedure that uses high frequency sound imaging waves to produce an image of an internal body structure

G. Branch of medicine that uses radioactive isotopes for the purpose of diagnosing and treating diseases

H. Unable to be penetrated by the x-ray beam (allows visualization of a structure)

I. X-ray of moving body structures in real time, similar to a movie

J. X-ray procedure that views the bile ducts within and outside of the liver and gallbladder

K. Device attached to the x-ray tube that controls the size and shape of the x-ray beam

L. Unit of measure that determines the amount of ionizing radiation that is absorbed during an x-ray procedure

Assignment 31-2: Sentence Completion

Fill in the blanks below with Essential Terms from this chapter.

1. A(n) _____ is a high-energy beam capable of penetrating the body to produce images on film.

2. The _____ is the structure located inside the bucky which is made up of alternating strips of radiolucent and radiopaque material.

3. A(n) _____ is a radiographic procedure that views the kidneys, uterus, and bladder after a contrast medium has been injected.

4. A(n) _____ is a radioactive substance, such as iodine or cobalt, which is administered to patients prior to a nuclear medicine study.

5. Another name for an x-ray is a(n) _____.

6. A radiographic procedure that produces cross-sectional images of the body is _____.

7. A(n) _____ is a medical specialist who uses radioactive substances for visualization of internal body structures and diagnosis and treatment.

CHAPTER REVIEW
Assignment 31-3: Acronym Review
Write what each of the following acronyms stands for.

1. AP: _____

2. PA: _____

3. IVP: _____

4. CT: _____

5. MRI: _____

6. KUB: _____

Assignment 31-4: Short Answer

1. Explain the advantage of using ultrasound over an x-ray during pregnancy.

   _____

2. Define the following patient positions used for x-rays.

   A. AP: _____

   _____

   B. PA: _____

   _____

   C. Lateral: _____

   _____

   _____

   D. Oblique: _____

   _____

   E. Erect: _____

   _____

   F. Supine: _____

   _____

3. List patient risks associated with x-rays.

   _____

   _____

4. Explain patient preparation for an IVP and fluoroscopy.

   A. _____

   _____

   B. _____

   _____

5. List the safety precautions used by health care personnel and patients during x-ray procedures.

Safety Procedures to Protect the Health Care Worker　　*Safety Procedures to Protect the Patient*

_____　　_____

_____　　_____

_____　　_____

_____　　_____

_____　　_____

_____　　_____

_____　　_____

_____　　_____

_____　　_____

_____　　_____

6. List side affects associated with radiation therapy.

_____

_____

_____

_____

_____

_____

7. List medical assistant duties regarding radiographic procedures.

A. _____

B. _____

C. _____

D. _____

E. _____

F. _____

G. _____

H. _____

I. _____

J. _____

K. _____

L. _____

M. _____

N. _____

8. List and define the different types of contrast media used to perform x-rays.

A. _____

_____

_____

B. _____

_____

_____

C. _____

_____

_____

Assignment 31-5: Certification Practice

Choose the best answer and place the corresponding letter in the blank.

____ 1. Which of the following radiological procedures would require *no* patient preparation?

A. Fluoroscopy

B. IVP

C. Upper GI

D. X-ray of the hand

____ 2. In which of the following positions would the patient's back be against the film?

A. AP

B. PA

C. Lateral

D. Oblique

____ 3. All of the following are side effects of radiation therapy *except:*

A. vomiting.

B. hair loss.

C. increase in appetite.

D. nausea.

____ 4. Which of the following radiological procedures provides cross-sectional images of the body?

A. MRI

B. CT scan

C. Bone scan

D. Nuclear medicine study

____ 5. Which of the following controls the size and shape of the x-ray beam?

A. Grid

B. Cassette

C. Bucky

D. Collimator

____ 6. Which part of the x-ray equipment is designed to prevent scattering of the x-ray beam?

A. Grid

B. Processor

C. Cassette

D. Bucky

____ 7. In which of the following x-ray positions does the x-ray beam pass from the back to the front?

    A. Lateral

    B. AP

    C. PA

    D. Supine

____ 8. All of the following positions may be used for an x-ray of a fractured ankle *except:*

    A. AP.

    B. lateral.

    C. oblique.

    D. erect.

____ 9. Which of the following imaging procedures never requires film?

    A. CT scan

    B. Bone scan

    C. Digital radiograph

    D. All of the above

____ 10. How long must x-rays be kept on file?

    A. Patient preference

    B. Provider preference

    C. 5–7 years

    D. 2–3 years

____ 11. Which of the following units of measure is used to measure the amount of ionizing radiation that is absorbed during the procedure?

    A. Ionization

    B. Rad

    C. Unit x

    D. Ohm

____ 12. From which of the following types of radiation must the health care worker protect himself?

    A. Ionizing

    B. Primary

    C. Secondary

    D. Ultra

____ 13. In which of the following locations is the level of secondary radiation at its highest?

    A. Near the x-ray tube

    B. Directly in front of the lead shield

    C. In areas closest to the patient

    D. Near the control panel

____ 14. Which of the following statements is true regarding the radioactive materials used in x-ray procedures?

    A. Radioactive materials must be stored in lead containers.

    B. Radioactive materials should never be handled with bare hands.

    C. Special forceps must be used when handling radioactive materials.

    D. All of the above

____ 15. When instructing a patient about special preparation for an x-ray procedure, the medical assistant would do all of the following, *except:*

    A. review instructions verbally.

    B. provide the patient with written instructions.

    C. explain to the patient the importance of strict adherence to preparation guidelines.

    D. provide the patient with information regarding his own personal experience with this type of procedure.

___ 16. Which of the following imaging procedures would be ordered if the provider wanted to ascertain the presence of a blood clot in the brain?

    A. Arthrography

    B. Angiography

    C. Cholangiography

    D. Ultrasound

___ 17. A female who is breast-feeding is scheduled for an IVP. What should she be told regarding the procedure?

    A. The procedure can be painful.

    B. There may be adverse reactions during and after the procedure.

    C. The contrast medium used can be excreted in her breast milk.

    D. It is permissible to continue to breast-feed.

___ 18. Which of the following imaging procedures would be used to pinpoint the area to which radiation should be administered for treatment of a tumor or mass?

    A. MRI

    B. Flat-plate film

    C. CT scan

    D. Ultrasound

___ 19. Which of the following is a drawback regarding magnetic resonance imaging?

    A. Patients with pacemakers or metal implants cannot undergo an MRI.

    B. Patients must remove items that contain metal such as jewelry, belts, etc.

    C. Credit cards containing magnetic strips must be removed from patients' pockets.

    D. All of the above

___ 20. Which of the following imaging procedures uses no radiation?

    A. CT scan

    B. MRI

    C. Cholangiogram

    D. Arteriogram

SKILL APPLICATION CHALLENGE

Assignment 31-6: Web Activity

Using the Internet to gather information, design a patient information form for one of the following diagnostic imaging procedures:

- MRI

- KUB

- Upper GI

- Cholangiograph

- Fluoroscopy

COMPLETING SPECIAL FORMS

Assignment 31-7: X-Ray Request Form

Work Form Necessary: FORM 31-1

Directions: Complete the x-ray request form (Work Form 31-1) with the scenario information given below.

Complete the x-ray request form with the following information: Patient name: Nancy Tinksy, 5879 Parkside Road, Parkview NY 01652, (123) 259-6632, DOB: 05/22/55, Payer info: Name of insured: Nancy Tinksy, Insurance ID #: 5698AC1, Name of company: Meditel Insurance Company, Address of insurance company: 2345 Long Street, Anytown, OH 43256, (740) 236-9865, Clinical findings: Productive cough x 2 weeks, (nonsmoker), Referring provider: Dr. Corey Cook, Douglasville Medicine Associates, 5076 Brand Blvd, Douglasville, NY 01234 (123) 456-7890, X-rays ordered: PA and lateral of the chest to be performed at XYZ Radiology. The provider would like the results e-mailed to *ccook@douglasvillemed.org*.

You contact XYZ Radiology and speak with Kim Grossman. Date of order: 05/19/11, Date of appointment: 05/19/11 @ 3:00 p.m.

Assignment 31-8: Documentation/Charting Exercise

On the following progress note, document that you set the patient up to have a PA and lateral chest x-ray today at 3:00 p.m. at XYZ Radiology and that you spoke with Kim Grossman (date of entry: 05/19/11, time of entry: 12:45 p.m.) Document that you gave the patient the requisition form to take with her and that the office will call her with the results. Be sure to include an order for the x-ray in your documentation.

FIELD APPLICATION CHALLENGE

Assignment 31-9

Read the following Field Application Challenge and respond to the questions following the scenario.

You are excited because you just received your x-ray certification and are able to take x-rays in your facility. A 27-year-old patient, Claudia Green, has an order from her provider to have a chest-ray because of a possible broken rib.

1. What is the first question you should ask Claudia?

_____

2. What clothing and other articles should she remove prior to the x-ray ?

_____

3. After performing the x-ray, you notice that the patient has a necklace on in the x-ray. Which of the following should you do?

   A. Retake the x-ray.

   B. Check with the provider to see how he wants you to proceed.

   C. Scold the patient for not removing the necklace.

4. How will you make certain that this never occurs again?

_____

_____

JOURNALING EXERCISE
Assignment 31-10

What content within this chapter was most meaningful to you? Why? List some examples of how you might apply information contained in this chapter, both during your training and after you enter the health care industry.

Work Form 31-1

<table>
<tr><td colspan="3" align="center">**XYZ RADIOLOGY**
4598 HIGH STREET
DOUGLASVILLE, NY 01234
(123) 456-9874</td></tr>
<tr><td>Patient Name:
Address:

Phone #:
DOB:</td><td>Insured's Name:
Payer Info:</td><td>Referring Physician Info:</td></tr>
</table>

ULTRASOUND PROCEDURES	X-RAYS/RADIOGRAPHIC PROCEDURES	
Abdomen:	**Abdomen:**	**Upper Extremities**
☐ Complete Abdomen	☐ Plain Film (KUB)	R L AC Joints
☐ Both Abdomen & Pelvic	☐ Acute (2 Views)	R L Clavicle
☐ Other	**Barium Studies:**	R L Digits 1 2 3 4 5
Joint:	☐ BA Swallow	R L Elbow
☐ Sholder	☐ Upper GI Series	R L Forearm
☐ Knee	☐ GI Small Bowel	R L Hand
☐ Other +Fluid +Mass	☐ BA Enema (Colon)	R L Humerus
Neck:	**Chest:**	R L Scapula
☐ Neck & Thyroid	☐ PA & Lateral	R L Shoulder
Pelvic Female:	☐ Ribs: R L	R L Wrist
☐ Pelvic Routine (Only)	☐ Chest PA	**Lower Extremities**
☐ Transvaginal	☐ Sternum	R L Ankle
☐ Transvaginal & Kidneys	**Head and Neck:**	R L Femur
☐ Obstetrical	☐ Facial	R L Foot
☐ Biophysical	☐ Mandible	R L Hip
Pelvic Male:	☐ Mastoid	R L OS Calcius
☐ Prostate/Bladder	☐ Orbits	R L Toes 1 2 3 4 5
☐ Prostate/Bladder/Kidnes	☐ Orbits for MRI	**Spine and Pelvic**
☐ Scrotal	☐ Nasal Bones	☐ Cervical Spine
Vascular Diseases:	☐ Skull	☐ Lumpo-Sacral Spine
☐ Arterial Leg Doppler	☐ Sinuses	☐ Pelvis
☐ Carotid Doppler	☐ Soft Tissue of Neck	☐ Pelvis & Joints
☐ Venous Leg Doppler	☐ TM Joints	☐ Sacrum & Coccyx
☐ Other Doppler		☐ Thoracic Spine
Clinical Data or ICD-9	☐ Email Results: E-Mail Address: ☐ Fax Report: Fax #:	
Date of Order:	Date of Appointment:	Time of Appointment:
Physician's Office Rep:	**XYZ Radiology Rep:**	

C H A P T E R **32**

Fundamentals of Pharmacology

FIELD RELEVANCY AND BENEFITS

The medical assistant is quite often responsible for administering and dispensing medications and for preparing prescriptions. A general knowledge of basic pharmacology, including pharmacodynamics, drug classification, drug actions, and different forms of drug administration, are vital to the success of the medical assistant and the health care of the patient. Medical assistants must be familiar with laws regarding controlled substances and with medication delegation rules as they relate to medical assistants. The contents of this chapter are applicable to the many different types of offices in which medical assistants work.

NOTE SHEET

Drug Origins

_____

_____

_____

_____

Medicinal Uses of Drugs

_____

_____

_____

_____

Drug Classifications

_____

_____

_____

_____

Pharmacodynamics

_____

_____

_____

_____

Pharmacokinetics

_____

_____

_____

_____

Drug Names

_____

_____

_____

_____

Medication Tasks

_____

_____

_____

_____

Regulations and Legal Classifications of Drugs

_____

_____

_____

_____

The Medication Order/Prescription Writing

_____

_____

_____

_____

Drug Resources

_____

_____

_____

_____

Safe Drug Administration

_____

_____

_____

_____

Routes of Medication Administration

_____

_____

_____

_____

VOCABULARY REVIEW

Assignment 32-1: Matching

Match the term with its definition and place the corresponding letter in the blank.

_____ 1. Affinity

_____ 2. Anaphylaxis

_____ 3. Bioavailability

_____ 4. Drug

_____ 5. Drug ceiling

_____ 6. Drug interaction

_____ 7. Efficacy

_____ 8. Pharmacodynamics

_____ 9. Pharmacology

_____ 10. Receptors

_____ 11. Side effect

_____ 12. Therapeutic effect

_____ 13. Therapeutic index

A. Bonding proteins or sites in which a drug attaches; each has a unique structural design

B. Comparing a drug's benefits to its risks

C. Secondary effect in addition to the therapeutic effect

D. Measurement of how tightly a drug attaches or binds to a receptor

E. Advanced systemic reaction; may include bronchial constriction, swelling of the tongue or throat, and an inability to breathe

F. Range between the therapeutic dose of a drug and the dose at which the drug becomes toxic

G. Fraction of the drug that is released and the rate at which it is released into circulation and made available at the site of action

H. Any substance that produces a change in function of a living organism

I. When one drug diminishes or increases the affects of another drug

J. The study of the effects of drugs on living organisms

K. Maximum dose at which a drug will provide its greatest effect

L. Study of drugs, including their origin, nature, properties, and effects upon living organisms

M. Desired effect that a drug has on the body

Assignment 32-2: Definitions

Define the following terms.

1. Agonists: _____

   _____

2. Antagonists: _____

   _____

3. Buccal: _____

   _____

4. Enteral: _____

   _____

5. Parenteral: _____

   _____

6. Pharmokinetics: _____

   _____

7. Sublingual: _____

_____

8. Topical: _____

_____

9. Transdermal patches: _____

_____

CHAPTER REVIEW

Assignment 32-3: Acronym Review

Write what each of the following acronyms stands for.

1. OTC: _____

2. FDA: _____

3. APhA: _____

4. ®: _____

5. DEA: _____

6. CSA: _____

7. USP: _____

8. ISMP: _____

9. PDR: _____

10. USP/NF: _____

11. LASA: _____

12. SR: _____

Assignment 32-4: Short Answer

1. List five different sources of drugs.

    A. _____

    B. _____

    C. _____

    D. _____

    E. _____

2. List and describe four processes that affect drug plasma levels.

    A. _____

    _____

    _____

    B. _____

    _____

    _____

C. _____

_____

_____

D. _____

_____

_____

3. List and describe three different names by which a drug may be referred.

A. _____

_____

_____

B. _____

_____

_____

C. _____

_____

_____

4. Describe the following terms and designate which health care professionals can perform each task.

A. Prescribe: _____

_____

B. Administer: _____

_____

C. Dispense: _____

_____

D. Physicians: _____

_____

E. Nurse practitioners and physician assistants: _____

_____

F. Medical assistants: _____

_____

_____

5. Describe the potential for abuse for each of the five drug schedules.

Schedule	Potential for Abuse
I	_____
II	_____
III	_____
IV	_____
V	_____

6. How often should a full inventory be completed of controlled substances in the medical office?

   _____

7. How often should inventories be performed in areas in which staff has access?

   _____

8. How long should controlled substances logs be kept?

   _____

9. Define the term prescription and list its parts.

   Prescription: _____

   _____

   Parts of a prescription: _____

   _____

   _____

   _____

   _____

   _____

10. List and describe the seven rights of drug administration.

Right	Description
1. _____	_____
2. _____	_____
3. _____	_____

4. _____ _____

_____

_____

5. _____ _____

_____

_____

6. _____ _____

_____

_____

7. _____ _____

_____

_____

_____

11. List the two major routes of drug administration and the list and describe all the routes within each major route.

Route   *Examples*

_____   _____

_____   _____

_____   _____

_____   _____

_____   _____

_____   _____

_____   _____

_____   _____

_____   _____

_____   _____

12. Describe the following forms and list their uses:

A. DEA Form 222: _____

_____

_____

B. DEA Form 224: _____

_____

_____

C. DEA Form 106: _____

_____

_____

D. DEA Form 41: _____

_____

_____

Assignment 32:5: Fill in the Blank

Fill in the missing components to drug classifications.

Drug Classification	*Action*	*Example*
Anti-inflammatory	_____	ibuprofen
_____	Prevents cough	Benylin cough syrup
Miotic	Contracts pupils of the eyes	_____
Vasodilator	_____	nitroglycerin
_____	Relieves mild to moderate fever, pain, and inflammation	Celebrex, Relafen, naproxen, ibuprofen
Muscle relaxant	Aids in relaxation of skeletal muscles	_____
_____	Reduces nasal congestion and swelling	Sudafed
Emetic	Facilitates vomiting	_____
Laxative	_____	Dulcolax, Senokot
Antimanic	_____	lithium
_____	Eases breathing by dilating the bronchial tubes	Atrovent, Combivent, albuterol
Cardiogenic	Strengthens the heart muscle	_____
Antihypertensive	_____	Accupril, Altace, atenolol
_____	Relieves pain	Tylenol, Advil, Motrin
Antiacne	Prevents or works against acne	_____
_____	Prevents or delays blood clotting	Coumadin, heparin sodium, Lovenox
Antidepressant	_____	Celexa, Effexor XR
Antidiabetic	Helps to lower blood glucose levels	_____
_____	Helps to decrease cholesterol or lipid levels	Lescol, Lipitor, Zocor

Assignment 32-6: Certification Practice

Choose the best answer and place the corresponding letter in the blank.

____ 1. Which of the following drug classifications produces a calming effect?
   A. Sedative
   B. Hypnotic
   C. Tranquilizer
   D. All of the above

____ 2. Once a drug reaches the therapeutic level in the blood plasma, the dose is usually tapered off to maintenance dose.
   A. True
   B. False

____ 3. Drugs may be grouped by the type of action they produce in the body. The application of topical medication to a joint to relieve pain is an example of a:
   A. local action.
   B. remote action.
   C. systemic action.
   D. nerve action.

____ 4. All of the following would be factors that affect drug actions *except:*

    A. body weight.

    B. disease processes.

    C. blood type.

    D. age.

____ 5. Which of the following is the name under which a drug is registered with the U.S. Patent Office?

    A. Generic name

    B. Trade name

    C. Chemical

    D. Brand name

____ 6. Which of the following is the drug's formula which includes letters and numbers?

    A. Generic name

    B. Trade name

    C. Chemical

    D. Brand name

____ 7. To apply for a DEA number, the provider will need to complete and submit which of the following forms?

    A. DEA Form 222

    B. DEA Form 224

    C. DEA Form 106

    D. DEA Form 41

____ 8. Which of the following sections of the *PDR* provides full-color photographs of the tablets and capsules and is arranged alphabetically by manufacturer?

    A. Section 1 Gray

    B. Section 2 White

    C. Section 3 Gray

    D. Section 4 Gray

    E. Section 5 White

    F. Section 6 White

____ 9. Which of the following sections of the *PDR* is the main section of the book and includes product information arranged alphabetically by manufacturer (indications, contraindications, warnings, precautions)?

    A. Section 1 Gray

    B. Section 2 White

    C. Section 3 Gray

    D. Section 4 Gray

    E. Section 5 White

    F. Section 6 White

____ 10. How long should the patient wait following drug administration?

    A. 10–15 minutes

    B. 15–20 minutes

    C. 20–30 minutes

    D. 1 hour

____ 11. Which of the following is the total number of times a medical assistant should read a label before administering the medication?

    A. Once

    B. Twice

    C. Three times

    D. Four times

____ 12. A medication that is mixed with special binding powder and pressed and molded into a particular shape is called a:
   A. caplet.
   B. capsule.
   C. gel cap.
   D. tablet.

____ 13. Of the following minerals which are suspended in water, which should be well-mixed before use?
   A. Sprays
   B. Magmas
   C. Elixers
   D. Syrups

____ 14. Which of the following is a medical preparation that is rubbed into the skin and usually mixed with a quick drying solvent?
   A. Lotion
   B. Ointment
   C. Liniment
   D. Transdermal patch

____ 15. Which of the following comes in liquid form and is applied externally to the skin?
   A. Lotion
   B. Ointment
   C. Liniment
   D. Transdermal patch

____ 16. Which of the following is an example of type of drug developed from a plant source?
   A. Insulin
   B. Silver nitrate
   C. Digitalis
   D. Epogen

____ 17. The purpose of which of the following types of drug is to help detect abnormalities?
   A. Therapeutic
   B. Diagnostic
   C. Curative
   D. Replacement
   E. Preventive

____ 18. The purpose of which of the following drugs is to provide a remedy for the patient?
   A. Therapeutic
   B. Diagnostic
   C. Curative
   D. Replacement
   E. Preventive

____ 19. Each of the following abbreviations is correctly defined *except:*
   A. tid (three times a day).
   B. QID (four times a day).
   C. BID (two times a day).
   D. NPO (take by mouth).

____ 20. Each of the following abbreviations is correctly defined *except:*
   A. DAW (dispense as written).
   B. OTC (over-the-counter).
   C. pc (before meals).
   D. hs (bedtime).

___ 21. Of the following drugs, which one can be dispensed only with a written prescription?

    A. Morphine

    B. Benadryl

    C. Valium

    D. Tylenol

___ 22. Which of the following schedules includes some drugs that can be dispensed by the pharmacist without an order from the provider?

    A. Schedule III

    B. Schedule IV

    C. Schedule V

    D. None of the above

___ 23. Controlled substances contain which of the following letters followed by the drug's schedule?

    A. A capital A

    B. A capital C

    C. A capital S

    D. A capital X

___ 24. Security features for tamper-resistant drugs include:

    A. the prescription paper must be both heat and chemically sensitive.

    B. the paper must have anticopy features that cause the word "void" to appear if someone tries to make a copy of the prescription.

    C. Rx symbol disappears if someone tries to lighten the form.

    D. all of the above.

SKILL APPLICATION CHALLENGE

Assignment 32-7: Flash Card Connection

1. Make flash cards for all of the medication abbreviations listed in Appendix A of the textbook.
2. Make flash cards for all of the drug classifications listed in Table 32-1 in this chapter.

COMPLETING SPECIAL FORMS

Assignment 32-8: Prescription Practice

Work Forms Necessary: FORMS 32-1, 32-2, 32-3, and 32-4

Directions: Using the prescription abbreviations in Appendix A of the textbook, write prescriptions for the orders given in the following case studies.

Case study information: All of the refills are to be dispensed as written; no generics are to be used. (Note: Remember to write out the quantity.) Use the following patient information for each prescription. The patient's name is Kevin Heller, 5106 Springdale Court, Columbus OH 43227, DOB: 05/07/66, Provider's name, Dr. Paul Timmons.

1. Using Work Form 32-1, write a prescription for Augmentin, tablets, 250 mg strength, Dispense amount 30, patient should take one tablet by mouth three times a day for 10 days. No refills are to be given.

2. Using Work Form 32-2, write a prescription for Prilosec tablets, 20 mg strength, Dispense amount 90, patient should take one tablet three time a day before meals. Refill amount three.

3. Using Work Form 32-3, write a prescription for Vicoden ES Capsules, Dispense amount 20, patient should take one to two every four to six hours as needed for pain. No refills are to be given. DEA # B2462810

4. Using Work Form 32-4, write a prescription for Procardia capsules, 10 mg strength, Dispense amount 60, patient should take one every morning and one at bedtime. Refill amount one.

Assignment 32-9: Reading Prescriptions

Rewrite the following prescriptions in lay terms.

1. Rx: Alprazolam 0.25 mg, sig 1 tab tid. Disp #90, 0 refills

_____

_____

2. Rx: Tussionex Susp 5 mg/5 mL, sig 5 mL. q 12 hours prn cough. Disp 50 mL , 0 refills.

_____

_____

3. Rx: Ventolin Inhaler, 90 mcg/actuation, sig 1–2 puffs prn for asthma. Disp 1 inhaler /c 2 refills.

_____

_____

FIELD APPLICATION CHALLENGE

Assignment 32-10

This Field Application Challenge has two parts. In Part A, read the scenario presented and respond to the questions following. In Part B, role play with a partner as instructed below, followed by a documentation exercise.

Part A: Mrs. Peterson has been placed on digoxin 1.5 mg daily due to congestive heart failure (CHF). Digoxin has a narrow therapeutic index and can cause organ toxicity if the blood plasma level exceeds the therapeutic index. The test must be conducted in a very narrow time line (six to eight hours following her last dose). Mrs. Peterson takes her single dose of digoxin at 7:00 a.m. every morning.

1. Based on the above criteria regarding when the blood must be tested and the time that Mrs. Peterson regularly takes her digoxin, what timeline can be used to schedule her testing?

_____

2. Because it may take awhile to get the patient back to the drawing station and processed, what time ideally would the patient need to be scheduled by in order to have the blood drawn within the correct timeline?

_____

Part B: Amy from XYZ lab calls the office to state that Mrs. Peterson's digoxin level is 2.8 ng/mL (elevated) and that the provider, Dr. Butcher, will need to be notified right away of the patient's result. You notify the provider and he tells you to call the patient and tell her that she will need to reduce her dose by cutting her 1.5 mg tablets in half for the next seven days. The patient will need to return to the office for another digoxin level on day seven at the new dose. With a lab partner playing the role of Mrs. Peterson, practice calling the patient to give her the provider's instructions. Set the patient up for her next appointment. Remember that the provider wants the patient to be tested on day seven of taking the new dose. (Recall what time of day Mrs. Peterson takes her dose so that you can determine what date and time she will need to be tested.) Chart both the call from the lab and the phone call to the patient on the following progress note. Date both entries as 11/04/11 and use 9:00 a.m. as the time the lab called and 9:30 a.m. as the time you called the patient with the provider's instructions. Be certain to document the instructions given to the patient, the patient's apparent comprehension of the instructions, and the date of the new appointment.

PROGRESS NOTE

Patient Name: DOB:

DATE/TIME	PROGRESS NOTES	ALLERGIES

JOURNALING EXERCISE

Assignment 32-11

What content within this chapter was most meaningful to you? Why? List some examples of how you might apply information contained in this chapter, both during your training and after you enter the health care industry.

Work Form 32-1

Douglasville Medicine Associates
5076 Brand Blvd.
Douglasville, NY 01234
(123)456-7890

Patient Name:

Address:

DOB: Date:

R_X

    Disp:

    Sig:

Signature:

DEA # _____

☐ **Dispense as Written/Do Not Substitute**

Refills: none   1   2   3   4   5

Work Form 32-2

Douglasville Medicine Associates
5076 Brand Blvd.
Douglasville, NY 01234
(123)456-7890

Patient Name:

Address:

DOB: Date:

R_X

    Disp:

    Sig:

Signature:

DEA # _____

☐ **Dispense as Written/Do Not Substitute**

Refills: none   1   2   3   4   5

Work Form 32-3

Douglasville Medicine Associates
5076 Brand Blvd.
Douglasville, NY 01234
(123)456-7890

Patient Name:

Address:

DOB: Date:

R_X

Disp:

Sig:

Signature:

DEA # _____

☐ **Dispense as Written/Do Not Substitute**

Refills: none 1 2 3 4 5

Work Form 32-4

Douglasville Medicine Associates
5076 Brand Blvd.
Douglasville, NY 01234
(123)456-7890

Patient Name:

Address:

DOB: Date:

R_X

Disp:

Sig:

Signature:

DEA # _____

☐ **Dispense as Written/Do Not Substitute**

Refills: none 1 2 3 4 5

C H A P T E R **33**

Dosage Calculations

FIELD RELEVANCY AND BENEFITS

One of the most important responsibilities that you will incur as a medical assistant is the task of administering medications. In order to properly administer medications, you must be able to correctly read a medication label and to calculate the correct dosage. Incorrect dosage calculations can cause serious complications for the patient and even death in some instances. The information in this chapter will assist you in learning important formulas for calculating medication dosages. It will also provide you with important information for learning how to properly read a medication label. Because medication administration is regularly performed in many types of practices, the information in this chapter will be applicable to most positions that you will possess as a medical assistant.

NOTE SHEET

Medication Order

_____

_____

_____

Medication Math Fundamentals

_____

_____

_____

Calculating Drug Dosages for Administration

_____

_____

_____

Calculating Insulin Dosages

_____

_____

_____

Reading Medication Labels

_____

_____

_____

_____

VOCABULARY REVIEW

Assignment 33-1: Sentence Completion

Fill in the blanks below with Essential Terms from this chapter.

1. A pharmacist or chemist was formerly known a(n) _____.

2. The _____ was the original or primary system used for calculating and measuring medication dosages.

3. A(n) _____ is the unit that is used when measuring anything that has mass or weight.

4. A(n) _____ is the fundamental unit for volume and is used when measuring liquids.

5. A(n) _____ is the fundamental unit for length and is used when measuring distance.

6. The _____ is used throughout the world and is the primary system for measuring weight, volume, and length (area).

7. A(n) _____ is a graph that illustrates a relationship between two known values.

Assignment 33-2: Matching I

Match the term with its definition and place the corresponding letter in the blank.

____ 1. Drug dosage

____ 2. Expiration date

____ 3. Generic name

____ 4. Lot control

____ 5. Medication label

____ 6. Prescription

____ 7. Product name

A. An order for a prescribed drug

B. The strength of the drug or amount to be given

C. Gives vital information about the product. Medications normally come with an insert, which has additional information that may be helpful in the administration of the medication.

D. Refers to the trade name or brand name of the medication

E. A drug's official name; can also be a listing of active and nonactive ingredients within the medication

F. Batch number used to track medications in the event that a bulk production of the drug must be recalled due to numerous reports of severe adverse reactions or product contamination

G. Guarantees the effectiveness and safe use of the medication up to the date posted on the drug package or container

CHAPTER REVIEW

Assignment 33-3: Acronym Review

Write what each of the following acronyms stands for.

1. BSA: _____

2. NDC: _____

3. PDR: _____

Assignment 33-4: Matching II

Match the term with its definition and place the corresponding letter in the blank.

___	1. Centi	A.	One-millionth of the base unit
___	2. Milli	B.	One thousand units
___	3. Micro	C.	One-thousandth of the base unit
___	4. Kilo	D.	One-hundredth of the base unit
___	5. Gram	E.	kg
___	6. Meter	F.	g
___	7. Kilogram	G.	mg
___	8. Milligram	H.	cc
___	9. Milliliter	I.	mm
___	10. Centimeter	J.	cm
___	11. Microgram	K.	m
___	12. Millimeter	L.	L
___	13. Liter	M.	mL
___	14. Cubic centimeter	N.	mcg

Assignment 33-5: Short Answer

1. Describe how insulin is measured and what type of syringe is used to administer insulin.

   _____

2. List and describe the types of insulin that are available.

   A. _____

   _____

   B. _____

   _____

   C. _____

   _____

3. List the important parts of a medication label.

   A. _____

   B. _____

   C. _____

   D. _____

   E. _____

   F. _____

   _____

Assignment 33-6: Certification Practice

Choose the best answer and place the corresponding letter in the blank.

____ 1. The patient is to receive 10 mL of Amoxicillin. How many teaspoonfuls should the patient take?

     A. 1.5 teaspoons

     B. 2 teaspoons

     C. 2.5 teaspoons

     D. 3 teaspoons

____ 2. If a physician prescribes 2 tbsp. twice a day, how many days will an 8 oz. bottle last?

     A. 2 days

     B. 3 days

     C. 4 days

     D. 1 week

____ 3. A child weighs 45.9 kg. Convert her weight to pounds (round to the nearest hundredth).

     A. 132.64 lb

     B. 69.58 lb

     C. 87.65 lb

     D. 100.98 lb

____ 4. 2 cups = _____

     A. 8 ounces

     B. 16 tablespoons

     C. 1 quart

     D. 1 pint

     E. None of the above

____ 5. Dosages of insulin are always measured in which of the following?

     A. Cubic millimeters

     B. Grams

     C. Micromilligrams

     D. Units

____ 6. Metric prefixes should be written in lowercase letters.

     A. True

     B. False

____ 7. Which of the following is the unit for length?

     A. Liter

     B. Gram

     C. Meter

____ 8. Which of the following is the unit for volume?

     A. Liter

     B. Gram

     C. Meter

____ 9. Which of the following is the unit for weight or mass?

     A. Liter

     B. Gram

     C. Meter

____ 10. A child weighs 66 pounds and the physician has ordered a daily dose of 30 mg/kg of body weight. The daily dose should divided into three equal doses. Which of the following dosages will be given to the patient per dose?

    A. 300 mg

    B. 600 mg

    C. 900 mg

    D. None of the above

____ 11. The physician orders Amoxicillin 0.05 g. Available is Amoxicillin 150 mg/5 mL. How many milliliters will you give the patient (round to the nearest tenth)?

    A. 1.5 mL

    B. 1.7 mL

    C. 2 mL

    D. 1 mL

____ 12. The physician orders 5 mg of Coumadin. On hand are 5 mg tablets. How many tablets will you give the patient?

    A. ½ tablet

    B. 1 tablet

    C. 1.5 tablets

    D. 2 tablets

____ 13. The physician orders 1.5 mg of Compazine, IM. Available is Compazine 5 mg/mL provided in 10 mL multidose vials. How many milliliters will you give the patient?

    A. 0.2 mL

    B. 0.3 mL

    C. 1.5 mL

    D. 3 mL

____ 14. When a metric measurement/symbol is named after a person, you should:

    A. capitalize the measurement.

    B. capitalize the symbol.

    C. not capitalize any metric measurements.

    D. both A and B.

    E. none of the above.

____ 15. Metric units do not have a singular or plural form.

    A. True

    B. False

____ 16. The Arabic number always follows the metric unit of measurement.

    A. True

    B. False

____ 17. According to the international convention, there should be no commas when writing long numbers: 25 232 (not 25,232).

    A. True

    B. False

____ 18. Which of the following persons is credited with developing the metric system?

    A. Gabriel Mouton

    B. Wilhelm Mouton

    C. Gabriel Wilhelm

    D. None of the above

SKILL APPLICATION CHALLENGES

Assignment 33-7: Math Review

1. Convert the following measurements. The conversion factor is 1 kg 5 2.2 lb (round your answers to the nearest hundredth when applicable).

   A. 38 lb = _____ kg

   B. 14 kg = _____ lb

   C. 67 kg = _____ lb

   D. 45 lb = _____ kg

   E. 113 lb = _____ kg

2. Convert the following units.

   A. 1,000 mcg = _____ mg

   B. 0.6 g = _____ kg

   C. 15.6 L = _____ mL

   D. 8 oz = _____ mL (there are 30 mL in 1 ounce)

   E. 1 cup = _____ oz

Assignment 33-8: Dosage Calculations

Calculate the correct number of tablets or capsules to be administered per dose. Tablets are scored. Show your work!

1. Order: 0.5 g of Duricef p.o.

   Supply: Duricef 500 mg tablets

   Answer: Give the patient _____ of Duricef (500 mg strength)

2. Order: Motrin 600 mg

   Supply: Motrin 300 mg tablets

   Answer: Give the patient _____ of Motrin (300 mg strength)

3. Order: Inderal 15 mg

   Supply: Inderal 10 mg tablets

   Answer: Give the patient _____ of Inderal (10 mg strength)

4. Order: Tylenol 0.5 g

   Supply: Tylenol (acetaminophen) liquid 500 mg in 5 mL

   Answer: Give the patient _____ of Tylenol

Assignment 33-9: Calculations Using Drug Labels

Read the following drug labels and calculate the following medication to be administered per dose. Show your work!

1. Order: Carafate 500 mg

   Answer: Give the patient _____ of Carafate

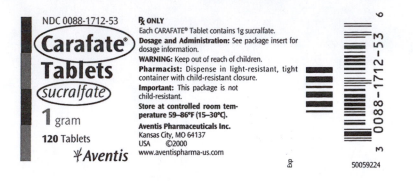

2. Order: 7.5 mg of Terbutaline

   Answer: Give the patient _____ of Terbutaline

3. Order: Promethazine 12.5 mg

    Answer: Give the patient _____ of Promethazine

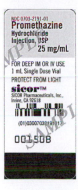

4. Order: Synthroid 0.3 mg

    Answer: Give the patient _____ of Synthroid

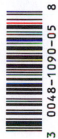

5. Order: Butorphanol 0.75 mg (round to the nearest hundredth)

   Answer: Give the patient _____ of Butorphanol

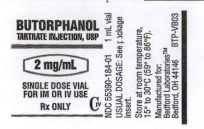

6. Order: 4 mg of Inaspine (round to the nearest tenth)

   Answer: Give the patient _____ of Inaspine

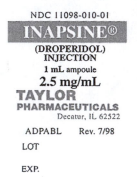

7. Order: 50 mg of Amoxil

   Answer: Give the patient _____ of Amoxil

   AMOXIL®
   125mg/5mL

   125mg/5mL
   NDC 0029-6008-22

   Directions for mixing: Tap bottle until all powder flows freely. Add approximately 1/3 total amount of water for reconstitution (total=116 mL); shake vigorously to wet powder. Add remaining water; again shake vigorously. Each 5 mL (1 teaspoonful) will contain amoxicillin trihydrate equivalent to 125 mg amoxicillin.
   Usual Adult Dosage: 250 to 500 mg every 8 hours.
   Usual Child Dosage: 20 to 40 mg/kg/day in divided doses every 8 hours, depending on age, weight and infection severity. See accompanying prescribing information.

   Keep tightly closed.
   Shake well before using.
   Refrigeration preferable but not required.
   Discard suspension after 14 days.

   AMOXIL®
   AMOXICILLIN
   FOR ORAL
   SUSPENSION

   R_x only

   150mL
   (when reconstituted)

   gsk **GlaxoSmithKline**

   Net contents: Equivalent to 3.75 grams amoxicillin. Store dry powder at room temperature.
   GlaxoSmithKline
   Research Triangle Park, NC 27709

   3 0029-6008-22 4

   LOT
   EXP.
   9405813-G

8. Order: 40 mg of Gentamicin

   Answer: Give the patient _____ of Gentamicin

   NDC 63323-010-02   1002
   GENTAMICIN
   INJECTION, USP
   equivalent to 40 mg/mL
   Gentamicin
   80 mg/2 mL
   For IM or IV Use.
   Must be diluted for IV use.
   2 mL Multiple Dose Vial
   Sterile
   Usual Dosage: See insert.
   APP AMERICAN PHARMACEUTICAL PARTNERS, INC.
   Los Angeles, CA 90024
   401896A

   SAMPLE

Assignment 33-10: Pediatric Dosage Calculations

1. The 12-year-old patient is to receive 5 mg/kg of Quivadil every 8 hours. The patient weighs 132 pounds.

   A. How much of the Quivadil should the patient receive per dose?

   Answer: The patient should receive _____ of the medication per dose

   B. How many total mg should the patient receive of the Quivadil per day? (Show your work.)

   Answer: The patient should receive _____ per day.

2. Referring to the above problem, if the label on the Quivadil bottle reads 250 mg/mL, how many mL should the patient receive per dose?

   Answer: The patient should receive _____of Quivadil.

3. A 2-year-old child has a BSA of 0.5. The adult dose of medication is 25 mg. What dosage should be given to the child? (Round to the nearest whole number.)

   Answer: The child should receive _____ of the medication.

4. A 4-year-old child has a BSA of 0.7. The adult dose of medication is 250 mg.
   A. What dosage should be given to the child? (Round your answer to the nearest whole number, but do not round answers until the final step.)
   Answer: The child should receive _____ of the medication

   B. The medication comes available in tablets of 75 mg, 100 mg, 125 mg, and 250 mg. What strength would be the most appropriate strength based on the physician's order?

   _____

   C. Why did you select the strength that you did?

   _____

   D. Should you check with the physician just to make certain before giving the patient the available dose?

   _____

   _____

FIELD APPLICATION CHALLENGES

Assignment 33-11

Read the following Field Application Challenges and respond to the questions following each scenario.

1. You just administered an oral medication to a child, and within five minutes the child vomits. Should you re-administer the drug?

   _____

   _____

2. You are explaining dosage instructions to a 12-year-old patient and her father. You explain that the medication is in capsule form. The father tells you that his daughter (the patient) has a difficult time swallowing any type of pills. What should you do?

   _____

   _____

   _____

   _____

   _____

JOURNALING EXERCISE

Assignment 33-12

What content within this chapter was most meaningful to you? Why? List some examples of how you might apply information contained in this chapter, both during your training and after you enter the health care industry.

C H A P T E R   **34**

Administration of Parenteral Medications

FIELD RELEVANCY AND BENEFITS

Administering parenteral medications is a rather common task performed by medical assistants in today's health care settings. Learning how to properly administer parenteral medications will help ensure that the medication is deposited within the correct tissue and prevent the patient from experiencing any needless complications or injuries. Gaining the skills introduced in this chapter will be beneficial for the majority of health care settings where medical assistants work including family practice, urgent care, specialty offices, and clinics.

NOTE SHEET

Administration of Parenteral Medications

_____

_____

_____

_____

Routes of Administration

_____

_____

_____

_____

Parenteral Complications

_____

_____

_____

_____

Immunizations

_____

_____

_____

_____

Basics of Intravenous Therapy

_____

_____

_____

_____

Intra-articular Injections

_____

_____

_____

_____

VOCABULARY REVIEW

Assignment 34-1: Definitions

Define the following terms.

1. Ampule: _____

2. Aqueous: _____

3. Bolus: _____

4. Cannula: _____

5. Diluent: _____

6. Gauge: _____

7. Occlusion: _____

8. Parenteral: _____

9. Phlebitis: _____

10. Precipitate: _____

11. Taut: _____

12. Vial: _____

Assignment 34-2: Misspelled Words

Underline the correctly spelled term.

1. Aspirate   Asporate   Asipirate

2. Hypudermic   Hyperdermic   Hypodermic

3. Infilration   Infiltrashion   Infiltration

4. Patency   Patoncy   Patiency

5. Thrombisis   Thrombosis   Thormbosis

6. Viscocity   Viscosity   Visocity

7. Wheal   Wheel   Weal

Assignment 34-3: Matching I

Match the term with its definition and place the corresponding letter in the blank.

____	1. Cartridge unit	A. The second drug to be drawn up; usually the cloudier medication
____	2. Cubic centimeter	B. Within the muscle
____	3. Extravasation	C. Threaded end in which the needle can be locked by twisting
____	4. Intra-articular	D. First drug to be drawn up when combining two drugs into one syringe; often the clearer medication
____	5. Intradermal	E. Within a joint
____	6. Intramuscular	F. Pertaining to under the dermis
____	7. Luer-Lok	G. Disposable prefilled cartridge of medication that slips into a nondisposable injection device
____	8. Primary drug	H. Unit used for the calibration of syringes (no longer used in charting because cc is considered a dangerous abbreviation; mL is used in its place)
____	9. Secondary drug	I. Medication fluid that leaks from the cannula or from the vein into the tissues surrounding the site
____	10. Subcutaneous	J. Pertaining to within the skin

CHAPTER REVIEW

Assignment 34-4: Short Answer

1. List five separate routes used for delivering parenteral medications.

   _____

   _____

2. List four common parenteral routes by injection and mark those that are routinely performed by the medical assistant with an X.

   Performed by Medical Assistant

   A. _____   _____

   B. _____   _____

   C. _____   _____

   D. _____   _____

3. Describe factors that help determine the size of the syringe, length of needle, and the gauge of needle to be used.

   A. _____

   _____

   B. _____

   _____

   C. _____

   _____

4. List several complications that may occur when administering IV therapy.

   _____

   _____

   _____

5. Explain why Z-track injections are not massaged after injection.

_____

_____

6. What protocol should be followed when upon aspiration there is blood in the syringe?

_____

_____

_____

7. The purpose of forcing air into the vial is to equalize the pressure within the vial after the medication has been removed.

A. What happens if the proper amount of air is not inserted?

_____

_____

B. What happens when too much air is inserted?

_____

_____

8. What two vaccines should not be given to pregnant patients?

_____

Assignment 34-5: Matching II

Match the type of injection to the description. Answers may be used more than once.

____ 1. Deltoid, gluteus, ventrogluteal,
         dorsogluteal, vastus lateralis   A. Intradermal injection

____ 2. 10- to 15-degree angle   B. Subcutaneous injection

____ 3. TB testing   C. Intramuscular injection

____ 4. 23–25 G   D. Intravenous injection

____ 5. Upper, fleshy part of arm

____ 6. No more than 1.0 mL

____ 7. Normally 20–23 G (may use larger gauge for really viscid medications)

____ 8. 20–21 G

____ 9. 45- to 90-degree angle

____ 10. Thicker medications

____ 11. 26–27 G

____ 12. No aspiration

____ 13. ½- to ⅝-inch

____ 14. 90 degree

____ 15. ⅜- to ⅝-inch

____ 16. No more than 3 mL

Assignment 34-6: True or False

Fill in the blank with a "T" for true statements and an "F" for false statements. Rewrite the false statements to make them true.

____ 1. The larger the gauge, the smaller the diameter of the needle.

_____

_____

____ 2. IM injections will require a longer needle than subcutaneous or intradermal injections because muscles are deeper.

_____

_____

____ 3. Unit is the amount of a substance necessary to stimulate a systematic effect.

_____

_____

____ 4. The stopper of the vial must be cleansed with alcohol each time medication is withdrawn.

_____

_____

____ 5. When giving an intradermal injection, one should aspirate.

_____

_____

____ 6. When administering a subcutaneous injection, one should hold the skin taut.

_____

_____

Assignment 34-7: Certification Practice

Choose the best answer and place the corresponding letter in the blank.

____ 1. What type of diluent is typically used to reconstitute powders?
   A. Sterile peroxide
   B. Sterile alcohol
   C. Sterile saline
   D. Sterile chloride

____ 2. All of the following are types of medication that are single-dose and available in prefilled cartridges *except*:
   A. Penicillin G.
   B. Phenergan.
   C. DepoProvera.
   D. Albuterol.

____ 3. At what angle should an intradermal injection be given?
   A. 5-degree
   B. 10- to 15-degree
   C. 45-degree
   D. 90-degree

____ 4. At what angle should an intramuscular injection be given?

    A. 5-degree

    B. 10- to 15-degree

    C. 45-degree

    D. 90-degree

____ 5. At what angle should a subcutaneous injection be given?

    A. 5-degree

    B. 10- to 15-degree

    C. 90-degree

    D. None apply

____ 6. At what angle should an IV be started at?

    A. 25-degree

    B. 10- to 15-degree

    C. 45-degree

    D. 90-degree

____ 7. All of the following would be sites for subcutaneous injection *except:*

    A. inner forearm.

    B. upper arm.

    C. lower abdomen.

    D. thigh region.

____ 8. What nerve should be avoided when administering IM injection into the dorsogluteal site?

    A. Ulnar

    B. Sciatic

    C. Femoral

    D. Popiliteal

____ 9. All of the following would be common medications given subcutaneously *except:*

    A. MMR.

    B. insulin injections.

    C. allergy injections.

    D. allergy extracts for testing.

____ 10. Which of the following routes would you use for allergy testing?

    A. Intradermal

    B. Subcutaneous

    C. IM

    D. Z-track

____ 11. Which of the following routes would you use if the medication may cause irritation or discoloration to superficial layers of tissue or to the skin?

    A. Intradermal

    B. Subcutaneous

    C. IM

    D. Z-track

____ 12. Which of the following routes is used for most vaccinations?

    A. Intradermal

    B. Subcutaneous

    C. IM

    D. Z-track

____ 13. Which of the following routes is used for hormone injections?

    A. Intradermal

    B. Subcutaneous

    C. IM

    D. Z-track

____ 14. Which of the following routes should be used for the MMR vaccine?

    A. Intradermal

    B. Subcutaneous

    C. IM

    D. Z-track

____ 15. Which of the following routes should be used for TB testing?

    A. Intradermal

    B. Subcutaneous

    C. IM

    D. Z-track

____ 16. Which of the following are benefits of IV therapy?

    A. Hydration

    B. Homeostasis

    C. Fast results

    D. All of the above

____ 17. The term phlebitis means:

    A. blood clot.

    B. blood bruise.

    C. vessel collapse.

    D. inflammation of a vein.

____ 18. The most common joint for intra-articular injections would be the:

    A. shoulder.

    B. knee.

    C. elbow.

    D. hip.

____ 19. Which of the following types of IV solution is typically used for a patient who needs to be rehydrated?

    A. 5% Dextrose in water

    B. Normal saline

    C. Dextrose in saline solution

    D. Ringer's Solution

____ 20. All of the following statements are true about intramuscular injections *except:*

    A. insert at a 45-degree angle.

    B. use the deltoid, gluteal, and vastus lateralis muscles.

    C. aspirate to ensure the needle is not in a blood vessel.

    D. use a 20–23 G and 1- to 3-inch needle (a larger gauge may be necessary for really viscid medications).

____ 21. All of the following statements are true about subcutaneous injections *except:*

    A. use for allergy injections, some immunizations, and insulin.

    B. inject in the fatty portion of the upper arm, thigh, or abdominal area.

    C. use no more than 3.0 cc.

    D. insert at a 45- to 90-degree angle.

____ 21. Which of the following is the maximum dose that you can administer for intramuscular injections?

    A. 0.5 mL

    B. 2.0 mL

    C. 3.0 mL

    D. 4.0 mL

____ 22. The length of the needle is determined by the:

    A. route of administration and amount of adipose tissue.

    B. amount of medication to be delivered.

    C. viscosity of the medication.

    D. all of the above.

____ 23. The needle's gauge is determined by the:

    A. size of the patient's muscle/amount of fat.

    B. amount of medication to be delivered.

    C. viscosity of the medication.

    D. all of the above.

____ 24. Syringe size is determined by the:

    A. size of the patient's muscle/amount of fat.

    B. amount of medication to be delivered.

    C. viscosity of the medication.

    D. all of the above.

____ 25. Routine medications that are administered in the deltoid are:

    A. medications less than 1.0 cc.

    B. medications that are aqueous-based.

    C. routine immunizations.

    D. all of the above.

____ 26. Routine medications that are administered using the subcutaneous route include all but which of the following?

    A. Allergy shots

    B. Hepatitis B and flu vaccines

    C. Insulin shots

    D. MMR, IPV and VA vaccines

____ 27. All of the following statements are true about intravenous injections *except:*

    A. the medical assistant may prepare medications to be given.

    B. use a needle gauge of 20–21 G.

    C. state laws may vary as to who may administer intravenous medications.

    D. it provides the slowest absorption of all parenteral routes.

SKILLS APPLICATION CHALLENGES

Assignment 34-7: Labeling

1. Label the parts of this syringe.

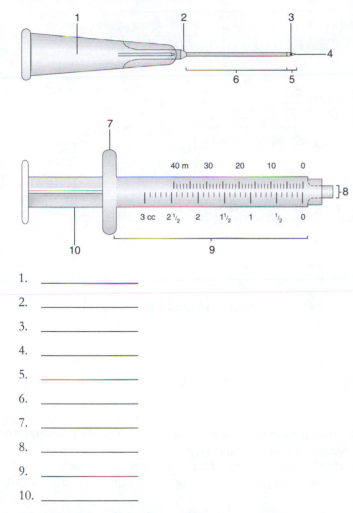

1. _____

2. _____

3. _____

4. _____

5. _____

6. _____

7. _____

8. _____

9. _____

10. _____

2. Label the angles of injections and list the type of injection that matches each angle (i.e., intradermal, subcutaneous, IM) in these pictures.

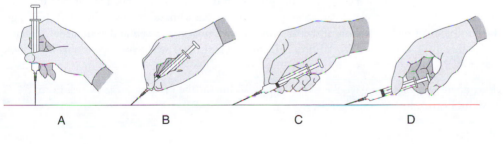

A. _____

B. _____

C. _____

D. _____

Assignment 34-8: Syringe Review

Illustrate the amount of medication that should be drawn up in each syringe by coloring the amount of medication requested with a colored pencil, marker, or crayon.

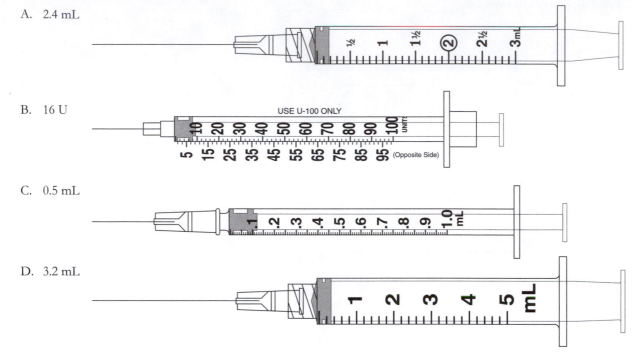

A. 2.4 mL

B. 16 U

C. 0.5 mL

D. 3.2 mL

COMPLETING SPECIAL FORMS

Assignment 34-9: Immunization Activity

Work Forms Necessary: FORMS 34-1, 34-2, 34-3, 34-4

Directions: This assignment has two parts. First, role play with another student to simulate preparing a patient to receive an immunization. Second, document the immunization in the patient's progress note and the immunization log. (Note: You wouldn't ordinarily need to document manufacturer, lot number, and expiration info on both the progress note and log, but for practice purposes, document this information on both forms.)

A. With one of your fellow students, role play as medical assistant and patient using Work Form 34-1 (a VIS form). The patient's name is Lori Wise. Once you have finished going over the form with the patient, have the patient sign the consent form (Work Form 34-2). Use 07/18/11 as today's date. Sign your name as the witness, followed by SMA. Now, go to the CDC Web site and print the most recent version of the flu VIS form. (Go to *www.cdc.gov* and search for "Vaccine Information Statement.") Give this form, along with Work Form 34-2, to your instructor when you turn in this workbook assignment.

B. Using the information below, document that you gave the patient a flu vaccine on the progress note (Work Form 34-3) and in the vaccination log (Work Form 34-4).

   • Today's date: 07/18/11

   • Time: 10:55 a.m.

   • Patient's name: Lori Wise

   • Amount given: 0.5 mL

   • Location: Right deltoid

   • Route: IM

   • Ordering provider: Dr. Pella

- Manufacturer's name: Glaxo-Smith

- Lot number: 39838

- Expiration date: 02/12

- Medical assistant: Your Name

- Postinjection observation: No reactions

- Vaccination consent form signed and patient signed a consent form

FIELD APPLICATION CHALLENGE

Assignment 34-9

Read the following Field Application Challenge and respond to the questions following the scenario.

You work for a busy family practice and are in charge of ordering all of the medications. Unlike most medications, flu vaccine has to be ordered early in the year (usually during the months of February and March). If you forget to order the vaccine during those months, when flu shot season rolls around (in October and November) the office may be unable to obtain the vaccine, leaving patients scrambling to find other places to get their vaccines.

1. Based on this scenario, what can you do to make certain that this same scenario doesn't occur in your office?

_____

_____

2. Flu vaccines are water-soluble and the amount that is given to each patient is 0.5 mL. These vaccines are to be given intramuscularly. What site would be best for adults? For children under the age of 5?

_____

_____

3. When giving an injection in the deltoid, which arm is the best arm to use and why?

_____

_____

4. What population of people seen in your office will receive the majority of flu vaccine?

_____

5. Based on the location of the injection, the viscosity of the medication, and the population of patients receiving the vaccine, what gauges and lengths of needles should you have onhand during flu vaccine season?

_____

_____

_____

_____

6. If there is a shortage of the flu vaccine, which patients should receive the vaccine before others?

_____

_____

7. Why is it important to document vaccines into a medication log?

_____

_____

_____

8. Explain why it is important to ask patients about drug allergies each time they come into your office?

_____

_____

9. What other allergies should you inquire about from patients receiving flu shots? (Hint: This information can be found in a Field Smart box in Chapter 32.)

_____

JOURNALING EXERCISE
Assignment 34-10

What content within this chapter was most meaningful to you? Why? List some examples of how you might apply information contained in this chapter, both during your training and after you enter the health care industry.

Work Form 34-1

INACTIVATED INFLUENZA VACCINE

(WHAT YOU NEED TO KNOW) 2007-08

1 | Why get vaccinated?

Influenza ("flu") is a contagious disease.

It is caused by the influenza virus, which spreads from infected persons to the nose or throat of others.

Other illnesses can have the same symptoms and are often mistaken for influenza. But only an illness caused by the influenza virus is really influenza.

Anyone can get influenza, but rates of infection are highest among children. For most people, it lasts only a few days. It can cause:

· fever	· sore throat	· chills	· fatigue
· cough	· headache	· muscle aches	

Some people get much sicker. Influenza can lead to pneumonia and can be dangerous for people with heart or breathing conditions. It can cause high fever and seizures in children. On average, 226,000 people are hospitalized every year because of influenza and 36,000 die – mostly elderly.

Influenza vaccine can prevent influenza.

2 | Inactivated Influenza vaccine

There are two types of influenza vaccine:

Inactivated (killed) vaccine, or the "flu shot" is given by injection into the muscle.

Live, attenuated (weakened) influenza vaccine, called LAIV, is sprayed into the nostrils. *This vaccine is described in a separate Vaccine Information Statement.*

For most people influenza vaccine prevents serious influenza-related illness. But it will *not* prevent "influenza-like" illnesses caused by other viruses.

Influenza viruses are always changing. Because of this, influenza vaccines are updated every year, and an annual vaccination is recommended. Protection lasts up to a year.

It takes up to 2 weeks for protection to develop after the vaccination.

Some inactivated influenza vaccine contains thimerosal, a preservative that contains mercury. Some people believe thimerosal may be related to developmental problems in children. In 2004 the Institute of Medicine published a report concluding that, based on scientific studies, there is no evidence of such a relationship. If you are concerned about thimerosal, ask your doctor about thimerosal-free influenza vaccine.

3 | Who should get inactivated influenza vaccine?

People 6 months of age and older can receive inactivated influenza vaccine. It is recommended for **anyone who is at risk of complications from influenza or more likely to require medical care:**

- **All children** from 6 months up to 5 years of age.
- Anyone **50 years of age or older.**
- Anyone 6 months to 18 years of age on **long-term aspirin treatment** (they could develop Reye Syndrome if they got influenza).
- Women who will be **pregnant** during influenza season.
- Anyone with **long-term health problems** with:
  - heart disease
  - lung disease
  - asthm
  - kidney disease
  - metabolic disease, such as diabetes
  - anemia, and other blood disorders
- Anyone with a **weakened immune system** due to:
  - HIV/AIDS or other diseases affecting the immune system
  - long-term treatment with drugs such as steroids
  - cancer treatment with x-rays or drugs
- Anyone with certain **muscle or nerve disorders** (such as seizure disorders or severe cerebral palsy) that can lead to breathing or swallowing problems.
- **Residents of nursing homes** and **other chronic-care facilities.**

Influenza vaccine is also recommended for anyone who lives with or cares for people at high risk for influenza-related complications:

- **Health care providers.**
- **Household contacts and caregivers of children** from birth up to 5 years of age.
- **Household contacts and caregivers** of people 50 years and older, and those with medical conditions that put them at higher risk for severe complications from influenza.

A yearly influenza vaccination should be *considered* for:

- People who provide **essential community services.**
- People living in **dormitories** or under other crowded conditions, to prevent outbreaks.
- People at high risk of influenza complications who **travel** to the Southern hemisphere between April and September, or to the tropics or in organized tourist groups at any time.

Influenza vaccine is also recommended for anyone who wants to **reduce the likelihood of becoming ill** with influenza or **spreading influenza to others.**

(Continues)

Work Form 34-1 *(Continued)*

4 When should I get influenza vaccine?

Plan to get influenza vaccine in October or November if you can. But getting vaccinated in December, or even later, will still be beneficial in most years. You can get the vaccine as soon as it is available, and for as long as illness is occurring. Influenza illness can occur any time from November through May. Most cases usually occur in January or February.

Most people need one dose of influenza vaccine each year. **Children younger than 9 years of age getting influenza vaccine for the first time** should get 2 doses. For inactivated vaccine, these doses should be given at least 4 weeks apart.

Influenza vaccine may be given at the same time as other vaccines, including pneumococcal vaccine.

5 Some people should talk with a doctor before getting influenza vaccine

Some people should not get inactivated influenza vaccine or should wait before getting it.

• Tell your doctor if you have any **severe** (life-threatening) allergies. Allergic reactions to influenza vaccine are rare.
  - Influenza vaccine virus is grown in eggs. People with a severe egg allergy should not get the vaccine.
  - A severe allergy to any vaccine component is also a reason to not get the vaccine.
  - If you have had a severe reaction after a previous dose of influenza vaccine, tell your doctor.

• Tell your doctor if you ever had Guillain-Barré Syndrome (a severe paralytic illness, also called GBS). You may be able to get the vaccine, but your doctor should help you make the decision.

• People who are moderately or severely ill should usually wait until they recover before getting flu vaccine. If you are ill, talk to your doctor or nurse about whether to reschedule the vaccination. People with a **mild illness** can usually get the vaccine.

6 What are the risks from inactivated influenza vaccine?

A vaccine, like any medicine, could possibly cause serious problems, such as severe allergic reactions. The risk of a vaccine causing serious harm, or death, is extremely small.

Serious problems from influenza vaccine are very rare. The viruses in inactivated influenza vaccine have been killed, so you cannot get influenza from the vaccine.

Mild problems:
• soreness, redness, or swelling where the shot was given
• fever • aches
If these problems occur, they usually begin soon after the shot and last 1-2 days.

Severe problems:
• Life-threatening allergic reactions from vaccines are very rare. If they do occur, it is usually within a few minutes to a few hours after the shot.

• In 1976, a certain type of influenza (swine flu) vaccine was associated with Guillain-Barré Syndrome (GBS). Since then, flu vaccines have not been clearly linked to GBS. However, if there is a risk of GBS from current flu vaccines, it would be no more than 1 or 2 cases per million people vaccinated. This is much lower than the risk of severe influenza, which can be prevented by vaccination.

7 What if there is a severe reaction?

What should I look for?
Any unusual condition, such as a high fever or behavior changes. Signs of a serious allergic reaction can include difficulty breathing, hoarseness or wheezing, hives, paleness, weakness, a fast heart beat or dizziness.

What should I do?
Call a doctor, or get the person to a doctor right away.

• **Tell** your doctor what happened, the date and time it happened, and when the vaccination was given.

• **Ask** your doctor, nurse, or health department to report the reaction by filing a Vaccine Adverse Event Reporting System (VAERS) form.

Or you can file this report through the VAERS web site at www.vaers.hhs.gov, or by calling 1-800-822-7967.
VAERS does not provide medical advice.

8 The National Vaccine Injury Compensation Program

In the event that you or your child has a serious reaction to a vaccine, a federal program has been created to help pay for the care of those who have been harmed.

For details about the National Vaccine Injury Compensation Program, call **1-800-338-2382** or visit their website at **www.hrsa.gov/vaccinecompensation.**

9 How can I learn more?

• Ask your immunization provider. They can give you the vaccine package insert or suggest other sources of information.

• Call your local or state health department.

• Contact the Centers for Disease Control and Prevention (CDC):
  - Call **1-800-232-4636 (1-800-CDC-INFO)**
  - Visit CDC's website at **www.cdc.gov/flu**

DEPARTMENT OF HEALTH AND HUMAN SERVICES
CENTERS FOR DISEASE CONTROL AND PREVENTION

Work Form 34-2

DOUGLASVILLE MEDICINE ASSOCIATES
5076 BRAND BLVD
DOUGLASVILLE, NY 01234
(123) 456-7890

IMMUNIZATION CONSENT FORM

I have read the Vaccination Information Statements(s) regarding the following immunizations listed below and am aware of the adverse reactions associated with the vaccine(s). I have had an opportunity to ask questions regarding the possible adverse reactions and benefits of each immunization. I believe that the benefits outweigh the risks and I assume full responsibility for any reactions that may occur.

1._____   2._____

3._____   4._____

I am requesting that the immunization (s) be given to me or the person listed below for whom I am the legal guardian.

_____   _____
Signature /Legal Guardian   Today's Date

_____   _____
Print Name   Witness

Work Form 34-3

Work Form 34-4

DOUGLASVILLE MEDICINE ASSOCIATES
5076 BRAND BLVD
DOUGLASVILLE, NY 01234
(123) 456-7890

FLU VACCINE LOG								
Today's Date	Patient's Name	Ordering Physician	Amt Given	Manufacturer's Name	Lot Number	Exp. Date	MA	Time
07/18/2011	Gunter, Thomas	Little	0.5 mL	Glaxo-Smith	39838	02/2012	NS	10:45 am

C H A P T E R **35**

Urgent Care and Emergency Procedures

FIELD RELEVANCY AND BENEFITS

Working in the medical industry is anything but mundane. Emergencies happen quite often and medical assistants must be prepared to appropriately respond. Urgent care is a newer specialty to the ambulatory community and is booming. Many urgent care centers are staffed with medical assistants. The medical assistant who has specialized training in urgent care procedures will be better prepared to work in these types of centers upon graduation. The information contained in this chapter will equip you to handle office emergencies and provide you with the edge that is necessary to obtain a position in urgent care.

NOTE SHEET

On the Scene Emergency Procedures

_____

_____

_____

_____

The Urgent Care Industry

_____

_____

_____

_____

Preparing Personnel for Emergencies

_____

_____

_____

Triaging in Ambulatory Care

_____

_____

_____

VOCABULARY REVIEW

Assignment 35-1: Definitions

Define the following terms.

1. Embolus: _____

2. Diaphoresis: _____

3. Paresthesia: _____

4. Syncope: _____

5. Thrombus: _____

6. Heat stroke: _____

_____

7. Heat exhaustion: _____

8. Ischemia: _____

Assignment 35-2: Matching I

Match the term with its definition and place the corresponding letter in the blank.

____ 1. Abrasions

____ 2. Acute abdomen

____ 3. Anaphylaxis

____ 4. AVPU scale

____ 5. Asthma

____ 6. Automated external defibrillator

____ 7. Cardiopulmonary resuscitation

____ 8. First responder

____ 9. Chest compressions

____ 10. Concussion

____ 11. Crash cart

____ 12. Defibrillation

____ 13. Diabetic coma

____ 14. DOTS

A. Injury in which the brain is jarred

B. Chronic lung disease which causes the bronchial tubes to constrict and block the flow of air

C. Drugs or electrical shock used to restore normal contractions to the heart

D. Superficial scrapes that may be very painful

E. Cart that stocks all of the medications and supplies used in an emergency

F. Sudden or abrupt onset of intense abdominal pain

G. Life-threatening condition in which patient's blood sugar is dangerously high

H. A procedure to restore heart and lung function

I. Scale used by medics to determine the patient's level of consciousness

J. Acronym used when checking for other disabilities following the ABCD portion of CPR

K. First person to arrive at the scene of an emergency (in the workplace, a person with specialized training to respond to emergencies)

L. Severe allergic reaction to an allergen usually in the form of food, medication, a chemical, or an insect sting or bite

M. Maneuver in which the rescuer pushes up and down on the lower half of the sternum several times to compress the heart

N. Automated unit that defibrillates the heart

Assignment 35-3: Matching II

Match the term with its definition and place the corresponding letter in the blank.

____	1. Frostbite	A.	Breaths given during CPR
____	2. Heat cramps	B.	Process in which patient's symptoms are ranked in terms of importance or priority
____	3. Hemorrhaging	C.	Fatal condition that can be brought on by disease, injury, decrease in circulation, and/or fluid loss
____	4. Hypothermia	D.	Irregular-shaped cuts with jagged edges; may appear as a tear
____	5. Insulin shock	E.	Cramping that occurs when the body becomes overheated; confined to the abdomen and legs
____	6. Incision	F.	Position used to manage victims until the EMS arrives
____	7. Laceration	G.	Occurs when the ventricles of the heart twitch or flutter with no organized movement
____	8. Ventilation	H.	Sudden attacks that result from a malfunction of the brain; the two types are petite mal and grand mal
____	8. Pulse oximeter	I.	Uncontrollable bleeding
____	9. Puncture	J.	Local injury of skin due to freezing or subfreezing conditions
____	10. Recovery position	K.	Life-threatening condition in which the patient's blood sugar is very low
____	11. Seizures	L.	Blood pressure that drops upon standing
____	12. Shock	M.	Cuts in the skin made from sharp instruments or glass
____	13. Traumatic brain injury	N.	A condition that occurs when body temperature falls below 95°F or 35°C
____	14. Triage	O.	Device to measure the oxygen saturation level of the blood
____	15. Orthostatic hypotension	P.	Penetrating wound that leaves a hole in the skin; may be superficial or deep
____	16. Ventricular fibrillation	Q.	Injury to the brain caused by trauma

CHAPTER REVIEW

Assignment 35-4: Acronym Review

Write what each of the following acronyms stands for.

1. PPE: _____

2. DOTS: _____

3. TIA: _____

4. CVA: _____

5. AED: _____

Assignment 35-5: Short Answer

1. List the meaning or step for each letter in the mnemonic ABCDDR.

   A _____

   B _____

   C _____

   D _____

   D _____

   R _____

2. What is the purpose of cardiopulmonary resuscitation?

   _____

3. List common medications and supplies that can be found on a crash cart.

   Equipment and Supplies   *Respiration Devices*

   _____   _____

   _____   _____

   _____   _____

   _____   _____

   _____   _____

   _____   _____

4. Define triage and discuss the role of the medical assistant in triaging patients in the medical office.

   A. Triage is: _____

   B. The medical assistant's role is: _____

   _____

   _____

   _____

   _____

5. Discuss what signs the medical assistant should observe both before and after splinting a patient's limb.

   A. Before splinting: _____

   _____

   B. After splinting: _____

   _____

6. Explain the purpose of the AVPU scale and what each letter represents

   _____

   _____

   _____

7. State what each of the letters in the RICE and MICE acronyms stand for.

   _____

   _____

9. When would you use the RICE or MICE treatments?

_____

_____

_____

_____

Assignment 35-6: True or False

Fill in the blank with a "T" for true statements and an "F" for false statements. Rewrite the false statements to make them true.

____ 1. The order in which patients are seen in an urgent care facility is first determined by the seriousness of their symptoms and then on the order of their arrival.

_____

_____

____ 2. Acute episodes of hyperglycemia are usually more serious than acute episodes of hypoglycemia

_____

_____

____ 3. Chest compressions assist in delivering the oxygen that was ventilated into the patient's lungs during the breathing phase of CPR to cells throughout the body.

_____

_____

____ 4. Defibrillators can be used on infants.

_____

_____

____ 5. Exercise lowers blood sugar.

_____

_____

____ 6. If cervical spine injuries are likely, the rescuer should use the head tilt/chin lift maneuver to open the airway.

_____

_____

____ 7. If unsure whether a victim is suffering from hyperglycemia or hypoglycemia, treat for hyperglycemia.

_____

_____

____ 8. Fainting is not a disease but rather a symptom of an underlying condition or disease.

_____

_____

____ 9. The legs and arms are the most vulnerable sites to frostbite.

_____

_____

____ 10. Defibrillation should not be performed on someone with a pacemaker.

_____

_____

Assignment 35-7: Insulin Shock and Diabetic Coma Activity

Indicate whether the following symptoms would be experienced by someone who is more likely to slip into a diabetic coma (C) or for someone who is more likely to slip into insulin shock (S).

_____ 1. Confused and disoriented

_____ 2. Headache

_____ 3. Gradual onset

_____ 4. Skin is pale, cool, and clammy

_____ 5. Drowsiness

_____ 6. Thirst is intense

_____ 7. Fruity odor from the mouth

_____ 8. Pulse is full and pounding

_____ 9. Low blood sugar

_____ 10. High blood sugar

Assignment 35-8: Bleeding Emergency Activity

Indicate whether the following symptoms are Artery (A), Vein (V), or Capillary (C).

_____ 1. Bright red blood

_____ 2. Hard to control

_____ 3. Easy to control

_____ 4. Dark red blood

_____ 5. Steady flow of blood

_____ 6. Blood oozes

_____ 7. Blood spurts

_____ 8. Is not life-threatening

_____ 9. May cause great blood loss

Assignment 35-9: Certification Practice

Choose the best answer and place the corresponding letter in the blank.

____ 1. Which of the following drugs would not likely to be found on an emergency cart?

    A. Epinephrine injection

    B. Imitrex injection

    C. Lidocaine

    D. Dopamine

____ 2. All of the following are PPE *except:*

    A. gloves.

    B. gowns.

    C. mask.

    D. surgical cap.

_____ 3. If a victim has a pacemaker, in which of the following locations should the rescuer place AED electrode pads?

A. No change in placement

B. 3 inches from the pacemaker

C. 2 inches from the pacemaker

D. 1 inch from the pacemaker

_____ 4. All of the following symptoms are true for a patient experiencing hypoglycemia *except:*

A. skin is red, hot, and dry.

B. poor coordination.

C. headache.

D. confusion and disorientation.

_____ 5. Another term for heart attack is:

A. ischemic attack.

B. myocardial infarction.

C. ventricular fibrillation.

D. angina.

_____ 6. Epitasis is another term for:

A. artery.

B. diabetes.

C. nose bleed.

D. abdomen.

_____ 7. Poisons can enter the body through which of the following routes?

A. Inhalation

B. Ingestion

C. Injection

D. Absorption

E. All of the above

_____ 8. A severe, potentially life-threatening allergic reaction is called _____ shock.

A. neurogenic

B. cardiogenic

C. psychogenic

D. anaphylactic

_____ 10. Which of the following is the first step used to control external bleeding?

A. Elevation

B. Pressure points

C. Direct pressure

D. Tourniquet

_____ 11. Treatment of epistaxis includes all of the following *except:*

A. pressure to the upper lip and gum.

B. tilting the head forward.

C. cold compress.

D. lying the patient down.

E. pinching the nostrils.

_____ 12. Which of the following is common for an arterial bleed?

A. Bright red blood that spurts

B. Dark red blood that flows steadily

C. Dark red blood that oozes

D. Bright red blood that oozes

___ 13. A burn that is consistent with pain and blistering is a _____ burn.
A. first degree
B. second degree
C. third degree
D. fourth degree

___ 14. The proper first aid treatment for dry chemical burns to the skin includes all the following *except:*
A. remove any clothing in the area.
B. brush off dry chemicals.
C. rinse off dry chemicals with water.
D. Rinse skin after dry chemicals have been completely brushed away from the skin.

___ 15. Which of the following is the initial treatment for a sprain?
A. Casting
B. Surgery
C. Apply heat
D. Apply ice

___ 16. An injury to a muscle due to overworking or overstretching that muscle is called a:
A. dislocation.
B. sprain.
C. fracture.
D. strain.

___ 17. A patient enters the urgent care center with a severe burn to the hand. If available, what room should the patient be placed in?
A. Basic examination room
B. Cardiac bay/trauma room
C. Procedure room
D. None of the above

___ 17. When a patient comes in with a painful burn, what can be done until he or she can be seen by the provider to help ease pain?
A. Place sterile gauze over the burn and rinse with sterile saline.
B. Apply burn ointment with anesthetic over the burn.
C. Give the patient some Demerol IM, while the patient is waiting.
D. Wrap the burn in a sterile gauze dressing.

___ 18. A patient comes into the urgent care center with a gaping wound that has moderate bleeding. Which of the following steps should *not* be included while waiting for the provider?
A. Place patient in procedure room.
B. Apply direct pressure, elevate affected area, and apply pressure to pressure points if necessary to stop the bleeding.
C. Place Steri-strips over wound to help stop the bleeding.
D. Set up suture tray in the event that the provider wants to suture the patient.

___ 19. A patient comes into the office with severe abdominal pain that came on suddenly. She is very nauseated, has a fever, and is quite thirsty. Which of the following steps should be performed until the provider is available?
A. Immediately place the patient in a basic examination room.
B. Get all IV supplies ready in the event that the provider wants to start an IV.
C. Give the patient some water to quench her thirst.
D. Perform an EKG and chest x-ray.

____ 20. A patient enters the office with possible frostbite. Which of the following steps should you take until the provider is available?

    A. Allow frostbitten area to warm naturally; may also cover affected area with sheet or blanket.

    B. Wrap the area in an electric warming blanket.

    C. Gently rub the area to help assist with circulation and warming.

    D. Place affected area in very warm or hot water.

SKILL APPLICATION CHALLENGE
Assignment 35-10: Case Study

You are working for an urgent care center. Three patients arrive all about the same time. Patient 1 received an eye injury while at work. A tiny piece of wood flew in her eye, and she is unable to keep her eye open. Patient 2 has severe stomach flu-like symptoms and may be dehydrated, and Patient 3 is experiencing chest pain. In what order should these patients be seen? Why? What steps will you take for each patient to get them ready for the provider?

Patient	Priority (1, 2, 3)	Steps Taken to Prepare the Patient for the Provider
Patient 1	_____	
Patient 2	_____	
Patient 3	_____	

FIELD APPLICATION CHALLENGES
Assignment 35-11
Read the following Field Application Challenges and respond to the questions following each scenario.

1. When performing emergency assessment on a collapsed victim near your home, you notice the victim is wearing a medical identification bracelet. How is this information useful to a first responder?

   _____

   _____

2. You just administered an allergy injection and within a matter of minutes, the patient collapses on the floor.
   A. What could be wrong with the patient?

   _____

   B. What steps should you take in order to assist the patient?

   _____

   _____

   _____

   _____

   _____

   _____

   _____

3. A middle-aged man walks into your office, collapses onto the floor, and begins to shake uncontrollably. Coworkers state that the patient has a history of epilepsy. As you approach him, you see that he is breathing. His eyes are open but he does not respond when you call him by name.

   A. What could be wrong with the patient?

   _____

   B. What measures should you take to help the patient?

   _____

   _____

   _____

   _____

4. A father calls in to state that his 2-year-old daughter has gotten into the medicine cabinet and has chewed up and swallowed three Xanax tablets.

   A. What question should the medical assistant ask the father?

   _____

   B. If the daughter is unconscious or not breathing, what should be the medical assistant's course of action?

   _____

   _____

   _____

   _____

   _____

C. If the daughter is both conscious and breathing, what instructions should you give to the father?

_____

_____

JOURNALING EXERCISE
Assignment 35-12

What content within this chapter was most meaningful to you? Why? List some examples of how you might apply information contained in this chapter, both during your training and after you enter the health care industry.

PART 2

Exercises for SynapseEHR 1.1:
An Electronic Charting Simulation

INTRODUCTION TO SYNAPSE

SYNAPSE is an electronic charting program that simulates documenting information within an electronic medical record. SYNAPSE exercises incorporate many activities that mimic tasks the medical assistant will perform while working in an electronic medical record (EMR). SYNAPSE uses a variety of techniques to build chart notes, including:

- Entering free text in the chart note
- Clicking drop-down lists to populate information in the chart note
- Using standard templates

SYNAPSE allows students to get a feel of how the EMR works without getting into a great deal of extraneous technical content.

INSTRUCTIONS FOR INITIAL SETUP

1. The Sign-In screen is the first screen that will appear when SYNAPSE opens. You will notice a box labeled "Username" with the word "Student1" and a Password box that already has a password installed. These are the initial settings to get you into the program, so just click OK. You should now be in the main menu.

CHANGING YOUR USERNAME AND PASSWORD

1. You will notice an icon labeled "Change Password." This icon will open a screen to allow you to set up the software using your own name and password. Click the Change Password icon.

2. Enter your first name in the First Name box.

3. Enter your last name in the Last Name box.

4. Enter a username in the Username box. This may be a combination of your first and last name, or a name your instructor will assign you.

5. Next, enter a password. Write down this information so that it is handy in case you forget your username or password. The information is case-sensitive, so pay close attention to whether uppercase or lowercase letters are used.

6. Click the Save icon.

7. Click the Close icon.

8. Click the Quit icon.

9. Reopen the SYNAPSE software.

10. Clear the Username box and enter your username.

11. Clear the Password box and enter your last name.

12. You should now be in the Main Menu.

DESCRIPTION OF THE ICONS USED IN SYNAPSE

SYNAPSE uses a variety of icons that assist the user in navigating through each screen. Next is a description of the various icons found in this program.

Main Menu Screen

The Main Menu screen is the opening screen and contains icons that will allow the user to navigate throughout the software (Figure 1). Each icon represents a different section within SYNAPSE. Icons found on the Main Menu are described next.

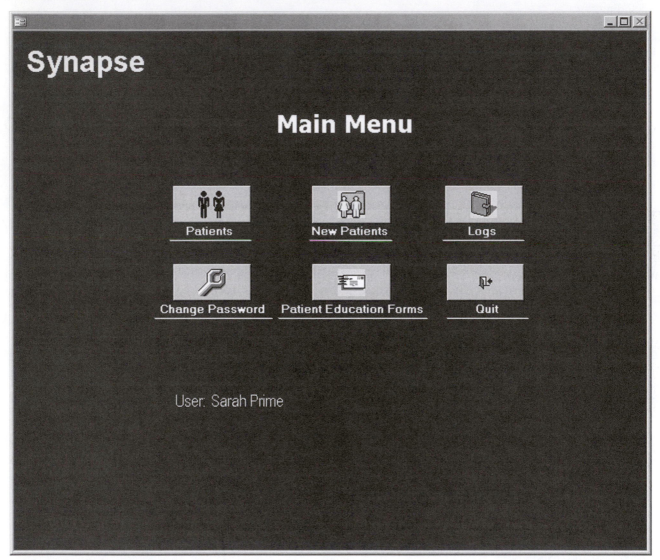

Figure 1   The Main Menu screen

PATIENTS ICON

When clicked, the Patients icon takes the user into a screen that lists all of the established patients in alphabetical order. There are only a few established patients within the software prior to beginning the SYNAPSE exercises; however, the patient population will grow with each exercise. Once a new chart is created, it will be stored in the patient database found on this screen.

NEW PATIENTS ICON

This icon is used when the user wants to create an electronic chart for a new patient. When the user clicks this icon, a series of tabbed screens appear, requesting the following patient information:

- Name and address
- Birth date

- Social Security number
- Telephone number
- Spouse information
- Responsible party information
- Payer information
- Allergy information
- List of the current medications, including over-the-counter medications

Once the chart has been created, the user will click the Demographics icon in the Patient Information Menu to make changes to this information. This screen should be accessed whenever there is a change in the patient's demographic information.

LOGS

The Logs icon takes the user to a screen that houses specific logs typically kept in paper form within the medical office. The following table includes a description of each type of log.

Name of Log	Description	Tracking Purpose
In-House Lab	This log tracks all tests performed in-house or within the medical office.	These logs track results of certain tests performed within the office and aid in tracking lot numbers of various testing reagents, kits, and strips. If the manufacturer sends out a recall notice for a specific lot number of reagents or test kits, the office will know which patients need to be retested.
Quality Control	This log tracks all of the controls used to check the accuracy of various test kits, strips, and instruments used for testing purposes.	The purpose of running lab controls is to confirm that test kits, strips, and lab equipment are working properly. Quality control logs confirm that the office institutes quality control measures, and may be reviewed when the medical office goes through a site evaluation.
Universal Narcotics	This log tracks narcotics that are dispensed or administered in the office.	The purpose of this log is to discourage employees tempted to steal narcotics. This log can also be used in reports to find trends within a specific patient population who use the drugs, or practitioners who prescribe the drugs.
Universal Immunization	This log tracks all immunizations administered in the office.	This log is useful in the event there is a recall on a specific lot number of a vaccine and is also useful for running reports for statistical data.

CHANGE PASSWORD ICON

This icon is used to set up a username and password, or to change an existing password.

PATIENT EDUCATION FORMS ICON

This icon takes the user to a screen that shows a series of educational forms used in the practice. Examples of educational materials include asthma, diabetes, smoking cessation, hypertension, IBS, and many other health-related materials.

QUIT ICON

This icon is used to quit SYNAPSE.

Patient Information Menu Screen

The Patient Information Menu screen is the initial screen within the patient's personal medical record (Figure 2). To get to this screen, the user clicks the Patients icon in the Main Menu. Next, the user clicks the name of the patient whose record is being accessed and clicks the Open Patient Record icon. The patient information screen then appears. A series of icons display in this screen, which allows the user to navigate within the patient's personal medical record. Icons found within this screen are listed next.

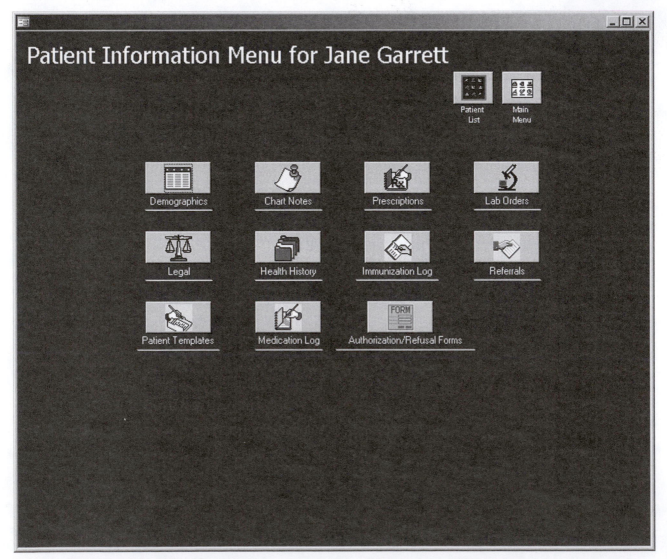

Figure 2   The Patient Information Menu screen

PATIENT LIST ICON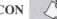

This icon is used to navigate from the current patient's record into the electronic record of another patient.

MAIN MENU ICON

This icon is used to return to the Main Menu, the starting point of SYNAPSE. This icon should be clicked whenever the user needs to document information in the Logs section, retrieve patient education forms, or to quit the program,

DEMOGRAPHICS ICON

This icon is used when the user wants to update the patient's demographic information. It can also be used to update allergy information, medication information, and the chronic problem list; however, these items can also be updated within progress notes. Because this information is private, more offices are now relying on clinical staff members to perform this task while the patient is behind closed doors.

CHART NOTES ICON

All previous chart notes for each patient are housed within this screen. The chart notes screen is also used to create a new office visit chart note or telephone note.

PRESCRIPTIONS ICON

This icon takes the user to the prescription screen. This screen allows the user to view the patient's prescription history and to create and discontinue prescriptions. Medication history should also be updated in the Allergies & Meds table found in the Patient Information screen in order for changes to be reflected in the patient's progress note.

LAB ORDERS ICON

The lab orders screen is used to create a lab requisition when the clinician orders a test. The user can also review the patient's lab history by clicking the Lab History icon found on this screen, and can update lab results by clicking the Update Lab Results icon.

LEGAL ICON

This screen has a list of topics frequently discussed between the clinician and patient that may have legal implications. Any time one of these topics is addressed, it should be documented within the patient's chart. Some of the listed items in this screen include privacy statement information, DNR orders, Power of Attorney information, and more. When patients complete and sign these forms, the forms should be scanned into the record for future use.

HEALTH HISTORY ICON

This icon takes the user into a series of tabs that display questions related to the patient's health. It is here that the user will record information about the patient's family history, hospitalization history, medical history, and social history. The lab and medication history can also be viewed from this section of the record. Any changes made in the lab and prescription screens will automatically populate into these screens.

IMMUNIZATION LOG ICON

This icon takes the user into the patient's personal immunization log. Any time a patient has an immunization performed, it should be documented in this log as well as the universal immunization log, which can be accessed by clicking the Logs icon on the Main Menu.

REFERRALS ICON

This icon takes the user to a referral letter template that can be used when the patient is referred to an outside physician. Names and addresses of physicians whom the practice routinely refers to are stored within this template to further simplify the referral process.

PATIENT TEMPLATES ICON

This icon takes the user to several letter templates that may be used in the medical office. Letter templates include Lab Results Are All Normal, Proof of Appointment, Lab Results (Unable to Reach by Phone), and a Return to Work Excuse. The user just clicks on the appropriate letter and completes the template information. Once the form is completed, it is either printed and given to the patient or sent to the patient, via email when appropriate.

MEDICATION LOG ICON

The Medication Log icon navigates the user to the patient's personal medication log. Any time an injection is administered or an oral medication is dispensed, it is documented within the patient's electronic medication log.

AUTHORIZATION/REFUSAL FORMS ICON

This icon takes the user to immunization consent forms, special procedure consent forms, and a refusal form that is completed when a patient refuses various treatments or tests. When working in the field, these forms will be scanned back into the patient's personal medical record.

SYNAPSE VERSION 1.1 EXERCISES

SYNAPSE is designed to simulate tasks the medical assistant typically performs within the electronic chart. The assignments for SYNAPSE are broken down into modules. Each module represents a portion of a new day in the medical office. Each module will include a variety of activities, including:

- Creating charts for new patients

- Documenting chief complaints and vital signs on existing charts

- Creating lab requisitions and prescriptions

- Documenting within a variety of electronic logs

Data for each new patient is listed within patient data tables. A variety of tasks will be assigned within each module. Modules I through III will end with a list of critical thinking questions that will challenge the user from both a software and clinical viewpoint. Each student should have a blank folder while performing SYNAPSE exercises. Any time the student is asked to print information, it should be printed, labeled, and placed in their SYNAPSE folder. Each module will have a different set of forms to print, so students should separate forms by module number. Module IV is a competency that is graded by the instructor to evaluate the student's comprehension of SYNAPSE. An EMR performance evaluation checklist is found at the end of this appendix, following Module IV.

MODULE I

Today's date: May 14, 2007
Appointments for May 14, 2007:

Patient's Name	Appointment Time	Reason for Appointment	Clinician	MA
Cindy Swaim	9:00 AM	Anxiety	Dr. Heath	Fauna Stout, CMA

Work Assignments

Module I has a total of ten tasks, and it lays the foundation for all other modules because it lists step-by-step instructions for the various tasks. Included throughout the exercises are Help boxes to assist the user what to do if he or she runs into problems while working in particular screens. The following tips may assist the user in finding information quickly when performing future SYNAPSE exercises:

1. Highlight all first-time instructions with a pink marker.

2. Highlight all Help boxes with a yellow marker.

3. Place a large paper clip on the pages that contain first-time instructions or Help boxes.

Task 1-1: Documenting in the Quality Control Log

Every morning, a different person is responsible for opening the lab and turning on the equipment. The person opening the lab also runs controls on various instruments and test kits. Today, it is Fauna Stout's turn to open the lab and run controls, and you will take on the role of this medical assistant.

1. Log in to SYNAPSE.

2. Begin documentation by clicking the Logs icon on the Main Menu screen.

3. Next, click the drop-down arrow under Quality Control Log. There will be a list of test kits or equipment on which you routinely perform controls. Yesterday, Fauna noticed that several of the patients had lower-than-normal glucose levels. Today she performed a control on the glucose unit to make certain it is functioning correctly. Start the documentation by clicking the word "Glucose."

4. Click Open Selected Log located at the top center of the screen.

5. Next, click the update button located at the bottom of the screen (Figure 3). Enter the information listed in Table 1 within the requested fields.

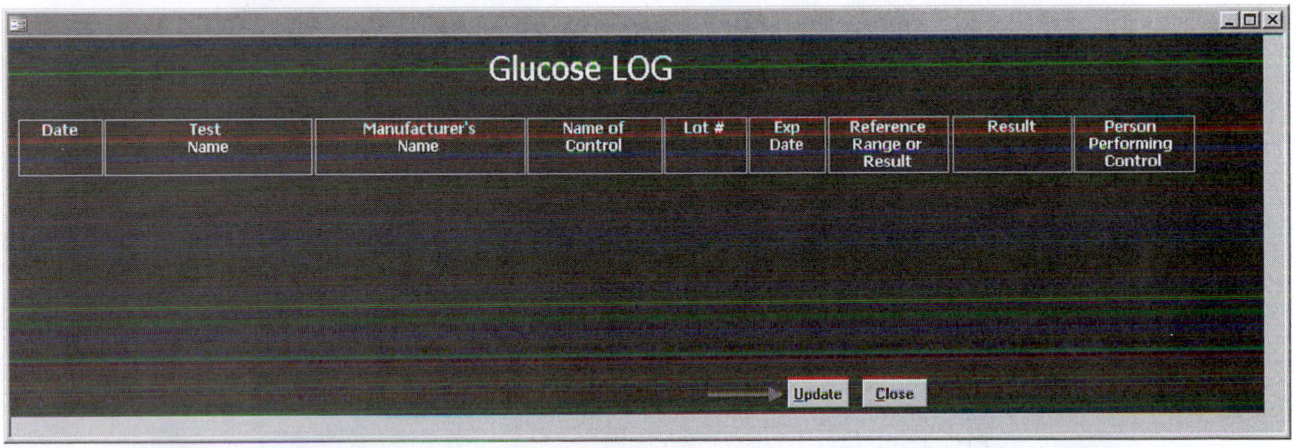

Figure 3 Glucose Log with Update button

TABLE 1   TASK 1-1 INFORMATION

Date	05/14/2007
Test Name	Glucometer Essential
Manufacturer's Name	Jefferson Diagnostics
Name of Control	High Control
Lot #	4890
Exp Date	02/01/2008
Reference Range or Result	250-300
Result	250 mg/dl
Person Performing Control	Fauna Stout, CMA

Help Box: Quality Control Logs

If the log you are working in has no prior entries, you can enter the data in Table 1 directly; however, if previous entries were made in the log, you need to click the Add Log icon before entering the information.

6. Once you have entered the requested information, compare your screen with Figure 4 to make certain it is correct.

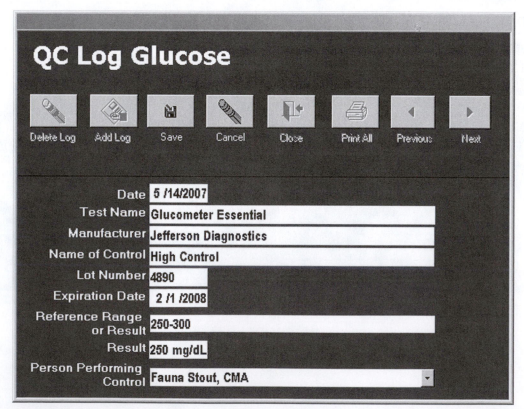

Figure 4   In-house glucose testing log for the glucose control

7. Click Save.

8. Next, click the Print All icon. Label your work as Task 1-1 and place it in your SYNAPSE folder.

9. Click Close. When you click Close, you should see the information you entered in the Glucose log. If the information does not match, delete the log by clicking the Update tab. This brings you back to the original screen in which you recorded the log entry. Make the appropriate changes and, once again, click Save. Click Print All, and click Close.

10. Close the Glucose log by clicking the Close tab next to Update.

11. Navigate out of the Open Selected Log screen by clicking Close, which is the little red box with the white X in the upper-right corner of the screen.

12. You should now be back in the Main Menu.

Task 1-2: Creating a New Chart and Progress Note for the Patient

The first patient of the day is Cindy Swaim. You greet the patient and take her back to the examination room. First, you will need to create a chart for Ms. Swaim. Information necessary to create the chart and progress note can be found in Table 2.

TABLE 2   CINDY SWAIM'S PATIENT DATA TABLE

Patient's Name	Cindy L. Swaim
Patient's DOB	04/14/1965
Patient's Chart Number	268506784
Patient's Address	429 Kingston Drive, Louis Center, NY, 01287-1111
Patient's Telephone Numbers	Home: 123-842-8421 Work: 123-652-9874
Patient's Employer Info	Lakeside Memorial Hospital Fostoria, NY, 01254-6543
Gender, Marital Status, Blood Type & Smoking Status	Gender: Female Marital Status: Single Blood Type: A+ Smoking Status: Smoker
Spouse Name, DOB, & Address	N/A
Responsible Party Info	Patient
Primary Payer Info	Signal HMO, 135 Carriagehill Lane, Douglasville, NY, 01268506784-00, Policy Holder: Self
Secondary Payer	None
Patient Drug Allergies	Tetracycline
Patient Other Allergy	Dust, Pollen
Current Mediation List	None
Preferred Pharmacy	Family Pharmacy Inc., 865 Livingston Ave, Fostoria NY, 01254
Lab Provider	National Diagnostics
Privacy Statement	Date the Privacy Statement was signed: 05/14/2007; note to be entered in the Notes box. April Patrick (mother of patient) can receive private information if unable to contact the patient directly. April Patrick's cell phone number is 123-328-9874.

Family Health History Info	Father: Age 62, Health: Fair
	Mother: Age 60, Health: Good
	Brother: Age 37, Health: Good
	Sister: Age at Death 6, Cause of Death: Leukemia
	Familial Diseases:
	Cancer: Enter the following note: Paternal grandfather died of liver cancer at age 72.
	Other: Father has emphysema.
Hospitalizations, Blood Transfusions, and Serious Injuries	Hospitalizations: 1984, Lakeside Memorial Hospital, emergency appendectomy (no complications)
	Blood Transfusions: The patient has not received any blood transfusions.
	Serious Injuries: None
Pregnancies	None
Medical History	Place checkmarks in the boxes for chicken pox, diabetes, and high cholesterol.
	Notes: Place the following in the Notes box:
	Chicken pox: 1970 (no complications).
	Diabetes: Diagnosed with borderline diabetes in 2003 (diet controlled)
	High cholesterol: Diagnosed in 2003 (diet controlled)
Health Habits	Check Caffeine: Two 12-ounce cups of coffee per day
	Check Tobacco: 1 to 1 1/2 packs of cigarettes per day × 22 years
	Check ETOH:
	Drink Type: Beer
	Drinks Week: Six 12-ounce cans per week
	Check the box for Heavy Lifting
	Occupation: Patient Care Associate
Subjective Information	Chief Complaint: Anxiety or stress
	Severity of symptoms is a 4 on a scale from 1 to 10.
	Duration of symptoms is 4 months.
	Associated symptoms: (Positives) Breathing irregularities, decrease in ability to concentrate, history of prior attacks, and increase in appetite or weight. (Negatives) Heart irregularities, and psychotic or delusional behavior
	Aggravating Factors: Crowded areas
	Relieving Factors: Eating and Sleeping
Objective Information	Vital Signs:
	Height: 64 inches
	Weight: 162 pounds
	Temperature: 99.8
	Blood Pressure: 150/98
	Pulse: 92
	Respiration: 20
	Pain: 0
	Subjective Information and Vital Signs Entered By: Fauna Stout, CMA

CREATING A CHART

1. Begin by clicking the New Patients icon on the Main Menu.

2. The first tabbed screen under Patient Information is the Patient Main screen. Using the information provided in Table 2 fill in the requested fields. When you are finished, click Save. Check your work with Figure 5.

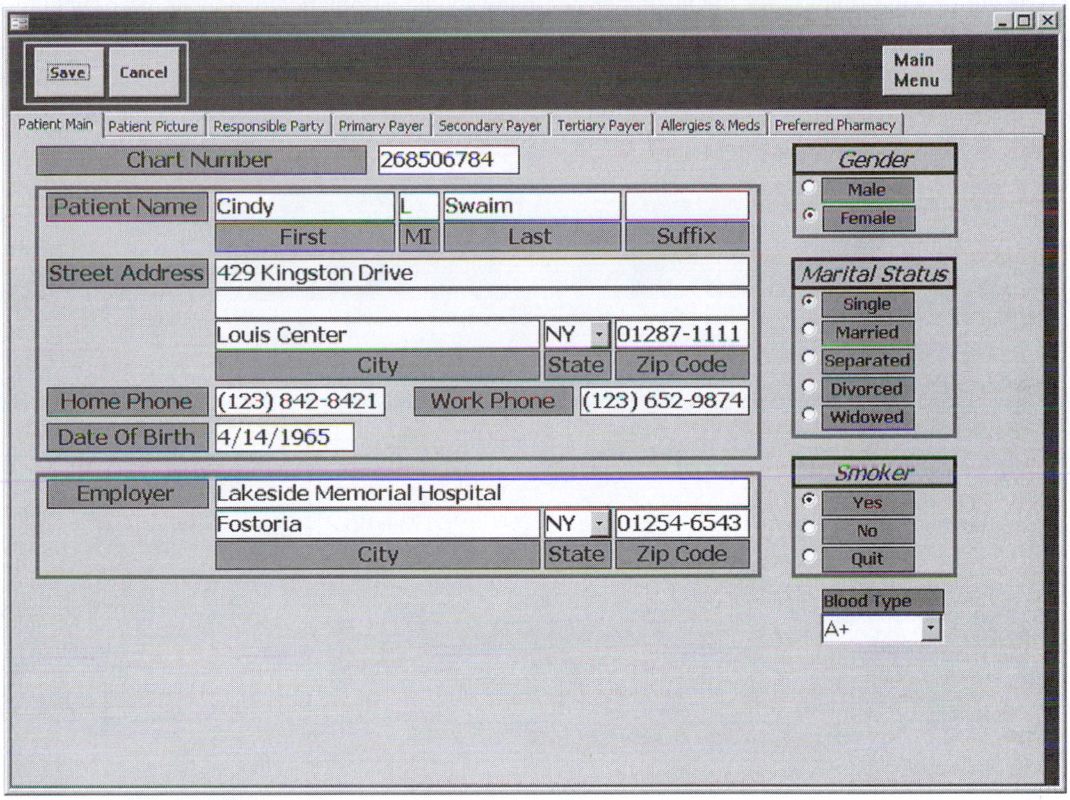

Figure 5   Patient Main screen completed for Cindy Swaim

Help Box: Navigating through Fields

Pressing the Tab key on your keyboard is an excellent way to move from one field to another. When you finish entering information in the field in which you are working, press the Tab key; this will move you to the next available field.

---

3. Next, click the Patient Picture tab. This is where you can attach a picture of a patient if you have a scanner or digital image. Check to make certain the patient's chart number is in the Patient Chart Number box. Under the Patient Picture box is another box labeled Patient Notes. This box serves as a reminder box. You will enter special facts about the patient in this box, such as how the patient wants to be addressed, special events in the patient's life (such as a wedding or graduation), or notes that remind you to take a certain action during the patient's next visit. These actions may include having the patient sign a specific form or making certain that the patient returned an X-ray that was borrowed from the office. You should look in this section of the record prior to rooming the patient to see if there are any specific notations directing you to take a specific action. Once the action has been applied, or the event has past, you should remove the note by deleting it and clicking Save. For this visit, enter the following information in the Patient Notes box: "The patient prefers to be addressed by her first name." Click Save.

4. Click the Responsible Party tab. The patient's chart number should have automatically populated in this screen, as well as the remainder of screens within the patient information section. Since Cindy is responsible

for her own bills, click Self. Note that all of Cindy's information automatically populates in this screen. Also notice that the numerals listed in the chart number is Cindy's Social Security number. Offices are currently moving away from using the patient's Social Security number as an identifier.

5. Click the Primary Payer tab. Click the drop-down menu arrow in the box next to the Name heading. Click Signal HMO. The address information for the insurance company should automatically appear after clicking Signal HMO. Next, enter the subscriber I.D. #, which is 268506784-00. There is no Policy/Group #, so leave that box empty. Under Policy Holder information, click Self. The remainder of the information should automatically populate within the Policy Holder section, except for Cindy's Social Security number. Enter 268-50-6784. Compare your work with Figure 6 and click Save.

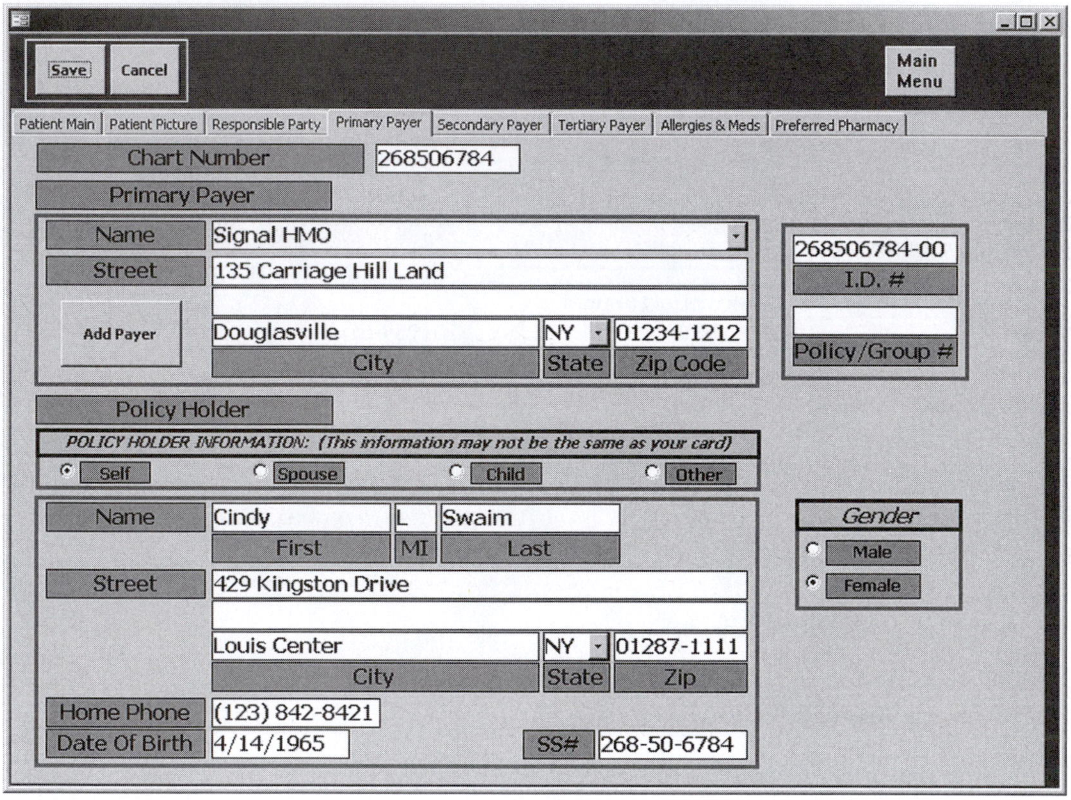

Figure 6   Primary Payer screen completed for Cindy Swaim

6. The patient does not have any secondary or tertiary insurance, so you can skip those tabs and go directly to the Allergy & Meds tab. The patient is allergic to Tetracycline. Begin this section by clicking the Click to Add tab within the Patient Drug Allergy List box. Another box will appear. Type Tetracycline in the Enter Patient Drug Allergy field. Next, click the Save button. Once you save your information, it should automatically appear in red in the Patient Drug Allergy List box. The patient is also allergic to dust and pollen, so click the Click to Add tab in the Patient Other Allergy List box. Type Dust in the Enter Patient Other Allergy field. Click Save. Repeat the same instructions for pollen. The patient is not taking any current medications, so click Save. Check your work with Figure 7.

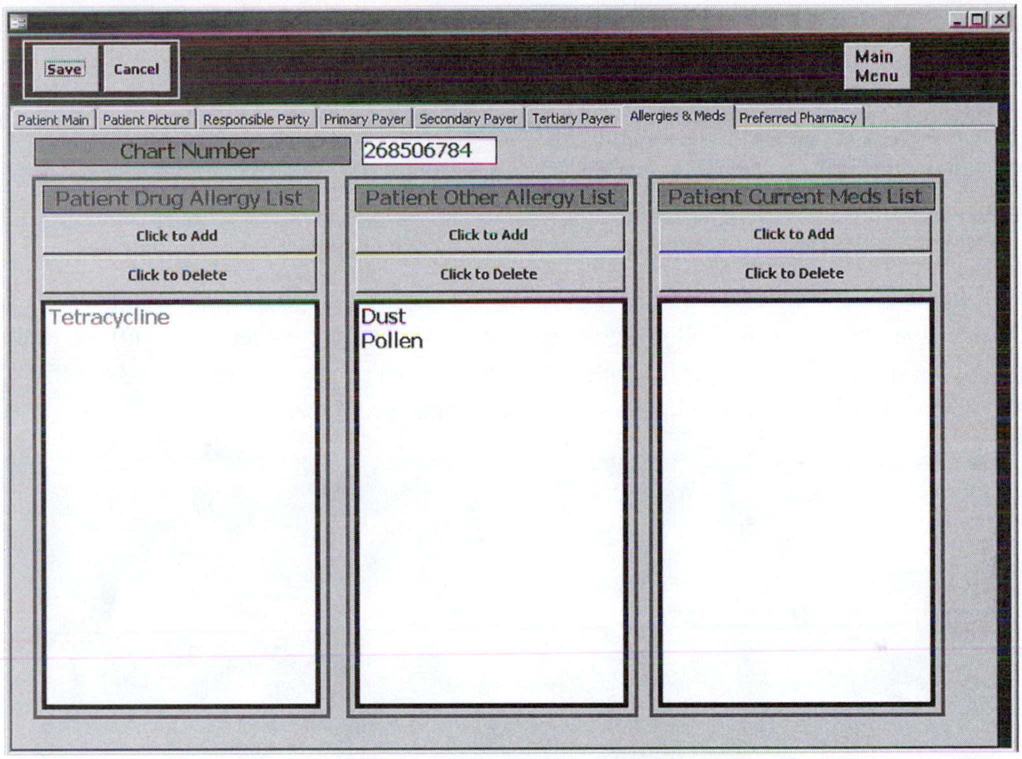

Figure 7   Allergies & Meds screen completed for Cindy Swaim

7. Next click the Preferred Pharmacy tab. Click Update Patient Preferred Pharmacies. The patient selected Family Pharmacy Inc., 865 Livingston Ave, Fostoria NY, 01254 as her preferred pharmacy. Click the Add/Remove button next to this pharmacy. A checkmark should appear in the box of the Add/Remove button. Click Close. The pharmacy you selected should now appear in the Patient Preferred Pharmacies box (see Figure 8). Click Save.

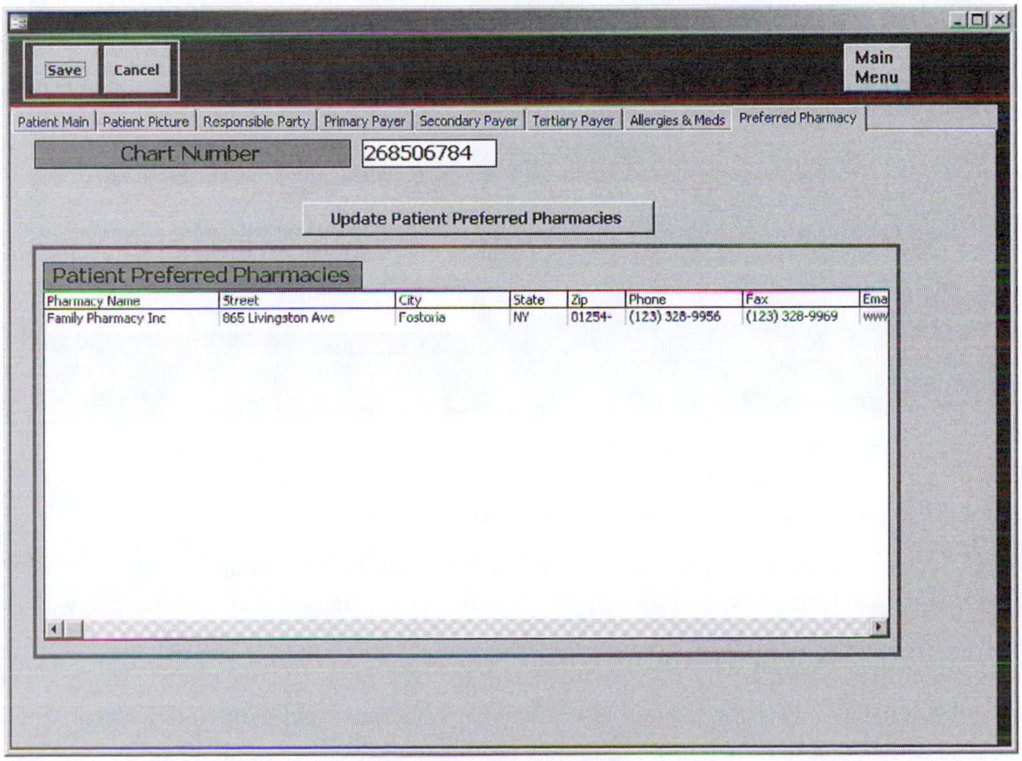

Figure 8   Preferred Pharmacy screen completed for Cindy Swaim

8. Review each tab and make certain that all of your information saved correctly.

9. Click the Main Menu icon.

10. Click the Patients icon. Cindy Swaim's name should now be listed within the alphabetical list of patients.

11. Highlight Cindy's name by clicking the patient selector column, which is the column just to the left of the patient's name. Click Open Patient Record. The Patient Information screen for Cindy Swaim appears.

12. Click the Legal Icon. You just finished reviewing the privacy statement with the patient. Now click the drop-down menu arrow in the Privacy Statement box. Click Yes. Enter today's date, May 14, 2007, in the box under the date column. In the Notes box, enter the following information: April Patrick (mother of patient) can receive private information if we are unable to contact the patient directly. Her cell phone number is 123-328-9874. Click Save, and check your work with Figure 9. Print the screen and label as Task 1-2A.

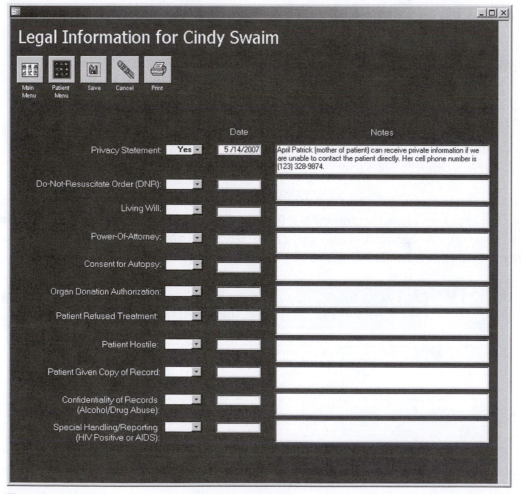

Figure 9   Legal Information screen completed for Cindy Swaim

13. Click Patient Menu and then click the Health History icon.

14. Using Table 2, enter all of the history information within the Health History sections. *Note: Save your information after completing each screen.* Make certain that you expound on any disease that was checked within the family history or past medical history tabs by entering information in the Notes sections of those particular screens. Do not enter any information within the lab history screen or the medication history screen. These screens will automatically populate when a prescription is written or a lab requisition is ordered. Refer to Figures 10, 11, and 12 to make certain that information was correctly entered in the corresponding screens.

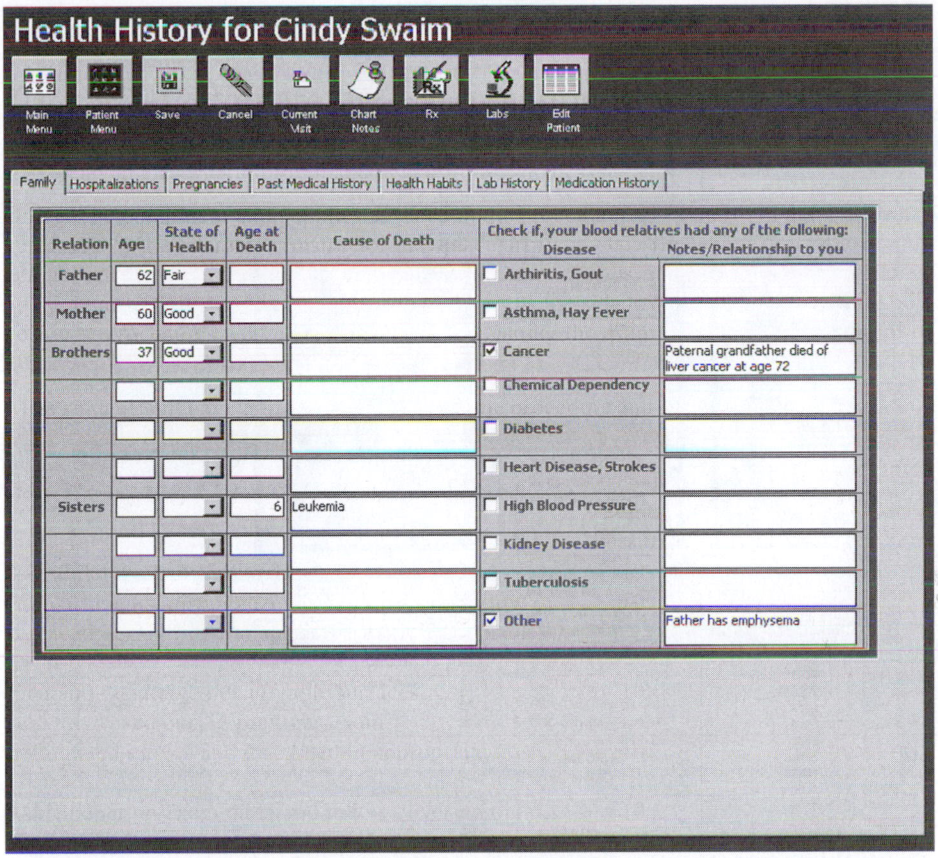

Health History for Cindy Swaim

Relation	Age	State of Health	Age at Death	Cause of Death	Check if, your blood relatives had any of the following: Disease	Notes/Relationship to you
Father	62	Fair			☐ Arthiritis, Gout	
Mother	60	Good			☐ Asthma, Hay Fever	
Brothers	37	Good			☑ Cancer	Paternal grandfather died of liver cancer at age 72
					☐ Chemical Dependency	
					☐ Diabetes	
					☐ Heart Disease, Strokes	
Sisters			6	Leukemia	☐ High Blood Pressure	
					☐ Kidney Disease	
					☐ Tuberculosis	
					☑ Other	Father has emphysema

Figure 10   Family History screen completed for Cindy Swaim

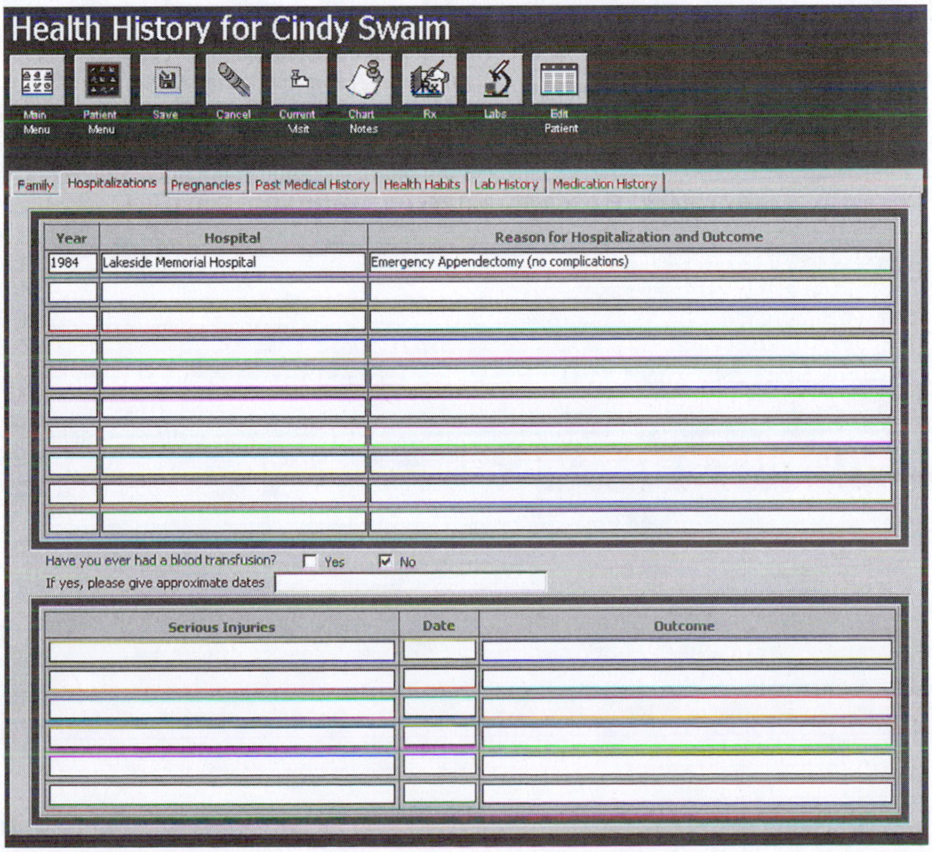

Health History for Cindy Swaim

Year	Hospital	Reason for Hospitalization and Outcome
1984	Lakeside Memorial Hospital	Emergency Appendectomy (no complications)

Have you ever had a blood transfusion?   ☐ Yes   ☑ No
If yes, please give approximate dates

Serious Injuries	Date	Outcome

Figure 11   Hospitalization screen completed for Cindy Swaim

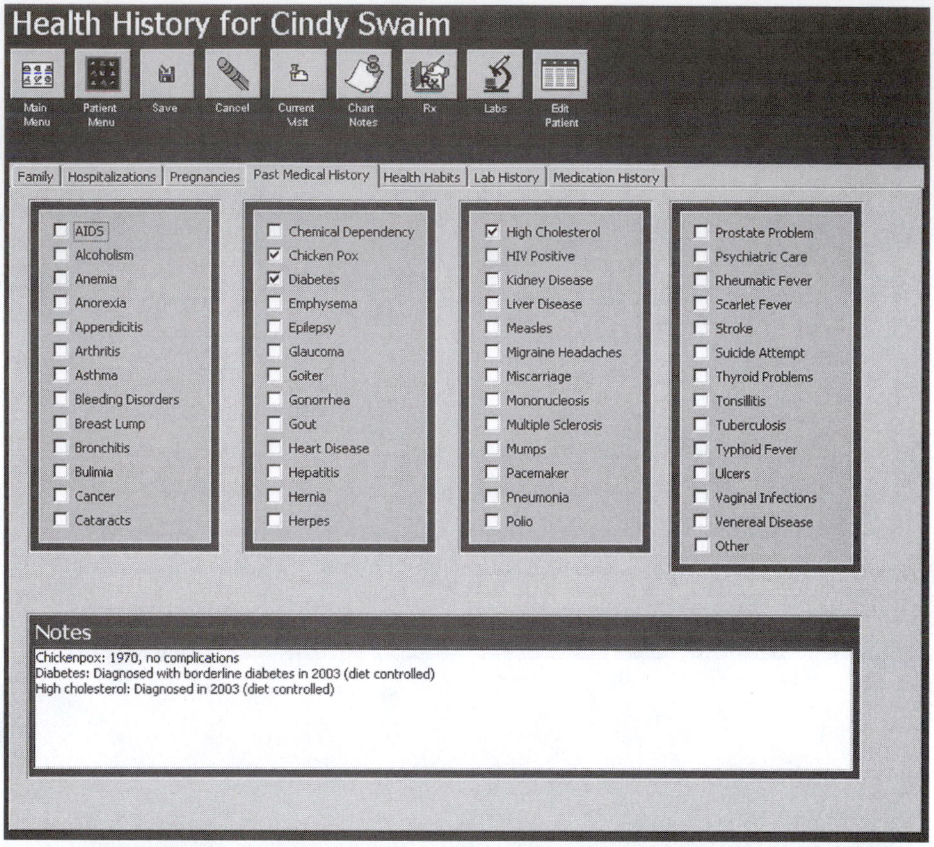

Health History for Cindy Swaim

| Main Menu | Patient Menu | Save | Cancel | Current Visit | Chart Notes | Rx | Labs | Edit Patient |

Family | Hospitalizations | Pregnancies | Past Medical History | Health Habits | Lab History | Medication History

☐ AIDS	☐ Chemical Dependency	☑ High Cholesterol	☐ Prostate Problem
☐ Alcoholism	☑ Chicken Pox	☐ HIV Positive	☐ Psychiatric Care
☐ Anemia	☑ Diabetes	☐ Kidney Disease	☐ Rheumatic Fever
☐ Anorexia	☐ Emphysema	☐ Liver Disease	☐ Scarlet Fever
☐ Appendicitis	☐ Epilepsy	☐ Measles	☐ Stroke
☐ Arthritis	☐ Glaucoma	☐ Migraine Headaches	☐ Suicide Attempt
☐ Asthma	☐ Goiter	☐ Miscarriage	☐ Thyroid Problems
☐ Bleeding Disorders	☐ Gonorrhea	☐ Mononucleosis	☐ Tonsillitis
☐ Breast Lump	☐ Gout	☐ Multiple Sclerosis	☐ Tuberculosis
☐ Bronchitis	☐ Heart Disease	☐ Mumps	☐ Typhoid Fever
☐ Bulimia	☐ Hepatitis	☐ Pacemaker	☐ Ulcers
☐ Cancer	☐ Hernia	☐ Pneumonia	☐ Vaginal Infections
☐ Cataracts	☐ Herpes	☐ Polio	☐ Venereal Disease
			☐ Other

Notes

Chickenpox: 1970, no complications
Diabetes: Diagnosed with borderline diabetes in 2003 (diet controlled)
High cholesterol: Diagnosed in 2003 (diet controlled)

Figure 12   Past Medical History screen completed for Cindy Swaim

Health History for Cindy Swaim

| Main Menu | Patient Menu | Save | Cancel | Current Visit | Chart Notes | Rx | Labs | Edit Patient |

Family | Hospitalizations | Pregnancies | Past Medical History | Health Habits | Lab History | Medication History

Check which substances you use and describe how much you use.

☑	Caffeine	2 12-ounce cups of coffee per day
☑	Tobacco	1 to 1-1/2 packs of cigarettes per day x22 years
☐	Drugs	
☑	ETOH	
	Drink Type	Beer
	Drinks Week	6 12-ounce cans per week
☐	Other	

Check if your work exposes you to the following:

| ☐ Stress | ☐ Hazardous Substances |
| ☑ Heavy Lifting | ☐ Other |

Occupation: Patient Care Associate

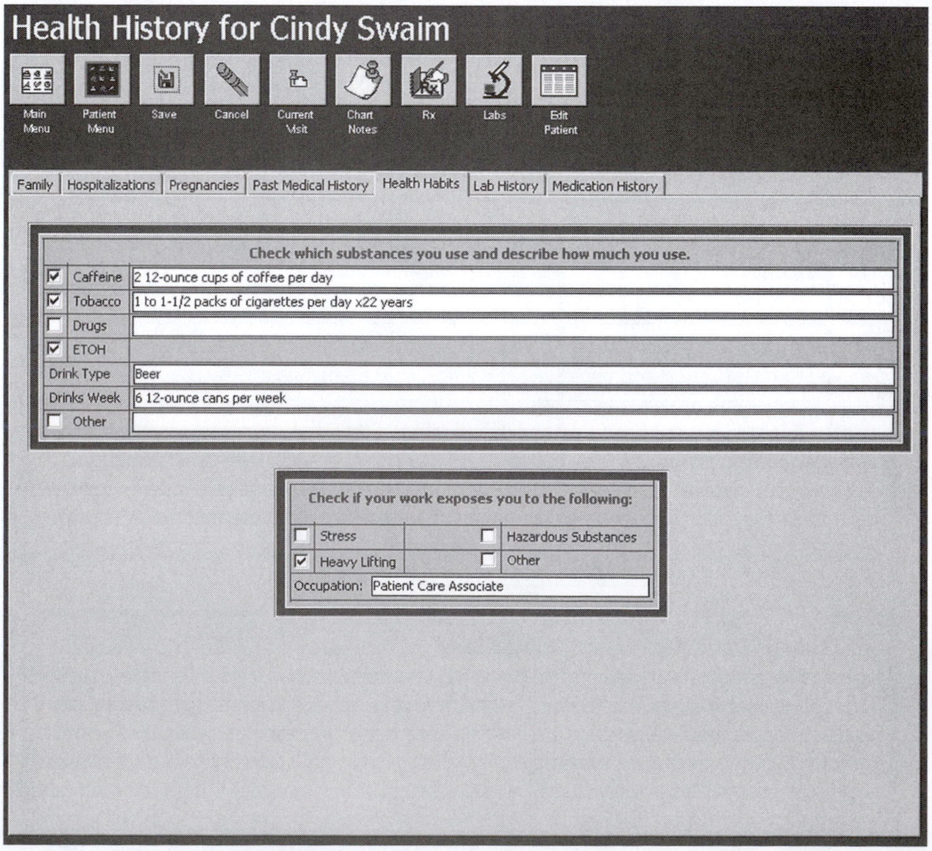

Figure 13   Health Habits screen completed for Cindy Swaim

Help Box: Entering Grandparent Information into the Family History Screen

When entering information about a grandparent, identify if it was the father's parents by placing the word "paternal" in front of the grandparent and by using the word "maternal" when referring to the mother's parents.

15. Click the Patient Menu icon. Next, click the Chart Notes icon.

   a. You should see four icons at the top of the screen and two long boxes below the four icons (Figure 14).

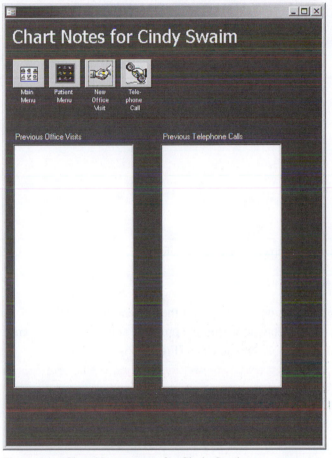

Figure 14   Chart Notes screen for Cindy Swaim

   b. The two boxes below the icons will include a listing of all previous office visits and telephone calls that the patient has had in the past. Your boxes should be blank because the patient has not been seen in the past. When you want to read a previous note of an established patient, just click the date in question and the note from that visit will appear. Each time a patient comes in for a new office visit, you should click the New Office Visit icon. When the patient calls the office for medical results or advice, you should click the Telephone Call icon. Cindy is here for a new office visit, so click New Office Visit.

16. Once you see the New Office Visit Screen, enter the date of Cindy's visit, which is May 14, 2007. Next, enter the time of Cindy's visit, 9:00 a.m.

17. Click the Update Progress Note button at the top of the toolbar and then click Save.

18. Next, click the Subjective Tab.

19. Click the drop-down menu in the box under Chief Complaint.

20. Click the words "Anxiety or Stress" from the drop-down list (Figure 15).

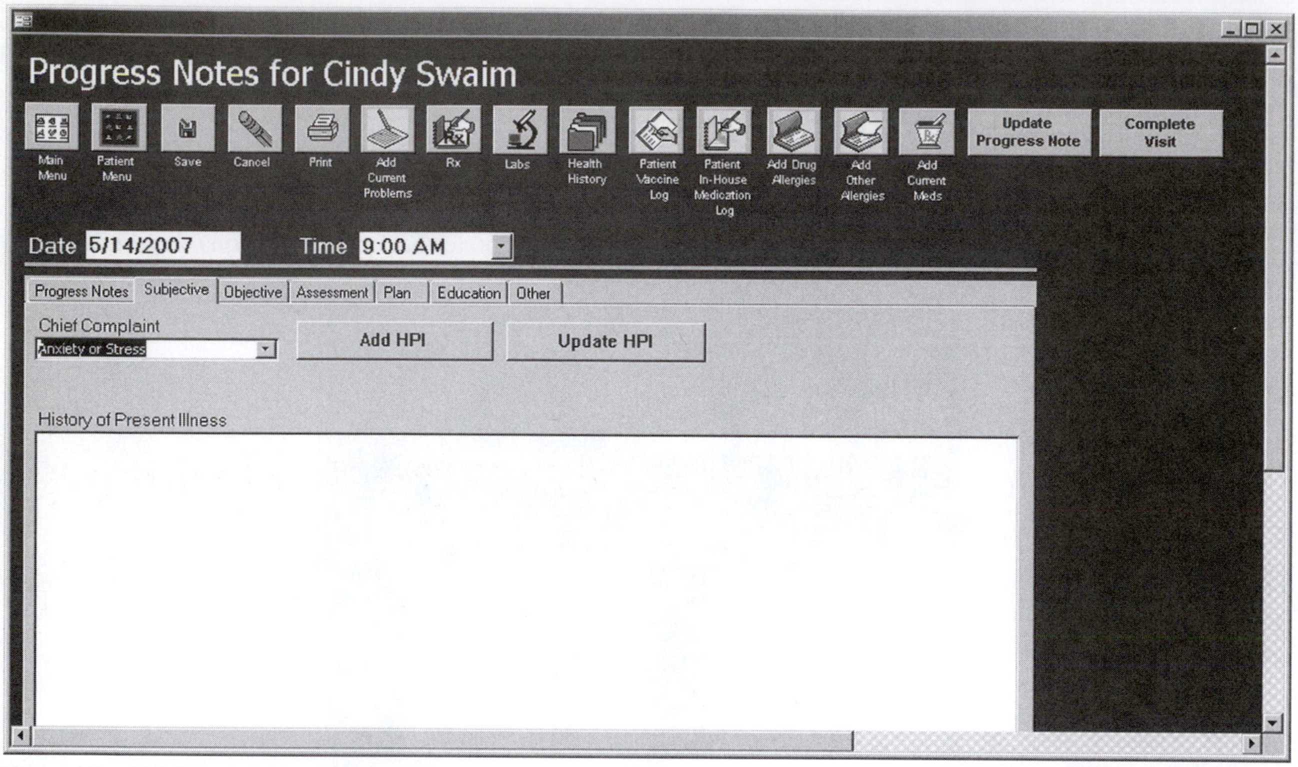

Figure 15   Chief Complaint screen completed for Cindy Swaim

21. Click Update Progress Notes and then click Save.

22. Most physicians will enter the patient's history of the present illness (HPI) information; however, you will enter it here to see how items populate within the progress note. Start by clicking the Add HPI button. The screen where HPI information is entered appears (Figure 16).

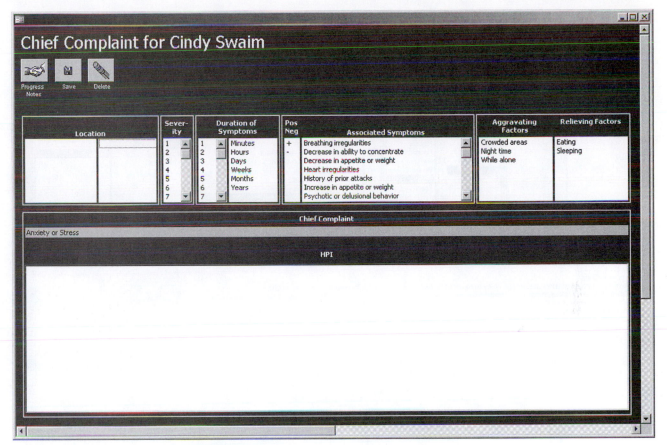

Figure 16   Chief Complaint screen that shows all of the HPI information for anxiety or stress

a. Since location is not a factor, the box is empty.

b. Under Severity of Symptoms, click 4. This signifies the severity of the patient's symptoms on a scale from 1 to 10.

c. In the row next to severity there is another set of numbers. Click 4 and then click Months. This signifies that the patient has had the symptoms for four months. All of this information should automatically populate within the white HPI box below the chief complaint.

d. Next is the Associated Symptoms box. Associated symptoms are symptoms that may be common with particular chief complaints. You will see a + symbol and – symbol. Click the + symbol first. Click all of the symptoms that are listed as positive in Cindy's patient data table. Positive symptoms included the following: *Breathing irregularities, Decrease in ability to concentrate, History of prior attacks,* and *Increase in appetite or weight.* Now click on the – symbol. Click the symptoms that do not apply, which include the following: *Heart irregularities and psychotic or delusional behavior.* You didn't click Decrease in appetite or weight because the patient already stated that she had an increase in appetite or weight.

e. Next is the Aggravating Factors box. Aggravating factors are factors that make the symptoms worse. Cindy stated that crowded areas make her symptoms worse, so click *Crowded areas.*

f. Next is the Relieving Factors box. Relieving factors are factors that seem to help the symptoms. Cindy stated that eating and sleeping seem to make her symptoms better, so click Eating and click Sleeping. Now that you are through entering the HPI information, click Save. Check your work with Figure 17.

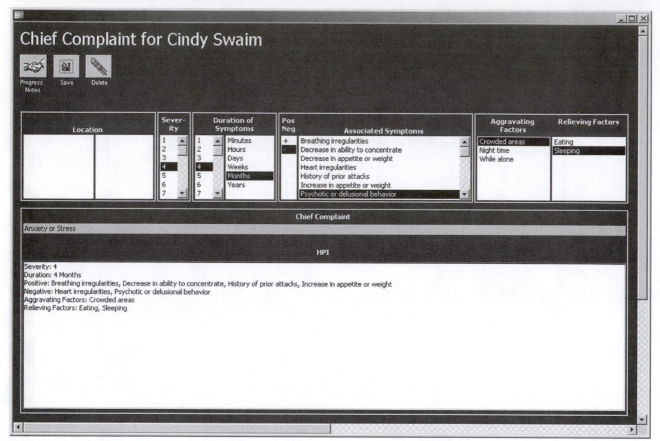

Figure 17   Cindy Swaim's completed HPI table

23. Next, click the Progress Notes icon. You should now be viewing the information within the Subjective Information tab. Click Update Progress Note and then click Save. Now click the Progress Notes tab. The subjective information should have automatically populated within the progress note. Refer to Figure 18 to make certain that your subjective information is correct.

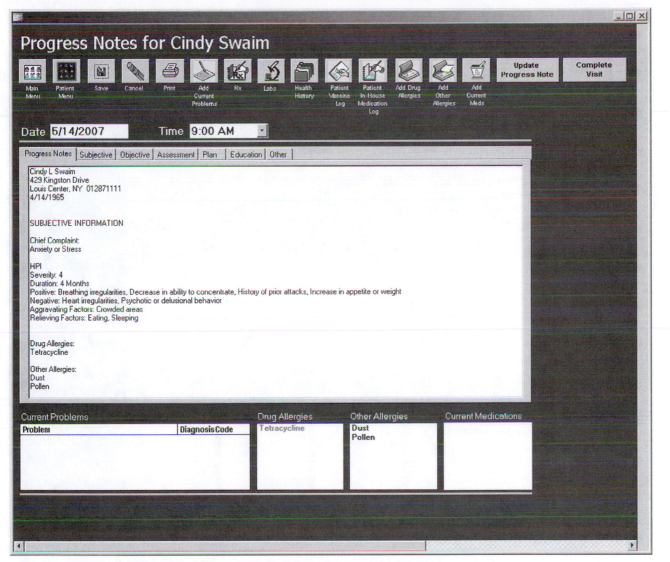

Figure 18   Progress Notes screen with the subjective information entered within the progress note

24. Click the Objective Tab. Enter the patient's vital signs in the requested fields:

Vital Signs:

Height: 64 inches

Weight: 162 pounds

Temperature: 99.8

Blood Pressure: 150/98

Pulse: 92

Respiration: 20

Pain: 0

25. Click the name of the medical assistant you are representing, which is Fauna Stout. This feature illustrates who entered the subjective findings and vital signs. Refer to Figure 19 to make certain that you entered the information correctly in the Objective screen.

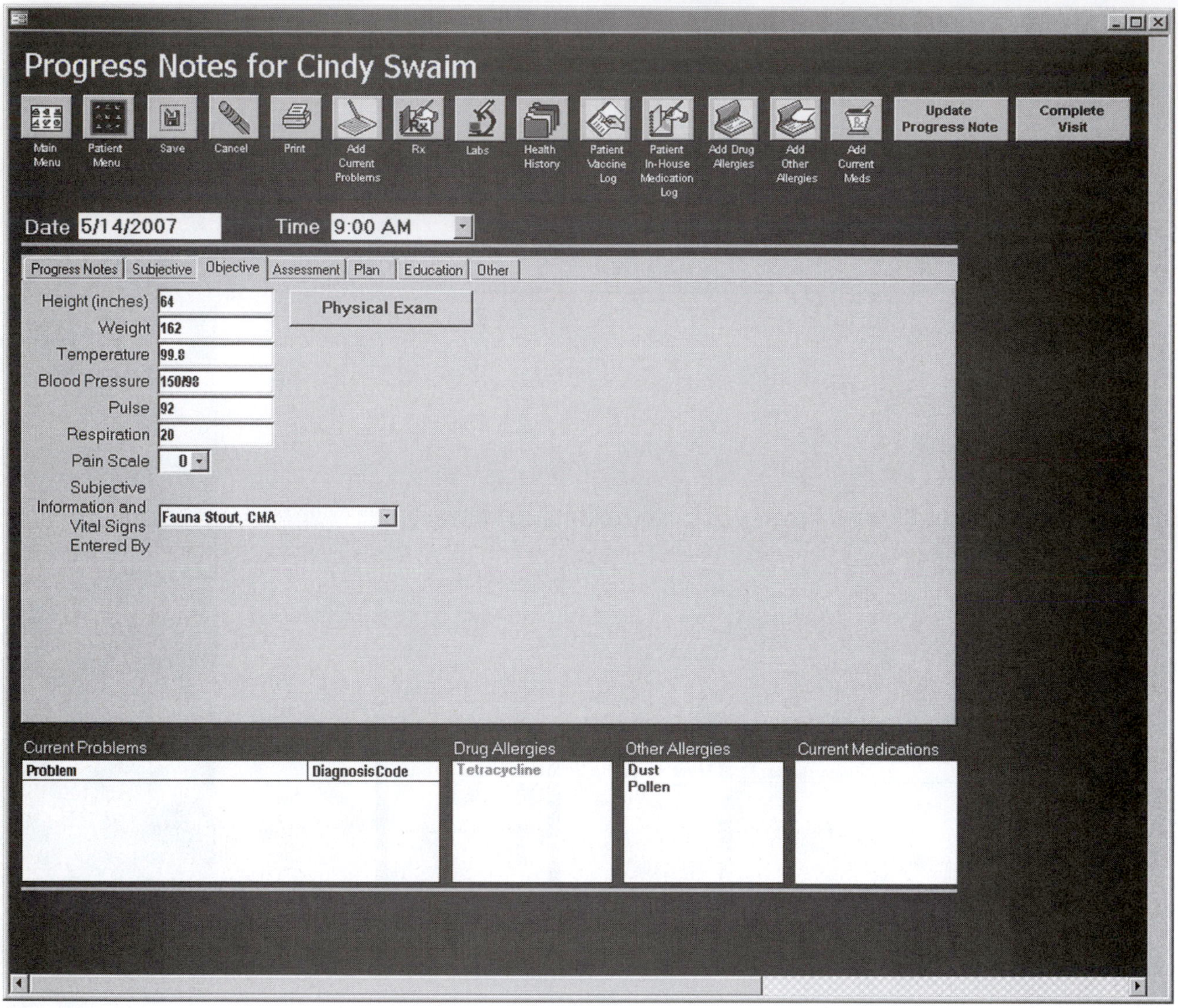

Figure 19   Objective screen completed with Cindy Swaim's vital sign information

26. Click the Update Progress Note icon at the top of the toolbar and then click Save.

27. Click the Progress Notes tab. Scroll down to view the objective information. You should see the information you entered within the Objective tab now populated within the progress note window. You should also see that the Patient's Drug Allergy Information and Other Allergy Information automatically populated within the note. You will also see the headings Physical Examination Findings, Assessment, and Plan. These headings illustrate the remainder of information to be added by the clinician. Check your work with Figure 20.

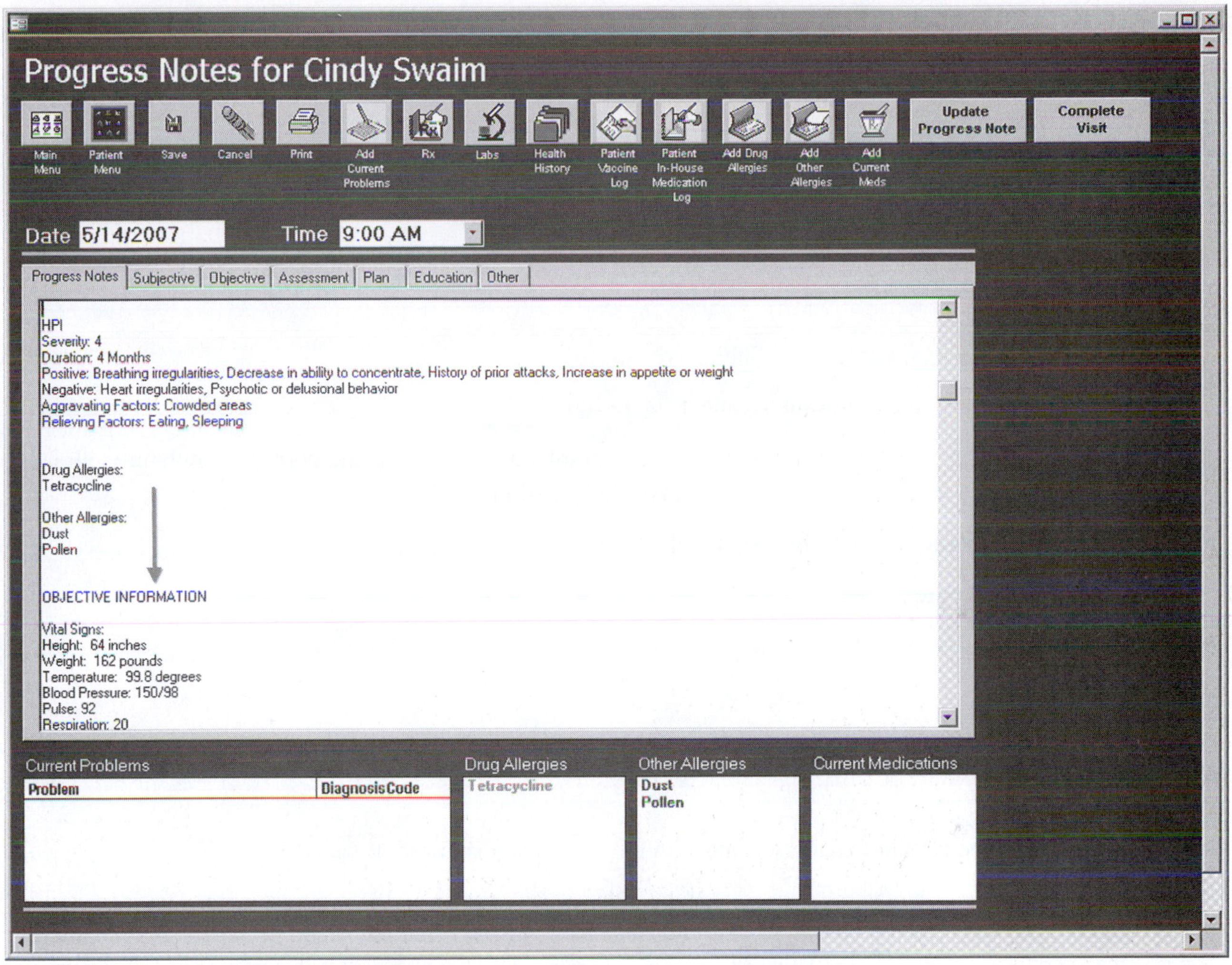
Progress Notes for Cindy Swaim
Main Menu
Patient Menu
Save
Cancel
Print
Add Current Problems
Rx
Labs
Health History
Patient Vaccine Log
Patient In-House Medication Log
Add Drug Allergies
Add Other Allergies
Add Current Meds
Update Progress Note
Complete Visit
Date 5/14/2007
Time 9:00 AM
Progress Notes
Subjective
Objective
Assessment
Plan
Education
Other
HPI
Severity: 4
Duration: 4 Months
Positive: Breathing irregularities, Decrease in ability to concentrate, History of prior attacks, Increase in appetite or weight
Negative: Heart irregularities, Psychotic or delusional behavior
Aggravating Factors: Crowded areas
Relieving Factors: Eating, Sleeping
Drug Allergies:
Tetracycline
Other Allergies:
Dust
Pollen
OBJECTIVE INFORMATION
Vital Signs:
Height: 64 inches
Weight: 162 pounds
Temperature: 99.8 degrees
Blood Pressure: 150/98
Pulse: 92
Respiration: 20
Current Problems
Problem
Diagnosis Code
Drug Allergies
Tetracycline
Other Allergies
Dust
Pollen
Current Medications

Figure 20 Completed progress notes for Cindy Swaim

28. Review the progress note and look for any errors. When you are satisfied the information is correct, click the Print icon. Print a copy of the progress note and label it Task 1-2B. Do not click the Complete Visit icon until the patient's visit is completed. Once you click this icon and leave the screen, you cannot enter any further information for this particular visit. The physician still has information to enter, so leave the screen for the physician.

Help Box: Progress Notes

If after viewing the progress note you notice any errors, take the following actions:

If the error occurs in the Subjective information:

1. You should return to the Subjective tab and make the appropriate corrections. Click Update Progress Note and then click Save. Make certain the information saved correctly.

2. If the updated subjective information does not save correctly after applying the above action, try the following:

    a. Click the Cancel icon while in the Subjective tab.

    b. Click Yes, you are sure you want to cancel.

    c. Click the drop-down menu arrow in the Chief Complaint box, even if the correct complaint is already displayed. (This should cause the previous HPI information to disappear.)

    d. Make certain that the correct complaint is displayed.

    e. Click Update Progress Note.

    f. Click Save.

    g. Click Add HPI.

    h. Click the appropriate symptoms.

    i. Click Save.

    j. Click the Subjective tab. The correct information should be displayed in the HPI box.

    k. Click the Progress Notes tab. You should be able to view the amended progress note. The information should now be correct. *Note: Remember, you will not click the Complete Visit tab until both you and the physician are completely finished with the patient. Once the note is completed, you will need to click the Complete Visit tab to complete the note; otherwise, the note will not save properly.*

If the error occurs in the Objective information:

1. Click the Objective tab.

2. Click Cancel.

3. Enter the corrected information in the appropriate boxes.

4. Click the Update Progress Note icon.

5. Click Save.

6. Click the Progress Notes tab.

7. You should be able to view the amended progress note now. The information should now be correct. *Note: Remember, you will not click the Complete Visit tab until both you and the physician are completely finished with the patient. Once the note is completed, you will need to click the Complete Visit icon to complete the note; otherwise, the note will not save properly.*

Now that the chart is created and all information is entered, you can alert the physician that the patient is ready to be seen.

When working in the field, the physician will typically exit the patient's room and instruct the medical assistant to read the Plan section of the progress note. Since this is not possible for these assignments, the plan will be provided in the instructions. The plan for Cindy Swaim states the following:

Plan: In-Office Glucose. Will send the patient's blood out for a Chem 12. Rx for Alprazolam, 0.5 mg, # 30, Take 1 tablet every day. One month prescription, no refills. Rx for Atenolol tabs, 50 mg, Take 1 tab each day before meals or at bedtime, One month prescription, no refills, Spoke to patient regarding hypertension, hypercholesterolemia, diabetes, and a smoking cessation program. Will give patient educational materials for hypertension, smoking cessation, heart disease, and diabetes. Re: Pt to follow up in one month for a thorough physical.

There are many things that you will need to do to finish with this patient. Time management will be very important. Let's start our tasks by creating all of the orders for the labs.

Task 1-3: Ordering Lab Tests

1. Since you should already be in the Progress Notes screen, click the Labs icon.

2. Click the drop-down menu arrow in the Laboratory box. A list of laboratories will appear. This box depicts which lab conducted the testing. Since the test will be performed in the office, select In-House Testing.

3. Next, click the drop-down menu arrow in the Ordering Provider box. Another drop-down list will appear. Click Dr. Heath.

4. Click the Payer drop-down menu arrow. Select Signal HMO.

5. Click the drop-down menu arrow in the General Lab Tests box. A drop-down list of tests will appear. Scroll and click Fasting Blood Sugar or FBS.

6. Leave the Number and Type of Specimens Sent box empty since we are not sending this test outside the office.

7. In the Today's Date box, enter the date of Cindy's appointment, which is 05/14/2007.

8. Next, click the Specimen Prepared By drop-down menu arrow. Click Fauna Stout, since she is the medical assistant taking care of the patient.

9. Click the drop-down menu arrow in the Was patient fasting? box. Click Yes. Check your work with Figure 21, and make the appropriate corrections before saving the information.

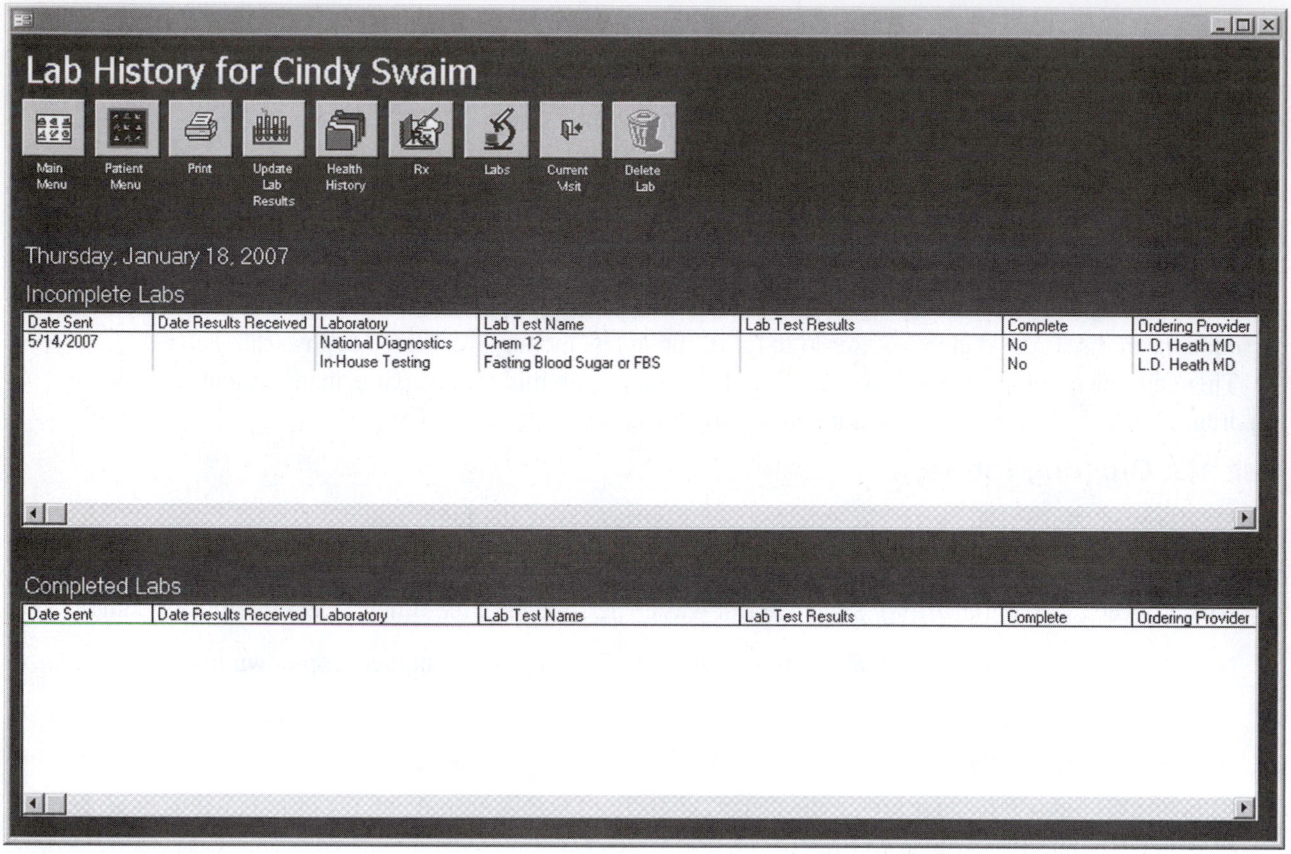

Figure 21   Completed Lab Requisition screen for Cindy Swaim illustrating the FBS order

10. Click Save.

11. Click the Preview Box to review the order. If you made an error, perform the steps in the Help Box: Correcting an Error in the Lab Preview Screen.

12. Once information is correct in the Preview box, click the Print icon in the upper-right corner of the lab requisition screen.

13. Label the requisition as Task 1-3A. Place it in your SYNAPSE folder. Close the screen by clicking the X in the upper-right corner.

14. Now click the Lab History icon. Your Fasting Blood Sugar order should be displayed in the Incomplete Labs table.

15. Since the doctor also ordered an outside test, which is the Chem 12, click the Labs icon. Since the patient is having an outside test as well, you should also create the requisition for that test. The patient's insurance company allows her to go to National Diagnostics, so select that name from the drop-down list.

16. Click Ordering Provider. Select Dr. Heath.

17. Click the Insurance box arrow. Select Signal HMO.

18. Click the General Lab Tests box arrow. Click Chem 12.

19. Type the following information within the Number of and Type of Specimens Sent box: One Red Top Tube.

20. Insert the date of the patient's appointment in the Today's Date box.

21. Next, click the Specimen Prepared By drop-down arrow. Select Fauna's name.

22. Click the drop-down arrow in the Was patient fasting? box. Click Yes. Click Save. Click the Preview Box to view the order.

23. Print a copy of this lab requisition by clicking the Print icon in the upper-right corner of the screen.

24. Label the form Task 1-3B and place it in your SYNAPSE folder. Close the screen by clicking the X in the upper-right corner.

25. Click the Lab History icon. Your order should be displayed in the Incomplete Labs table. Refer to Figure 22.

Lab History for Cindy Swaim

| Main Menu | Patient Menu | Print | Update Lab Results | Health History | Rx | Labs | Current Visit | Delete Lab |

Thursday, January 18, 2007

Incomplete Labs

Date Sent	Date Results Received	Laboratory	Lab Test Name	Lab Test Results	Complete	Ordering Provider
5/14/2007		National Diagnostics	Chem 12		No	L.D. Heath MD
		In-House Testing	Fasting Blood Sugar or FBS		No	L.D. Heath MD

Completed Labs

Date Sent	Date Results Received	Laboratory	Lab Test Name	Lab Test Results	Complete	Ordering Provider

Figure 22   Lab History table showing the requests for both labs for Cindy Swaim

---

Help Box: Correcting an Error in the Lab Preview Screen

1. If you observe any errors during the lab preview, click out of the preview by clicking the Close box (the white X in the red box in the upper-right corner of the screen).

2. Click the Lab History icon.

3. Click the lab test that has the error.

4. Click the Delete Lab icon.

5. Click the small selector box next to the Click to Delete the Lab heading.

6. Close the screen. The information should no longer be listed in the table.

7. Go to the labs section by clicking the Labs icon, and start the whole lab requisition over.

Now that the lab requisitions are completed, you will need to create the prescriptions.

Task 1-4: Creating a Prescription

The first prescription listed is for the patient's anxiety: Rx for Alprazolam, 0.5 mg, # 30, Take 1 tablet every day. One month prescription, no refills.

1. Click Patient Menu.

2. Click Prescriptions.

3. Click the Pharmacy box drop-down arrow. Select Family Pharmacy Inc. 865 Livingston Ave, Fostoria NY, 01254.

4. Click the Common Drug Formulary drop-down arrow. Select Alpazolam. The instructions that autopopulate on the right side of the screen should match the order above.

5. Next, click the Payer box drop-down arrow. Select Signal HMO.

6. Next, click the drop-down arrow in the Clinician Ordering Medication box. Select Dr. Heath.

7. Next, click the drop-down arrow in the Prescription Created By box. Select Fauna's name.

8. On the bottom right side of the screen, enter the Start Date as today's appointment date. Select the End Date as a month from today's appointment.

9. You will notice two little boxes above the Start Date and End Date boxes. One box is labeled Do Not Substitute and the other box is labeled New Common Drug. The Do Not Substitute box is checked when the doctor does not want the patient to have the generic or less-expensive form of the drug. The New Common Drug box is checked when you create a prescription for a drug that is not listed in the Common Drug Formulary. The doctor did not give instructions that the drug could not be substituted, and the drug is already in the Common Drug Formulary, so uncheck both boxes if they are not already unchecked.

10. Under Refills, select None.

11. Double-check each box to make certain all information is correct.

12. Click Save. The information should automatically populate within the Prescription History table (Figure 23).

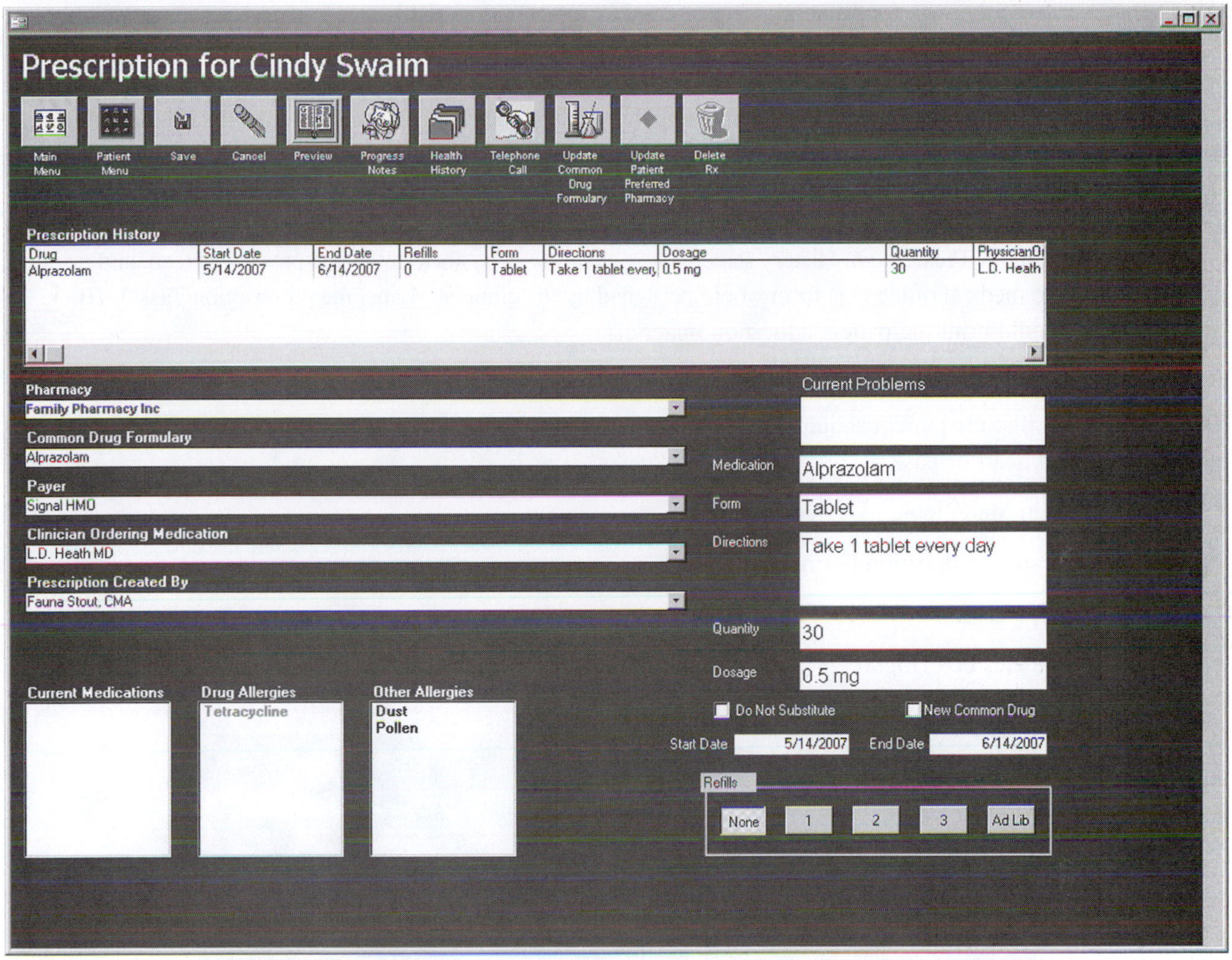

Figure 23   Prescription History screen for Cindy Swaim regarding the Alprazolam Rx

13. Click Preview. The Preview icon will allow you to view the prescription prior to printing it.

14. Click the Print icon in the Prescription Preview box and close the preview box.

15. In the medical office, the prescription would have been given to the physician to sign prior to giving it to the patient. Place the printed prescription in your folder and label it Task 1-4A.

Help Box: Correcting a Prescription Error after Saving

If you notice an error when previewing the information in the prescription screen after saving it, do the following:

1. Click the appropriate prescription within the Prescription History table.

2. Click the Delete Rx icon at the top of the toolbar.

3. Click in small empty box next to the Click to Delete the Prescription box.

4. Close the box.

5. Re-create the prescription and save.

The second prescription is for Atenolol, which is used to control the patient's blood pressure. The physician's order was for the following: Rx for Atenolol tabs, 50 mg, Take 1 tab each day before meals or at bedtime, One month prescription, no refills. This prescription should be easy to create because most of the necessary information was already entered for the first prescription. The only thing that needs to be changed is the name of the drug. Replace "Alprazolam" with "Atenolol." Make certain the information on the right matches the physician's order. The start date should be 05/14/2007 and the end date should be 06/14/2007. Be certain to click None under Refills. Take one final look at the information to make certain it matches the physician's order before clicking Save. Make certain the information saved in the Prescription History screen. Now click Preview, click out of the preview screen, and print the prescription. In the medical office, this form would be signed by the clinician. Label the prescription Task 1-4B.

Next, you should print the patient education materials.

Task 1-5: Printing Educational Handouts

The doctor stated that the patient should receive patient education materials for diabetes, smoking cessation, hypertension, and heart disease.

1. Click the Main Menu icon.

2. Next, click Patient Education Forms.

3. Next, click Education Letters.

4. Click the Diabetes box (Figure 24).

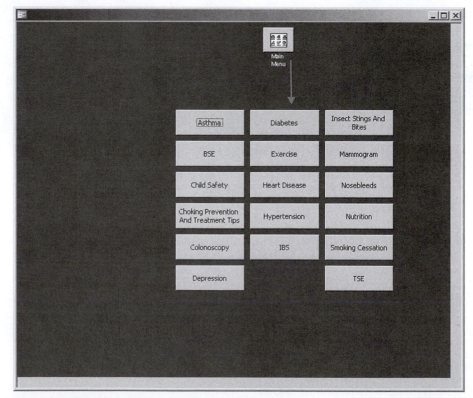

Figure 24   Education Letters screen

5. Choose Print from the File drop-down menu to print.

6. From the File drop-down menu, choose Close to return to the Education Letters screen.

7. Next, click Smoking Cessation tab.

8. Print the form and close the window, returning to the Education Letters screen.

9. Do the same for hypertension and heart disease.

10. Close the windows after printing.

11. After printing all of the handouts, label each handout as Task 1-5. Assign letters A through D for each individual handout. Place the educational handouts in your SYNAPSE folder.

Now you are ready to draw the patient's blood for outside testing and perform a finger stick for the in-house glucose testing. You finished the blood draw and blood glucose testing and are ready to log the information. The lab requisition forms have already been completed. Now you will need to record the glucose test in the In-House Test Log.

Task 1-6: Documenting an In-House Procedure within the In-House Test Log

1. Go to the Main Menu.

2. Click Logs.

3. Next, click the drop-down arrow in the In-House Log.

4. Select Glucose.

5. Click Open Selected Log.

6. Click Update.

7. Enter today's appointment date.

8. Choose the patient's name from the drop-down list in the Patient Name box.

9. Choose Dr. Heath's name from the drop-down list in the Ordering Provider box.

10. Enter the Manufacturer's Name, which is Jefferson Diagnostics.

11. Enter the Expiration Date from the test strips, which is 2/1/2008.

12. Enter the Lot Number, which is 4867.

13. Enter the results. Today's results are 204 mg/dl.

14. Click the drop-down arrow beside the Name of Person Performing the Test box. Click Fauna Stout's name.

15. Click Save. Refer to Figure 25 to make certain that you entered the information correctly.

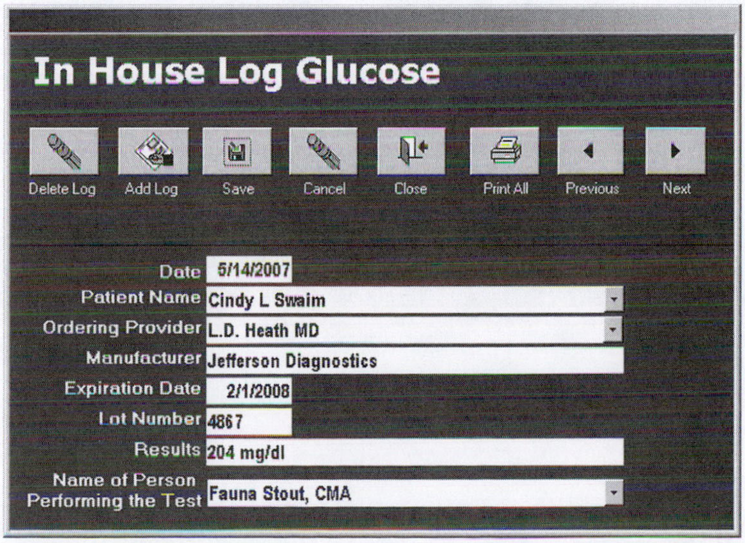

Figure 25 In-house log for Cindy Swaim's glucose

16. Print the glucose log by clicking the Print All icon. Label printout Task 1-6 and place it in your SYNAPSE folder.

17. Click Close.

18. The information should now appear on the In-House Glucose Test Log.

19. Click Close.

20. Close the Open Selected Log box by clicking the X in the upper-right corner of the window.

21. You should now be back in the Main Menu.

Help Box: In-House Logs

If the log you are working in has no prior entries, you can enter the information using the steps above; however, if other previous entries were made in the log prior to opening, you will need to click the Add Log icon before entering the information.

Task 1-7: Entering a Test Result in the Lab History Section

1. Select the Patients icon from the Main Menu.

2. Select Cindy Swaim's name.

3. Click Open Patient Record.

4. You should now be viewing Cindy's Patient Information Menu. Click the Lab Orders icon.

5. Click the Lab History icon.

6. Click the Fasting Blood Sugar test from the incomplete lab table.

7. Click the Update Lab Results icon (Figure 26).

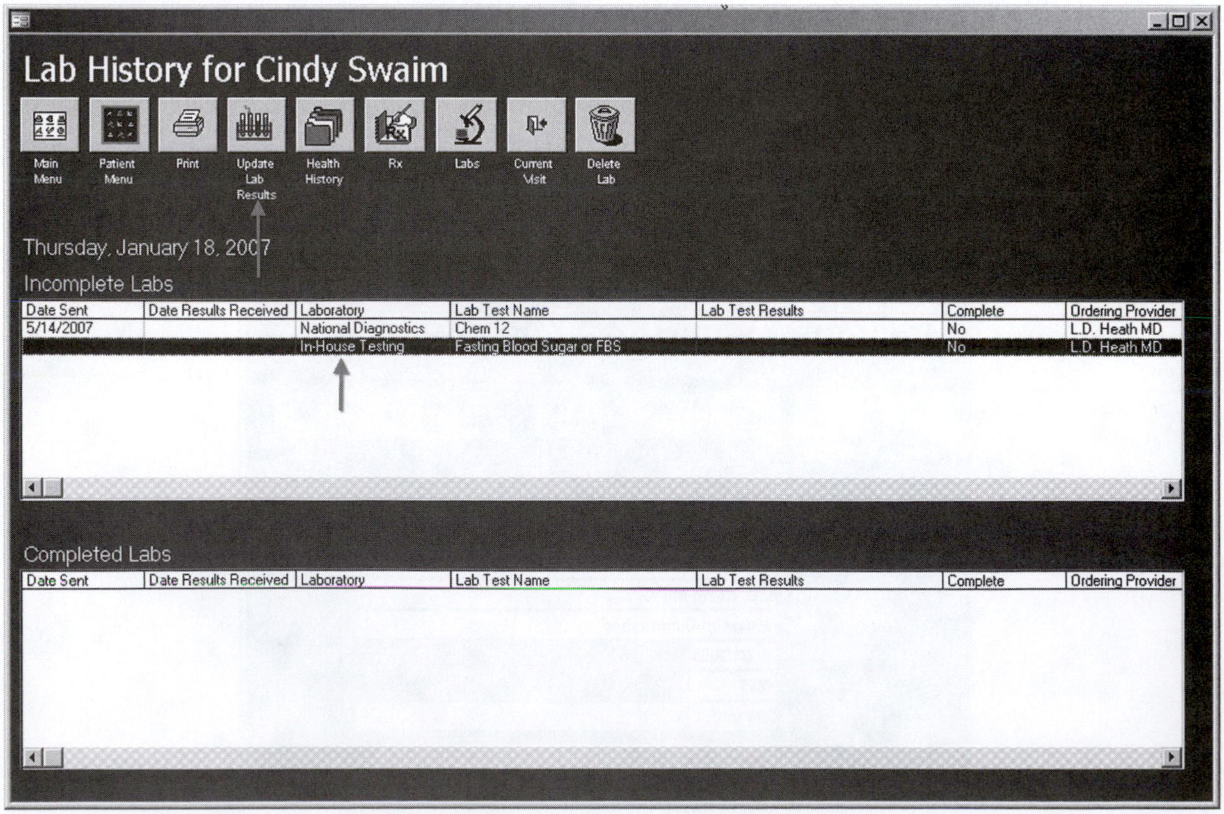

Figure 26   Lab History screen for Cindy Swaim

8. Type the lab result: 204 mg/dl.

9. Choose Fauna's name from the drop-down list in the Name of Person Who Recorded Results box.

10. Enter 5/14/2007 as the date the results were received. Check to make certain you entered the information correctly by comparing your information with Figure 27.

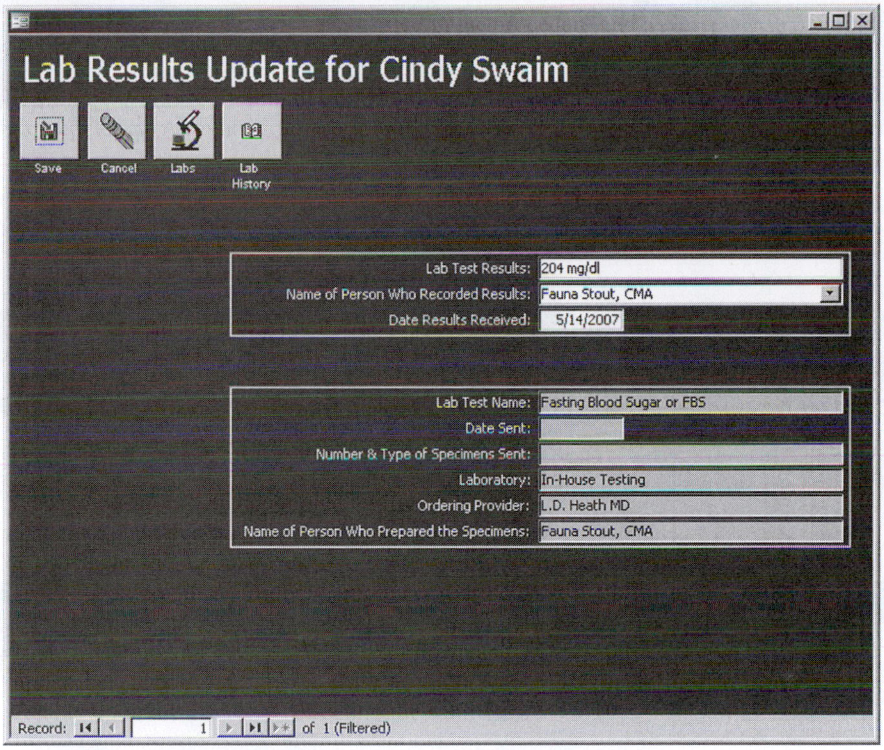

Figure 27   Lab Results Update screen for Cindy Swaim

11. Click Save.

12. Click Lab History.

13. The glucose results should have moved from the Incomplete Labs section to the Completed Labs section. (Figure 28).

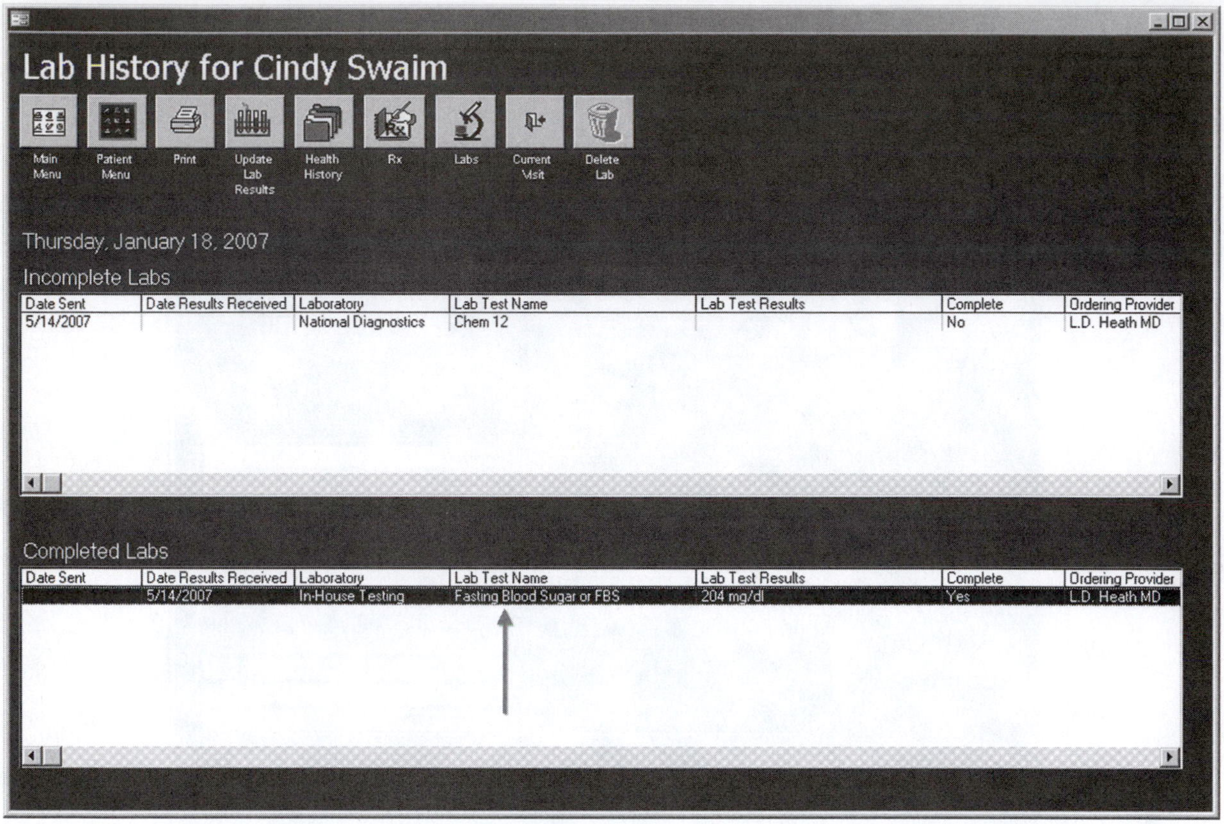

Figure 28   Lab History table for Cindy Swaim, illustrating how the glucose moved from the Incomplete Labs to the Completed Labs

14. Print the lab history tables by clicking the Print icon. Label the Incomplete Lab table as Task 1-7A and the Complete Lab table as Task 1-7B. Place both tables in your SYNAPSE folder.

Help Box: Printing Tables in the Lab History Screen

The Lab History Tables will not print unless there is data within the tables.

---

15. Click the Patient Menu icon.

Inform the physician of the patient's result and determine if he needs you to do anything else for the patient. The physician tells you he wants to go in and discuss the results with the patient, and that he will let you know when he is finished.

The physician re-enters the patient's examination room and discusses the findings. He notifies you that he is finished and informs you that you can complete the visit. You have already gathered all of the patient's prescriptions and educational handouts. You enter the patient's room and distribute and explain each prescription and educational handout. You ask the patient if she has any further questions. She asks you for a proof of appointment letter for her employer.

Task 1-8: Proof of Appointment Letter

1. Go to Cindy Swaim's Patient Information Menu, if you are not already there.

2. Click Patient Templates.

3. Click the Proof of Appointment button.

4. Insert the date of the appointment in the Date box.

5. Since Cindy's appointment was for 9:00, select 9:00 AM from the drop-down menu beside the appointment.

6. Click the Clinician drop-down list and select Dr. Heath. Refer to Figure 29 ensure you properly completed the template.

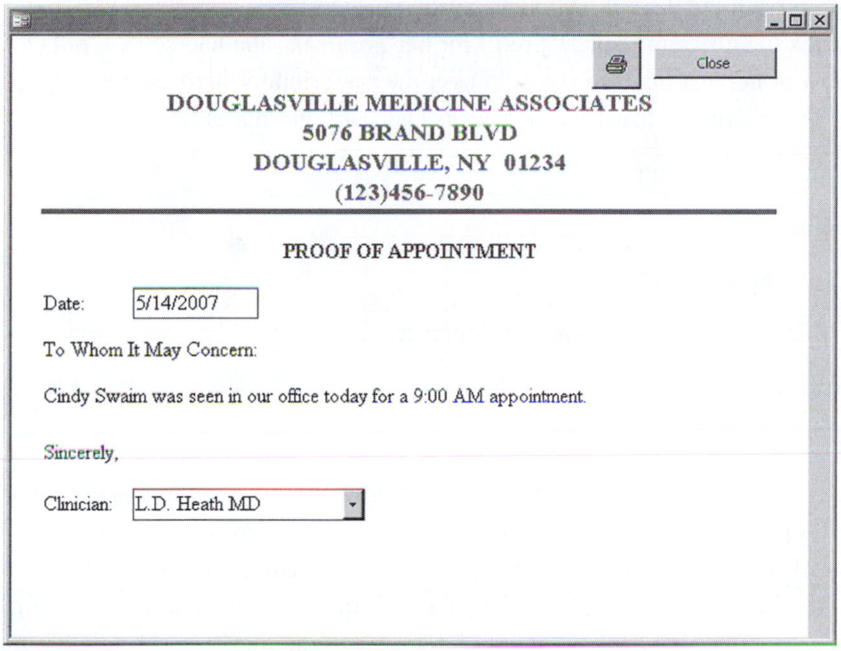

Figure 29   Proof of Appointment Letter template completed for Cindy Swaim

7. Print the letter and label it Task 1-8 and place it in your SYNAPSE folder.

8. Click Close.

9. Close the template letters by clicking the X in the upper-right corner of the window. You should now be in the Patient Information Menu for Cindy Swaim screen.

Task 1-9: Completing the Progress Note and Closing Out of the Patient's Record

Since the patient is gone and you are done working in the patient's personal EMR, you can now close the chart note.

1. Click the Chart Notes icon.

2. Click New Office Visit.

3. Click Save.

4. Click Update Progress Notes to make certain that all of the latest information was entered in the chart.

5. Click on the Complete Visit icon. *Note: When you leave this page, you will be unable to enter any additional data within the chart note.*

6. Click Patient Menu.

7. Click the Chart Notes icon.

8. Check to make certain that the date of your progress note saved to the Previous Office Visits box.

9. Click the visit and view the note.

10. Click Chart Notes.

11. Click Patient Menu.

12. Click the Main Menu.

Task 1-10: Phone Call from Blanche White

You will receive many phone calls, even while you are working in a clinical capacity. It is important that you document all encounters with the patient, including telephone calls.

Blanche White calls the office to request a refill for her Fosamax. She had several pills left from her previous prescription at the time of her last visit, so she didn't get the prescription filled. She lost the prescription and is now out of the drug. The pharmacy that Blanche uses is DanMart on Polaris Drive.

1. On the Main Menu, click Patients.

2. Select Blanche White.

3. Click Open Patient Record.

4. Now you should be in the Patient Information Menu screen.

5. Click Chart Notes.

6. Click the Telephone Call icon.

7. Notice there are four tabs in the center of this screen (Figure 30). The first tab is used when the patient is calling to request a prescription refill. When you click this tab, the Prescription History table will appear, which illustrates all of the medications the patient is currently taking. The second tab is labeled Follow-Up on Lab Test Results. You select this tab when the patient is requesting information regarding a lab test. This screen contains the patient's lab history for easy referencing. The third tab is labeled Symptoms. This tab is used when the patient has questions regarding symptoms he or she is currently experiencing, or when the patient has questions regarding his or her condition. The fourth tab is labeled Other Calls. This tab is used when the patient is calling about something other than the three previous tabs. Since the patient is calling regarding a prescription refill, keep the Prescription Refill tab current.

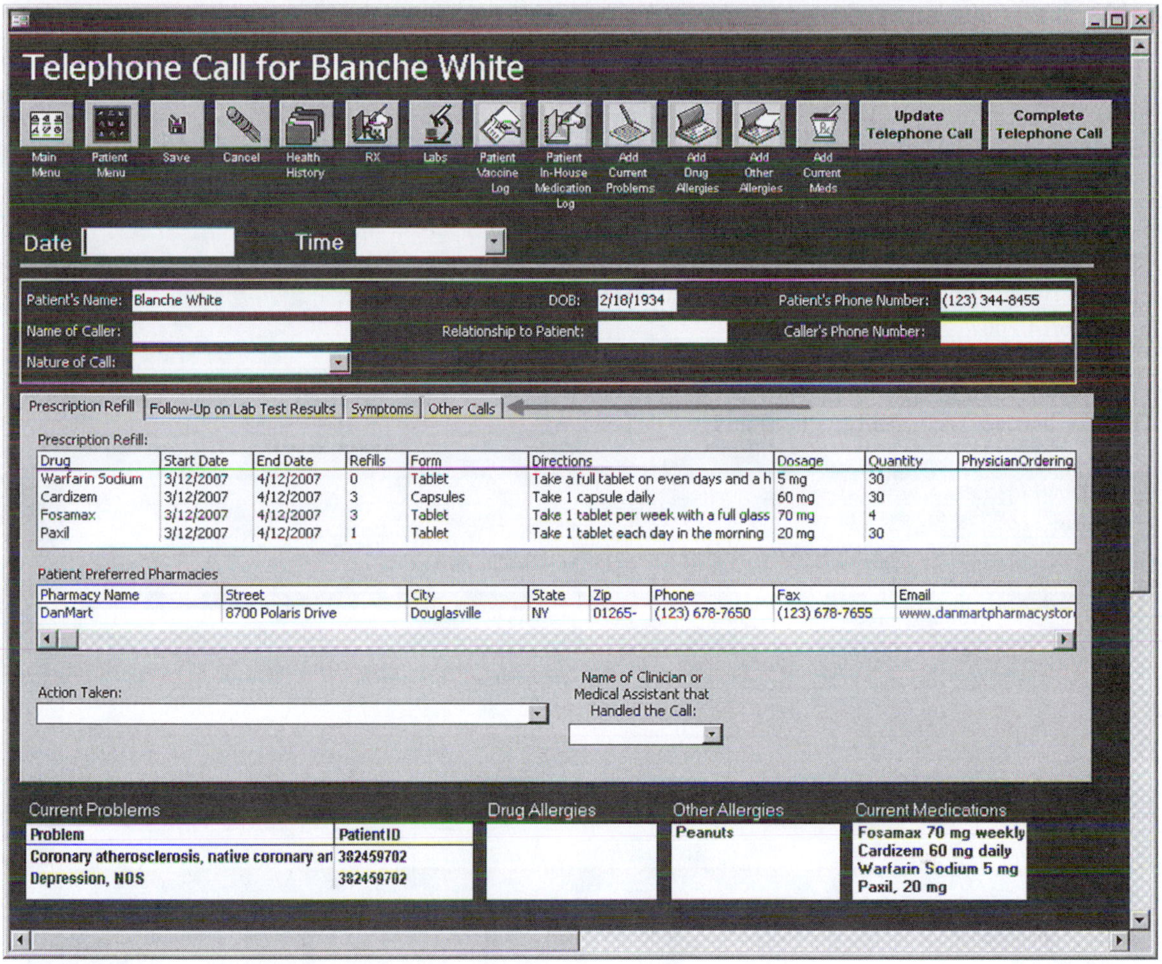

Figure 30   Telephone screen for Blanche White

8. Enter 05/14/2007 in the Date box.

9. Enter 9:45 AM in the Time box.

10. Enter Blanche White in the Name of Caller box.

11. Click the drop-down list arrow in the Nature of Call box, and select Prescription Refill.

12. The patient's birthday should have automatically populated in the DOB box.

13. In the Relationship to Patient box, enter Self.

14. The patient's home phone number should have automatically populated in the Patient's Phone Number box.

15. The caller's phone number is the same number as above, so type SAA in this box.

16. The patient's prescriptions will appear on the screen. Click Fosamax, since that is the prescription the patient is requesting.

17. Another box will appear. Place a checkmark in the box beside the Click to Indicate Telephone Inquiry box. Click out of the box by clicking the X on the upper-right corner of this window.

18. There is only one pharmacy, so you don't have to click in anything in that box.

19. Select the action you took from the drop-down list: Sent an Electronic Task to the Physician.

20. Select the person who handled the call (Fauna) from the drop-down list.

21. Double-check to make certain that you have all the information correct by comparing your screen with Figure 31.

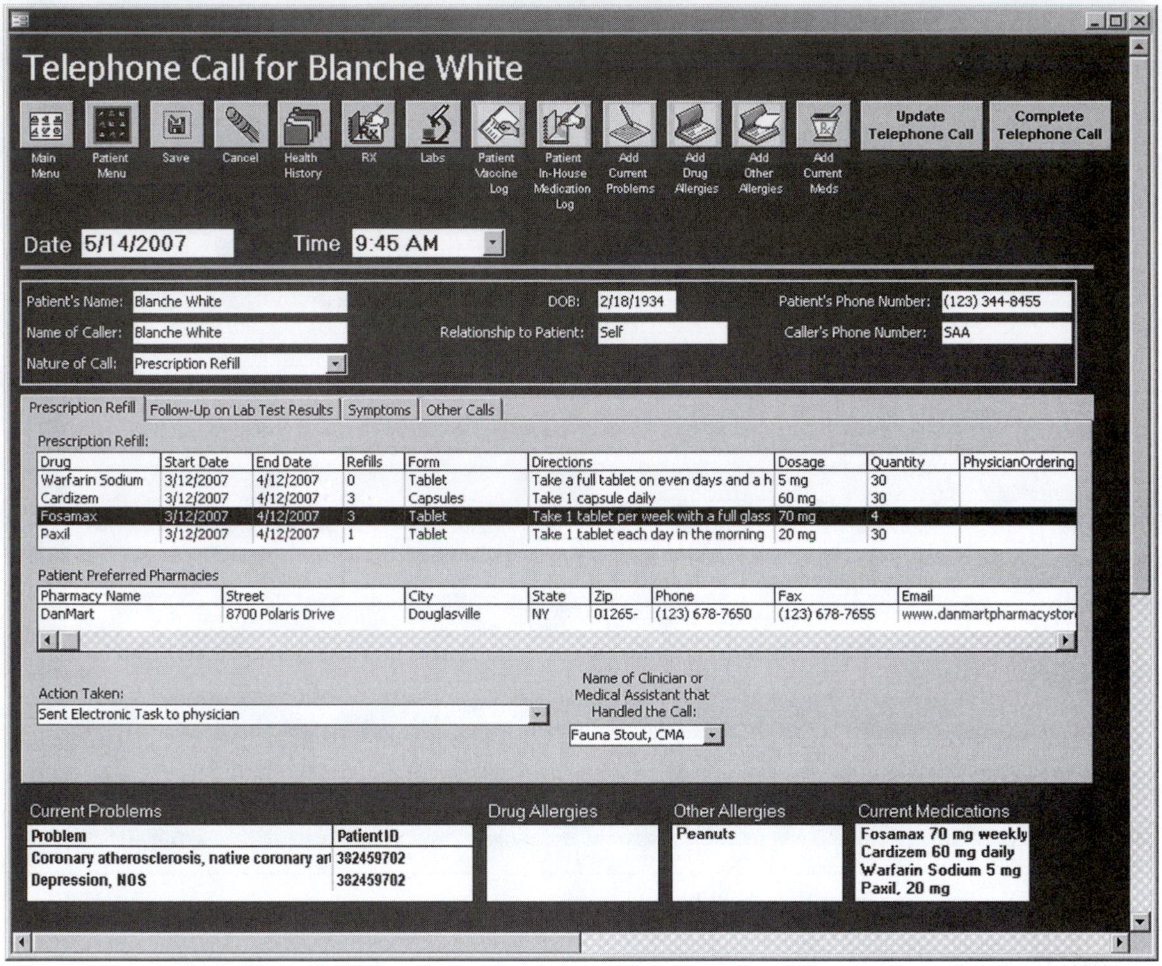

Figure 31   Completed Telephone Note for Blanche White

22. Click Update Telephone Call.

23. Click Save.

24. Click Complete Telephone Call. Once you click this icon and leave the screen, you will not be able to make any more adjustments, so make certain the information is correct before leaving the screen.

25. Click Patient Menu.

26. Click Chart Notes.

27. Click 5/14/2007 under Previous Telephone Calls.

28. Click the Print icon. Label your assignment as Task 1-10 and place in your SYNAPSE folder.

29. Click the Main Menu. The activities for Module I are now concluded.

Critical Thinking Questions for Module I

1. Cindy Swaim stated that she was a borderline diabetic and had high cholesterol during the health history portion of the interview. Her chief complaint was in regard to anxiety. Why shouldn't the medical assistant enter this information within the Current Problems screen? What information should be entered in the Current Problems screen? Whose responsibility would it be to enter such information?

2. Why is Cindy such a likely candidate for a heart attack?

3. What was the purpose of running a control on the glucometer? Why do you think that Fauna chose the High control?

4. Who may the office leave private information with when Cindy is not available?

5. What part of the chart should you check to find out how Cindy wants to be addressed for future visits? What other type of information may be entered in this section?

6. Cindy's complaint for today's visit was anxiety; however, after reading the history information and following her examination, Dr. Heath ordered patient education forms for diabetes, smoking cessation, hypetension, and heart disease. Explain the probable reason that each form was ordered. Dr. Heath did not order a patient education form for anxiety. This may be because there wasn't one stocked within the EMR. If Dr. Heath did order a patient education pamphlet that was not stocked in the EMR, what would be the next course of action?

MODULE II

Today's date: May 15, 2007
Appointments for May 15, 2007.

Patient's Name	Appointment Time	New Patient or Established Patient	Reason for Appointment	Clinician	MA
Morgan Penrose	9:00 AM	NP	UTI	Dr. Schwartz	Roger Wong, RMA

Work Assignments

You will be working as Roger Wong, RMA, for the next several tasks.

Task 2-1: Documenting in the Quality Control Log

After using the last rapid strep test in the rapid strep kit, Roger needs to open a new strep kit. He will need to run a control prior to using the new kit. Log information is found in Table 3.

TABLE 3   TASK 2-1 INFORMATION

Date	05/15/2007
Test Name	Two-Step Rapid Strep Test
Manufacturer's Name	Jefferson Diagnostics
Name of Control	+ Control
Lot #	6598
Exp Date	06/12/2008
Reference Range or Result	Positive
Result	Positive
Person Performing Control	Roger Wong, RMA

1. Go to the Main Menu and select Logs.

2. Go to the Quality Control Logs and click Rapid Strep Test. Open the selected log and click Update.

3. Enter the information from Table 3. **Do not forget to save the information.**

4. Print the log and label it Task 2-1.

5. Place the log in your SYNAPSE folder.

6. Close the log window. You should now see the information in the rapid strep log table. Close out of the log by clicking the Close box.

7. Close the Open Selected Log box by clicking the X in the upper-right corner of the window. You should now be back at the Main Menu screen.

Task 2-2: Creating a New Chart

Mrs. Morgan Penrose just arrived. You obtained her vitals and performed a medical history. You also obtained her chief complaint and reviewed the privacy statement with her. All responses to Mrs. Penrose's questions can be found in Table 4.

TABLE 4   MORGAN PENROSE'S PATIENT DATA TABLE

Patient's Name	Morgan A. Penrose
Patient's DOB	05/16/1960
Patient's Chart Number	257986523
Patient's Address	876 Honeycut Lane, Douglasville, NY 01234-1212
Patient's Telephone Numbers	Home: 123-457-9865 Work: None
Patient's Employer Info	None
Gender, Marital Status, Blood Type & Smoking Status	Gender: Female Marital Status: Married Blood Type: O– Smoking Status: Non-smoker
Patient Picture Screen: Patient Notes	Patient prefers to be addressed by her first name. Patient is getting ready to start nursing school (05/14/2007).
Spouse Name, DOB, & Address	Chad W. Penrose, DOB: 02/13/1955, Address: Same as patient
Responsible Party Info	Responsible Party: Spouse SS # or ID #: 365-84-9865 Address and Home: 876 Honeycut Lane, Douglasville, NY 01234-1212 Home Phone: 123-457-9865 Work Phone: 123-698-8888 Employer: Douglasville Textiles, 3658 City Park, N. Douglasville, NY 01236-1245
Primary Payer Info	Name: Flexihealth ID # 365849865-00 Policy/Group # 4ABDT DOB: 02/13/1955 Gender: Male SS # or ID #: 365-84-9865
Secondary Payer	None

Patient Drug Allergies	Codeine
Patient Other Allergy	Strawberries
Current Mediation List	Singulair, 10 mg/day, Albuterol Inhaler, and Clonazepam, 1 mg/day
Preferred Pharmacy	DanMart Pharmacy, 567 S. High Street, Douglasville, NY, 01234
Lab Provider	American Labs
Privacy Statement	Reviewed and signed May 15, 2007 Enter the following information in the Notes box: No one except the patient can receive private information. Do not leave any information on patient's answering machine.
Family Health History Info	Father: Age 69, Health: Good Mother: Age 68, Health: Fair Brother: Age 45, Health: Fair Brother: Age 41, Health: Good Sister: Age 39, Health: Good Heart disease: Mother has CAD. Had stent surgery in March 2001. High blood pressure: Mother, controlled with medication. Asthma: Brother has asthma. Controlled with steroids and breathing tx. Other: Stroke, maternal grandmother died of a stroke in 1992.

Hospitalizations, Blood Transfusions, and Serious Injuries	Hospitalizations:
	   1982, Lakeside Memorial Hospital, birth of oldest daughter
	   1986, Lakeside Memorial Hospital, birth of youngest daughter
	   1987, Lakeside Memorial Hospital, birth of son
	Blood Transfusions: No blood transfusions
	Serious Injuries: None

Pregnancies	1982, female, C-section (baby's heart rated dropped) 1986, female, C-section (no complications) 1987, son, C-section (no complications)
Medical History	Click the following diseases: asthma, chicken pox, and other. In the Note's box, list the following: Asthma: Diagnosed in 1966. Treated with Singulair 10 mg/day and Albuterol Inhaler. Averages 1 attack every 1–2 months. Chicken pox: 1965 (no complications) Other: Seizure disorder, diagnosed in 1975. Clonazepam, 1 mg capsule/day. (Seizure-free for past 2 years)
Health Habits	Caffeine, 1 8-ounce cup of coffee/day. Does not smoke or drink alcohol. Occupation: Going to nursing school

Subjective Information	Urinary tract symptoms: Severity of Symptoms: 7 Duration: 3 days Associated Symptoms: + Abdominal pressure or pain, back pain, fever, nausea/vomiting, and urinary frequency. - Hx of UTI, mucus in urine, or vaginal symptoms Aggravating Symptoms: Not urinating Relieving Factors: OTC pain reliever
Objective Information	Vital Signs: Height: 67 inches Weight: 135 pounds Temperature: 101.4 Blood Pressure: 142/86 Pulse: 90 Respiration: 18 Pain: 7 Subjective Information and Vital Signs Entered By: Roger Wong, RMA

CREATING A CHART

1. In the Main Menu, click New Patients.

2. Complete all of the information within each tab of the Patient Information screen and save. Use Table B-4 to complete each tab.

3. Save each screen as you complete each tab.

4. Go back through each tab and make certain your information is correct and saved.

5. Click Main Menu.

6. Click the Patients tab.

7. Highlight Morgan Penrose and click Open Patient Record.

8. You should now be in the Patient Information Menu for Morgan Penrose.

9. Click the Legal icon.

10. Click the drop-down arrow in the box next to Privacy Statement. Click Yes and enter the Date of today's visit in the date box. Enter the corresponding information in the Notes box from Table 4. Save your information.

11. Return to the Patient Menu and click the Health History icon.

12. Enter the corresponding information from Table 4 within each tab. Remember to save your information within each screen.

13. Click the Patient Menu, then Chart Notes.

14. Click New Office Visit. Enter the date and time of the patient's visit.

15. Click Update Progress Note and then Save.

16. You are now ready to enter the patient's subjective information. Start by clicking the Subjective tab.

17. Click the drop-down arrow in the Chief Complaint box.

18. Scroll and click Urinary Tract Symptoms.

19. Click Update Progress Note and then click Save.

20. Click Add HPI. Using the HPI information from Table 4, enter the appropriate information. Click Save after entering the HPI data.

21. Click Progress Note. You should now be on the Subjective tab.

22. Click the Objective tab.

23. Using the patient data table, enter the appropriate information.

24. List Roger Wong as the medical assistant who entered the subjective information and vital signs.

25. Click Update Progress Note, then click Save.

26. Click the Progress Notes tab. Make certain all of your information populated correctly within the progress note.

27. Print the progress note and label it Task 2-2. Place it in your SYNAPSE folder. Leave the screen for the physician. *Note: If you made an error in the progress note and do not recall how to correct it, refer to Help Box: Progress Notes.*

The doctor goes in to examine Mrs. Penrose. When he comes out of the patient's room, he instructs you to read the Plans section of the progress note. The plans state the following:

Plans: Complete UA and C&S. Rx for Septra DS Tab # 20, Take 1 tablet every 12 hours for 10 days, No refills. Rx for Singulair Tab, 10 mg, # 30. Take 1 tablet each day, 3 refills, Rx for Clonazepam Tablets, 1 mg, # 30. Take 1 tablet each day, 3 refills. Patient is getting ready to go to nursing school and needs the Hepatitis B series. Will give patient her first Hepatitis B shot today. Patient to return in 4 weeks for second Hepatitis B shot and a complete physical.

There are many tasks to perform, so time management is very important. Since the physician ordered a Complete UA and C&S, you will want to give the patient instructions for performing a clean-catch urine sample and hand the patient a labeled specimen container with cleansing towelettes. Inform the patient what to do with the sample once she collects it. While the patient is collecting the sample, you will create the electronic lab requisitions and prescriptions. Start by creating the lab requisition forms.

Task 2-3: Creating a Lab Requisition

1. You should still be in the Progress Note screen for the current visit.

2. Click the Labs icon.

3. Click the drop-down menu arrow in the Laboratory box and select American Labs. This is the lab that is listed as a provider for the patient's insurance company.

4. Click the Ordering Provider drop-down arrow. Click Dr. Schwartz, since he is the provider who saw Mrs. Penrose today.

5. Click the appropriate payer company.

6. Click the General Lab Tests arrow.

7. Scroll through the list and click UA Complete.

8. In the Number of and Type of Specimens Sent, type One Clean Catch Urine Sample (125 ml).

9. In the Today's Date box, enter the date of today's appointment.

10. In the Specimen Prepared By box, select Roger Wong.

11. Choose No in the Was patient fasting? drop-down list.

12. Click Save.

13. Preview the lab order. Make certain it is correct.

14. Click the Print icon. Label this Task 2-3A and place it in your SYNAPSE folder. Close the preview screen.

You now need to create a lab requisition form for the UA Culture & Sensitivity. The information for the last test should still be on the screen, so you will only need to change the name in the General Lab Test box to UA C&S, and change the Number of and Type of Specimens Sent to 1 UA Culture Swab in Liquid Media. Make certain all information is correct before saving. Click Preview. Click the Print icon. Label the requisition form as Task 2-3B and place it in your SYNAPSE folder. Close out of the print preview. Click Lab History and make certain that both tests populated within the Incomplete Labs table. Return to the Patient Menu.

Next, you will create the prescriptions.

Task 2-4: Creating Prescriptions

1. Start in the Patient Menu screen for Morgan Penrose.

2. Click Prescriptions.

3. Create prescriptions for all the prescriptions listed under the Plans section of the progress note. The patient's preferred pharmacy and payer information should automatically be loaded in the prescription screen. List the dosage for Septra as DS, which stands for double strength. Make certain you put today's date in the Start Date box and the end date for 30 days later on all the prescriptions. There shouldn't be any checks in the Start Date box or New Common Drug box.

4. Next click Save, Preview, and Print for each prescription. Label prescriptions as Task 2-4A through 2-4C and place in your SYNAPSE folder. *Note: If you made an error on one of the prescriptions and do not remember how to delete it, refer back to Help Box: Correcting a Prescription Error after Saving.*

Since the doctor also ordered a hepatitis B shot, you should print the vaccination information sheets form and consent form for that immunization.

Task 2-5: Printing Educational VIS Forms

1. Go to the Main Menu.

2. Click Patient Education Forms, and click Vaccination Information Sheets.

3. Click the Hepatitis B Form, and print it. Label it as Task 2-5 and place it in your SYNAPSE folder. Go to the File Menu and select Close.

4. Select Main Menu, then select Patients.

5. Select Morgan Penrose, and click Open Patient Record. You should now be in the Patient Information Menu for Morgan Penrose.

Task 2-6: Creating and Printing an Immunization Consent Form

1. Click the Authorization/Refusal Forms icon.

2. Click Immunization Consent Form.

3. Since the patient is only having one immunization today, click the drop-down arrow in the box beside 1. Click Hepatitis B. Do not do anything with the extra boxes.

4. Enter the name of the patient in the Typed Name box.

5. Enter the date of the visit in the Today's Date box. Refer to Figure 32 to make certain that the form is properly completed.

DOUGLASVILLE MEDICINE ASSOCIATES
5076 BRAND BLVD
DOUGLASVILLE, NY 01234
(123)456-7890

IMMUNIZATION CONSENT FORM

I have read the Vaccination Information Statement(s) regarding the following immunizations listed below and am aware of the adverse reactions associated with the vaccine(s). I have had an opportunity to ask questions regarding the possible adverse reactions and benefits of each immunization. I believe that the benefits out weigh the risks and I assume full responsibility for any reactions that may occur.

1 Hepatitis B   2

3   4

I am requesting that the immunization(s) be given to me or the person listed below for whom I am the legal guardian.

	05/15/2007
Signature/Legal Guardian	Today's Date
Morgan Penrose	
Typed Name	Witness

Figure 32   Immunization Consent Form for Morgan Penrose

6. Click Print.

7. In the medical office, both the patient and medical assistant would sign this form prior to scanning it back into the chart. This form must be signed. Label your work as Task 2-6 and place it in your SYNAPSE folder.

Once you have everything printed, take all of the paperwork into the patient's room. Give the patient all of her prescriptions and explain each one. Next, give the patient the VIS form for the hepatitis B immunization. Ask the patient to read the form thoroughly while you prepare the injection. After returning from preparing the injection, ask the patient if she has any questions. She states that she doesn't. Ask the patient to sign the consent form. Then, you give the patient the injection. Following the injection, you give the patient her prescriptions and tell her to schedule an appointment for a thorough physical. Dismiss the patient. You now need to enter the injection within the electronic chart.

Task 2-7: Entering Immunization Information in the Patient's Immunization Log

1. Go to the Patient Information Screen for Morgan Penrose.

2. Click Immunization Log.

3. Click the Update tab at the bottom of the screen. (If the patient had a previous vaccine, you will need to click Add Immunization before entering the information.)

4. Enter the information from Table B-5.

TABLE B-5   TASK 2-7 IMMUNIZATION INFORMATION

Date	05/15/2007
Time	9:30 AM
Ordering Physician	Dr. Schwartz
Immunization Name	Hepatitis B
Number in Series	#1
Amt. Given	0.5 ml
Location	R. Deltoid
Route	IM
Person Who Administered Injection	Roger Wong, RMA

5. Compare your screen to Figure 33, then click Save.

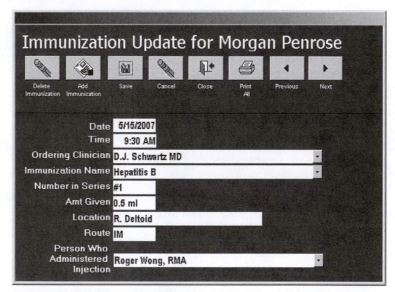

Figure 33   Immunization Update screen

6. Click Print All. Label the form Task 2-7 and place it in your SYNAPSE folder.

7. Click Close. You should now be in the Immunizations for Morgan Penrose log.

8. Close the screen. You should now be back in the Patient Information Menu screen.

Task 2-8: Closing the Chart Note for Morgan Penrose

Since the patient is finished and you are done working in the patient's personal EMR, you can now close the chart note.

1. Click Chart Notes.

2. Click New Office Visit.

3. Click Update Progress Note, and then click Save.

4. Click Complete Visit. After you leave this page, you will be unable to enter any additional data within this chart note.

5. Click Patient Menu.

6. Click the Chart Notes icon. Check to make certain that the date of your progress note saved to the Previous Office Visits box. Open the box and preview it.

7. Click Chart Notes. If the progress note is not listed in the Previous Office Visits box, you did not correctly exit the note. Return to the New Office Visit screen and review the information. If the information is correct, click the Update Progress Note button, click Save, and then click Complete Visit. Check to make certain that the information saved correctly this time. Click the Main Menu icon.

Task 2-9: Entering Immunizations on the Global Immunization Log

Now that you entered the information in the patient's personal information log, you will enter the information into the global immunization log. This log tracks all immunizations given in the office.

1. From the Main Menu, click Logs.

2. In the Global Immunization log drop-down list, choose Hepatitis B.

3. Click Open Selected Log, and then click Update.

4. Record the requested information. The only additional information you will need to complete this log is the Drug Form Injectable, Amt Given: 0.5 ml, Ordering Clinician: D.J. Scwartz MD, Manuf Name: CKD, Lot Number, 13698P, Exp Date: 06/15/2008, Who Administered: Roger Wong.

5. Click Save and then click Print All. Label the document Task 2-9. Click Close.

6. You should now see the Hepatitis B Immunization Log in the table.

7. Click the Close button at the bottom of the screen. Close the Open Selected Log screen. You should now be back at the Main Menu screen.

Critical Thinking Questions for Module II

1. Why do you think the physician ordered a culture and sensitivity in addition to the complete UA?

2. The patient arrived with urinary symptoms, so why do you think the physician ordered prescriptions for Clonazepam and Singulair in addition to the Septra DS? The patient also had Albuterol inhaler listed for her current meds. What might be a logical explanation as to why the physician didn't order a prescription for this medication?

3. What would you do if the patient refused to sign the immunization consent form?

4. Why did you have to record the immunization on two separate logs?

MODULE III

Today's date: May 16, 2007
Appointments for May 16, 2007

Patient's Name	Appointment Time	Reason for Appointment	Clinician	MA
Kevin Cook	1:00 PM	Sports physical	Megan Speck, NP	Roger Wong, RMA
Blanche White	1:15 PM	Complete physical	Dr. Schwartz	Roger Wong, RMA

TABLE 6   KEVIN COOK'S DATA TABLE

Patient's Name	Kevin R. Cook
Patient's DOB	03/12/1995
Patient's Chart Number	219365878
Patient's Address	1756 Edgeview Road, Douglasville, NY 01234-1212
Patient's Telephone Numbers	Home: 123-786-0098 No work number
Patient's Employer Info	None
Gender, Marital Status, Blood Type & Smoking Status	Gender: Male Marital Status: Single Blood Type: Leave blank (not known) Smoking Status: Non-smoker
Patient Picture Screen: Patient Notes	Patient prefers to be addressed by his middle name, which is Ryan.
Responsible Party Info	Responsible Party: Other (Father) Name: David M. Cook SS # or ID #: 356-98-5987 Address and Home: 1756 Edgeview Road, Douglasville, NY 01234-1212 Home Phone: 123-786-0098 Work Phone: 123-876-0987 Employer: Self-employed Douglasville, NY 01234-1212
Primary Payer Info	Name: Signal HMO ID # 356985987-00 Policy Holder Information: Other (father's information) Policy/Group: None Gender: Male DOB: 03/14/1967
Secondary Payer	None
Patient Drug Allergies	Aspirin
Patient Other Allergy	Dog and cat dander
Current Mediation List	None
Preferred Pharmacy	Douglasville Pharmacy, 7890 Cobblestone Place, Douglasville, NY
Lab Provider	Smith, Wright, & Kennedy
Privacy Statement	Reviewed and signed, May 16, 2007 Enter the following information in the Note's box: Father stated that private information may be left with him and the patient's mother.

Family Health History Info	Father: Age 40, Health: Good
	Mother: Age 39, Health: Good
	Brother: Age 16, Health: Good
	Sister: Age 9, Health: Good
	Heart disease: Maternal grandmother (heart attack at age 62).
	Other: Epilepsy, brother (onset at age 12, controlled with meds).
Hospitalizations, Blood Transfusions, and Serious Injuries	Hospitalizations: None
	Blood Transfusions: None
	Serious Injuries: None
Pregnancies	N/A
Medical History	Click the following disease: Chicken pox. In the Note's box, list the following: Chicken pox: 1998 (no complications)
Health Habits	Caffeine, 3 12-ounce cans of soda per day. Does not smoke or drink alcohol. Does not work.
Subjective Information	Patient here for sport's physical: Type "Sports Physical" in the Chief Complaint box.
Objective Information	Vital Signs:
	Height: 73 inches
	Weight: 165 pounds
	Temperature: 98.4
	Blood Pressure: 110/64
	Pulse: 64
	Respiration: 14
	Pain: 0
	Subjective Information and Vital Signs Entered By: Roger Wong, RMA

Task 3-1: Creating an Electronic Chart and Progress Note

You are acting as Roger Wong in these exercises.

1. Using Table 6, create an electronic chart and new progress note for Kevin Cook. Refer to Module I if you forget any of the specific components for creating a chart. The only difference in creating a progress note for this patient is that he is coming in for a sports physical instead of with symptoms.

2. Within the Subjective tab, type the words "Sports Physical" in the Chief Complaint box. You will not need to perform an HPI since the patient doesn't have any symptoms.

3. Click Update Progress Note, then click Save.

4. Next, click the Progress Notes tab. You should see the words "Sports Physical" under the Chief Complaint heading within the Subjective tab.

5. Click the Objective tab and enter the objective information.

6. Click Update Progress Note, then click Save.

7. Click the Progress Notes tab. Your subjective and objective information should populate in the progress note.

8. Click the Print icon and label the assignment Task 3-1.

You instruct Kevin on how to disrobe. Kevin's dad hands you a sports physical form from Kevin's school that needs to be completed. You give the form to Megan Speck, the nurse practitioner, before she examines the patient. Normally you would wait until the NP is finished with the patient to complete the record; however, you are finished recording this particular progress note, and you are ready to take a new patient to the room, so you complete and close the record at this time.

Task 3-2: Completing the Progress Note

1. Because you updated and saved the progress note information, you can now click the Complete Visit icon. *Note: Remember that once you leave the screen, you will be unable to make changes.*

2. Click the Patient Menu icon, and then click Chart Notes.

3. You should see the date of the visit in the Previous Office Visits box.

4. Click today's visit date to make certain the note saved properly.

5. Click the Chart Notes icon, and then click the Main Menu icon.

Task 3-3: Entering Information in a Previously Created Chart

While the nurse practitioner is in the room with Kevin Cook, Blanche White enters the reception area. She has an appointment with Dr. Schwartz. Since you are covering both Megan Speck and Dr. Schwartz, you will be taking care of Mrs. White.

1. Start by clicking the Main Menu icon, if you aren't already there.

2. Open Mrs. White's EMR by clicking the Patients icon, selecting her name, and then clicking Open Patient Record.

3. Click the Demographics icon. Read the information in the Patient Picture tab to see if Mrs. White has a preference on how she wants to be addressed, or to see if there are any other notes that may need attention before calling back the patient. You notice there is nothing entered in this section. When the patient enters the examination room, you ask her if she has a preference for the way she wants to be addressed. The patient states that she prefers to be addressed by her first name. The patient goes on to tell you that her granddaughter is getting married this weekend, on May 18. This is an important event in the patient's life, and you will want to ask her about the wedding on her next visit. Because of this, you should enter the information within the Patient Notes box as a reminder.

4. Enter the following notes in the Patient Notes box: Patient prefers to be addressed by her first name. Patient's granddaughter is getting married May 18, 2007. (The next time the patient comes in to the office, you may want to ask the patient about the wedding.) Click Save.

You ask Blanche if any demographic information has changed since her last visit. She states that it hasn't. Next, you ask if any legal information has changed since her last visit, such as privacy information, DNR information, etc. The patient once states it hasn't. Now you are ready to create a new progress note.

1. Click the Patient Main button at the top of your toolbar. You should now be in the Patient Information Menu for Blanche White.

2. Click the Chart Notes icon, and then New Office Visit.

3. Enter the date and time of the patient's appointment, and then click Update Progress Note. Click Save.

4. Click the Subjective tab. Enter "Complete Physical" in the Chief Complaint box. Click Update Progress Note, and then click Save.

5. Click the Objective Tab. Enter the following information:

Height: 60 inches

Weight: 164 pounds

Temperature: 97.8

Blood Pressure: 134/82

Pulse: 88

Respiration: 18

Pain: 0

Subjective information and vital signs entered by Roger Wong, RMA

6. Click the Update Progress Note button, then click Save.

7. Click the Progress Notes tab. Make certain that all of your information populated correctly in the progress note.

8. Click the Print icon at the top of the toolbar and label the assignment Task 3-3. Place the assignment in your SYNAPSE folder.

9. Do not click the Complete Visit icon until the clinician has finished entering the information. For now, click the Main Menu icon.

You are now finished entering the information within the patient's chart, and you instruct the patient how to disrobe. You leave the room and spot Megan, the nurse practitioner. Megan tells you Kevin Cook needs his second MMR shot because the parents cannot find records that prove he had the second immunization. The clinic in which he received the immunization is now closed. Mr. Cook and Kevin opted to have a second MMR instead of having a titer performed. Megan also tells you the patient needs a proof of appointment letter.

Task 3-4: Retrieving and Printing a VIS Form and a Consent Form

Since the patient needs an immunization, you will need to retrieve and print both a VIS form and an immunization consent form.

1. Click Patient Education Forms on the Main Menu screen.

2. Click Vaccination Information Sheets, then click MMR.

3. Print this form and label the assignment Task 3-4A.

4. Close the form and return to the Main Menu.

5. Click the Patients icon.

6. In the patient list, select Kevin Cook and click Open Patient Record.

7. Select the Authorization and Refusal Forms tab, and then click the Immunization Consent Form icon.

8. In box 1, choose MMR from the drop-down list.

9. Since the father is with the patient today, enter the father's name, David Cook, in the Typed Name box at the bottom of the form.

10. Enter the date of the appointment in the Today's Date box.

11. Print the form. Label the form Task 3-4B. In the medical office, the father would sign the form and the medical assistant would sign the witness box. Place Task 3-4A and Task 3-4B in your SYNAPSE folder.

12. Return to the Patient Information screen.

Now that you have printed the VIS and consent forms, you need to print a proof of appointment letter.

Task 3-5: Printing a Proof of Appointment Letter

1. Click the Patient Templates icon in the Patient Information screen. Choose Proof of Appointment.

2. Enter today's date, the time of the appointment, and the clinician's name.

3. Click the Print tab. Label the document Task 3-5 and place it in your SYNAPSE folder.

4. Return to the Main Menu.

You take the forms to the exam room, where the patient and his father are waiting. You ask the father to read over the VIS form and to sign the consent form while you go and prepare the immunization. You prepare the MMR immunization and re-enter the patient's room. You administer the injection in the subcutaneous tissue of the patient's left arm. The father of the patient asks if they can also have some kind of proof that the patient received his second MMR today. You tell the father that you can print him a copy of the immunization log from his electronic chart as soon as you enter the information.

Task 3-6 Documenting an Immunization in the EMR and Printing a Copy for the Patient

1. From the Patient Information Menu for Kevin Cook, click the Immunization Log icon.

2. Click the Update tab at the bottom of the box.

3. Complete the requested information by referring to Table 7.

TABLE 7   TASK 3-6 IMMUNIZATION TABLE

Date	May 16, 2007
Time	1:25 PM
Ordering Clinician	Megan Speck, NP
Immunization Name	MMR
Number in Series	2
Amt Given	0.5 ml
Location	Left Arm
Route	Sub Q
Person Who Administered Injection	Roger Wong, RMA

4. Save the information and print the form.

5. Label it Task 3-6 and place it in your SYNAPSE folder.

6. Click the Close icon. You should now see the immunization log for Kevin Cook. Close the immunization log for Kevin Cook.

You give the patient's father a copy of the immunization log so that they have verification that Kevin received the immunization. Kevin and his father leave after waiting the appropriate amount of time following the injection. You now need to enter the immunization information in the global immunization log within the Main Menu.

Task 3-7: Entering Immunization Information in the Global Immunization Log

1. From the Main Menu, click the Logs icon.

2. Click the Global Immunizations Log drop-down arrow, and select MMR.

3. Click Open Selected Log, and then select Update.

4. Enter the information found in the Table 8.

TABLE 8   TASK 3-7 GLOBAL IMMUNIZATION LOG TABLE

Date Administered	05/16/2007
Patient's Name	Kevin R. Cook
Drug Form	Injectable
Amt. Given	0.5 ml
Ordering Clinician	Megan Speck, NP
Manufacturer's Name	New York Pharmaceuticals
Lot Number	789451B
Exp Date	08/01/2008
Person Who Administered Injection	Roger Wong, RMA

6. Click Save and then print the form. Label the form Task 3-7.

7. Close the log and return to the Main Menu.

You just had a call sent back to you from the operator. It is Robert Green. He wants to know if he can have a prescription refill for his Cardizem.

Task 3-8: Documenting a Phone Call

You first need to bring up Robert Green's electronic chart. Follow the steps below.

1. Click the Patients icon on the Main Menu.

2. Select Robert Green, and then click Open Patient's Record.

3. Click Chart Note, and then click Telephone Call.

4. Enter 05/16/2007 in the Date box and 1:45 PM in the Time box.

5. Click Save.

6. Enter Robert Green's name in the Name of Caller box.

7. Enter "Self" in the Relationship to Patient box.

8. Enter abbreviation, SAA, in the Caller's Phone Number box.

9. In the Nature of the Call box, click Prescription Refill.

10. You should already be in the Prescription Refill tab, so check to see if the patient has any refills for Cardizem. The patient does not have any refills, so you will need to send an electronic task to the physician.

11. Click Cardizem in the Prescription Refill table.

12. A second box will appear. Put a check in the Click to Indicate Telephone Call Inquiry box. Close the box.

13. In the Action Taken box, click the drop-down arrow and select Sent Electronic Task to Physician.

14. Choose Roger Wong as the Name of Clinician or Medical Assistant that Handled the Call.

15. Double-check all of your information to make certain that the information is correct. Click Update Telephone Call, then Save.

16. Click Complete Telephone Call. Take one last look, because once you exit this screen, you will no longer be able to make any changes.

17. Click Patient Menu. Click Chart Notes.

18. Double-click the 05/16/2007 Previous Telephone Calls Entry to view the saved message. Click Print. Label the document Task 3-8 and file it in your SYNAPSE folder.

19. Return to the Main Menu.

Now that you have finished the call, you go to see if Dr. Schwartz is finished with Blanche. Dr. Schwartz is just exiting the patient's room when you arrive at the door. The doctor instructs you to read the Plans section of the progress note. The Plans section reads as follows:

Plans: In-Office PT and INR level today. After obtaining results, will adjust the patient's Wafarin Sodium medication if necessary. Depression much better; will continue to monitor over next couple of months. Patient to return in two weeks for another Pro-Time and INR.

You will need to perform a PT and INR level on the patient using your new CLIA-waived analyzer. Start by creating a lab requisition form for the patient.

Task 3-9: Creating a Lab Requisition Form

1. From the Main Menu, click the Patients icon.

2. Select Blanche White from the list of patients, and click Open Patient Record.

3. Click the Lab Orders icon.

4. Click In-House Testing in the Laboratory box, since we are performing this particular testing in the office.

5. Click D. J. Schwartz MD in the Ordering Provider box.

6. Click Medicare as the Payer, since Medicare is the primary payer.

7. Click Prothrombin Time in the General Lab Tests box.

8. Do not type anything in the Number of and Type of Specimens Sent box because we are performing the test in-house.

9. Enter today's date in the Today's Date box.

10. In the Specimen Prepared By box, select Roger Wong.

11. Select Yes in the Was patient fasting? box.

12. Click Save.

13. Click Preview, and then click the Print icon on the Preview screen. Label it Task 3-9A and place in your SYNAPSE folder. Close out of the preview.

14. Create a New Lab Requisition for the INR order. The only thing that will need to be changed is the name of the general lab test. Change the name of the general lab test to INR. Click Save.

15. Click Preview, and then click the Print icon. Label it Task 3-9B and place it in your SYNAPSE folder.

16. Next, click the Lab History icon. You should see both tests entered on the Incomplete Labs Log, as well as a previous test that was performed.

17. If you made an error, follow the instructions for deleting a log in Module I.

You enter the patient's room and perform the PT and INR via capillary stick. The results are as follows: PT 25.8 Seconds and INR 2.6. You will need to document this result in the Update Lab Results box.

Task 3-10: Entering Lab Results in the Electronic Medical Record

1. From the Lab Requisition for Blanche White screen, click Lab History.

2. Click the PT results, and then click Update Lab Results.

3. Enter 25.8 seconds in the Lab Test Results box.

4. Select Roger Wong as the Name of Person Who Recorded Results, enter the date of today's appointment, and click Save.

5. Click the Lab History icon.

6. You should notice that the result was sent from the Incomplete Labs box to the Completed Labs box.

7. Now repeat the same action for the INR results. There is no unit for INR, so you can enter 2.6 as the result.

8. Make certain that the test was sent to the Completed Labs box.

9. Print the screen and label the Incomplete Labs form Task 3-10A. Label the Complete Labs form Task 3-10B. File the forms in your SYNAPSE folder.

After completing the documentation, you immediately notify the physician of the result so that the physician can make any necessary adjustments in the patient's medication. If the physician was waiting on the result before finalizing the progress note, the physician would be responsible for closing the note. However, since you are finished with this project, you will complete the progress note.

Task 3-11: Finalizing the Progress Note

1. Click the Current Visit tab for Blanche White.

2. Click Update Progress Note, and then click Save.

3. Click Complete Visit. (*Note: Make certain that everything is correct before leaving this screen, because once you leave you will be unable to make changes.*)

4. Click the Patient Menu icon, then Chart Notes. Click the 05-16-2007 visit in the Previous Office Visits box to preview the note.

5. Return to the Main Menu.

Critical Thinking Questions for Module III

1. What was the purpose for writing down the date of Blanche's granddaughter's wedding?

2. Why do you think Kevin's father decided to have Kevin receive the second MMR instead of having a blood titer to determine Kevin's level of immunity?

3. In regard to the telephone call for Mr. Green, what information in the prescription history section caused you to send an electronic task to the physician instead of calling in a prescription for the Cardizem?

4. When you documented the labs in Blanche's electronic file, there was an outstanding blood test that was more than a month old? Which test was more than a month old. What would you do if you observed an outstanding test that was over a month old while working in the field?

5. What medication is Blanche taking that prompts the need to have Pro-Time and INR performed on a regular basis?

MODULE IV: PROCEDURE 1 CREATE AND MAINTAIN THE EMR

Module IV is an EMR competency, and it is designed to test your knowledge in performing tasks within the electronic chart. No step-by-step instructions are included; use the Competency Checklist for Procedure 3-1 as documentation of your competency in this skill.

Today's date: May 17, 2007
Appointments for May 17, 2007

Patient's Name	Appointment Time	Reason for Appointment	Clinician	MA
Paul M. Myers	2:00 PM	Cold/flu symptoms	Dr. Heath	Fauna Stout, CMA

Task 4-1: Creating an Electronic Chart and Progress Note

1. Refer to Table 9 for patient information. Create an electronic chart and new progress note for Paul Myers.

TABLE 9   PAUL MYERS'S DATA TABLE

Patient's Name	Paul M. Myers
Patient's DOB	08/12/1945
Patient's Chart Number	985632998
Patient's Address	2487 Springdale Court, Douglasville, NY 01234-1212
Patient's Telephone Numbers	Home: 123-786-6890 Work: 123-879-9865
Patient's Employer Info	Douglasville Steel Douglasville, NY 01234-1215
Gender, Marital Status, Blood Type & Smoking Status	Gender: Male Marital Status: Married Blood Type: O+ Smoking Status: Smoker
Patient Notes	Patient is hard of hearing in the left ear.
Responsible Party Info	Responsible Party: Self SS #: 985-63-2998 Address: SAA Home Phone: SAA Work Phone: SAA Employer: Douglasville Steel, Douglasville, NY 01234-1215

Primary Payer Info	Name: Flexihealth ID # 985632998-00 Policy/Group: 6532001 Gender: Male Policy Holder: Self SS#: 985-63-2998
Secondary Payer	None
Patient Drug Allergies	Penicillin
Patient Other Allergy	None
Current Mediation List	Accupril capsules, 20 mg Glyburide tablets, 2.5 mg Viagra tablets, 50 mg
Preferred Pharmacy	DanMart Pharmacy 8700 Polaris Drive, Douglasville, NY 01234
Lab Provider	American Labs
Privacy Statement	Reviewed and Signed, May 17, 2007 Enter the following information in the Note's box: Can leave information on the patient's home answering machine and with wife, Carol.
Family Health History Info	Father: Age at death: 72, Cause of death: Heart failure Mother: Age 84, Health: Poor Brother: Age 66, Health: Fair Sister: Age 54, Health: Good Diabetes: Type II diabetes both father and mother Heart disease: CHF, father High blood pressure: Mother, father, and brother
Hospitalizations, Blood Transfusions, and Serious Injuries	Hospitalizations: 1976, Riverside Hospital, hernia repair Blood Transfusions: None Serious Injuries: None
Pregnancies	N/A
Medical History	Click the following diseases: Chicken pox, diabetes, high cholesterol, measles, mumps, other In the Note's box, list the following: Chicken pox: UCHD (no complications) Diabetes: Type II, diagnosed in 1995, controlled with diet and oral medication High cholesterol: Diagnosed in 2001, diet controlled Measles: UCHD (no complications) Mumps: UCHD (no complications) Other: Hypertension, diagnosed in 1992. Controlled by low-sodium diet and Accupril.

Health Habits	Caffeine, drinks 1 10–12-ounce cup of coffee per day.
	Tobacco: Smokes ½–1 pack of low-filter cigarettes per day. Has been a smoker for 32 years.
	ETOH:
	Drink type: Beer
	Drinks per week: 6 pack
	Occupation: Steel worker
	Heavy lifting
Progress Notes: Date, Time, Clinician, and MA	Date: May 17, 2007
	Time: 2:00 PM
	Clinician: Dr. Heath
	MA: Fauna Stout, CMA
Subjective Information	Chief Complaint: Cold, flu, sore throat
	HPI:
	Severity: 6
	Duration of symptoms: 7 days
	+: Ear pain, fever, head or facial pain, nasal drainage, productive cough.
	–: Light sensitivity, nausea or vomiting or other GI distubances, sore throat.
	Relieving factors: OTC: Sinus/flu medication
Objective Information	Vital Signs:
	Height: 70 inches
	Weight: 215 pounds
	Temperature: 99.7
	Blood Pressure: 146/92
	Pulse: 92
	Respiration: 20
	Pain: 6
	Subjective Information and Vital Signs Entered By: Fauna Stout

2. When finished, print the note.

3. Label it Task 4-1 and place it in your SYNAPSE folder.

4. You will not complete the progress note until later.

Task 4-2: Creating and Printing an Electronic Prescription

1. Accupril, 20 mg Cap. Quantity: 30, Take 1 capsule each day, 0 refills

2. Atenolol, 50 mg, Tab, Quantity: 30, Take 1 tab each day before meals or at bedtime, 0 refills

3. Glyburide, 2.5 mg Tab, Quantity: 60, Take 1 tab in the morning and one tab in the evening, 0 refills

4. Viagra, 50 mg, Quantity: 10, Take 1–2 tabs 30 minutes before sexual intercourse, 0 refills

5. All prescriptions are considered one-month prescriptions.

6. Print and label the documents Tasks 4-2A through 4-2D and place them in your SYNAPSE folder.

Task 4-3: Creating and Printing Lab Requisition Forms

1. HgbA1c (in-house), patient was fasting.

2. Print and label it Task 4-3A and place it in your SYNAPSE folder.

3. Chem 12: American Labs, Patient was fasting, sent 1 SST tube.

4. Print and label it Task 4-3B and place it in your SYNAPSE folder.

Task 4-4: Entering Lab Results in the Patient's Electronic Medical Record

1. Result: HgbA1c: 8.2% on 5/17/2007.

2. Print and label the Incomplete Lab table Task 4-4A.

3. Print and label the Complete Lab table Task 4-4B.

4. Place both forms in your SYNAPSE folder.

Task 4-5: Printing Educational Forms and VIS Forms for the Patient

1. Diabetes and hypertension educational forms.

2. Shingles VIS form.

3. Print and label the forms Task 4-5A through 4-5C and place them in your SYNAPSE folder.

Task 4-6: Creating a Consent Form to go with Immunization

1. Print the form, label it Task 4-6, and place it in your SYNAPSE folder.

Task 4-7: Entering an Immunization in the Personal EMR

Date	May 17, 2007
Time	2:45 PM
Ordering Physician	Dr. Heath
Immunization Name	Shingles
Number in Series	1
Amt Given	0.5 ml
Location	Left Arm
Route	Sub-Q
Person Who Administered Injection	Fauna Stout, CMA

1. Print and Label the form Task 4-7.

Task 4-8: Entering an Immunization in the Global Immunization Log

Date Administered	05/17/2007
Patient's Name	Paul Myers
Drug Form	Injectable
Amt Given	0.5 ml
Ordering Physician	Dr. Heath
Manuf Name	New York Pharmaceuticals
Lot Number	2365879 C
Exp	12/10/2008
Person Who Administered Injection	Fauna Stout, CMA

1. Print and label it Task 4-8 and place it in your SYNAPSE folder.

Task 4-9: Creating and Printing a Proof of Appointment Letter

1. Label it Task 4-9 and place it in your SYNAPSE folder.

Task 4-10: Properly completing Paul Myer's Progress Note from 05/17/2007

1. Label it Task 4-10 and place it in your SYNAPSE folder.

Task 4-11: Creating and Printing a Telephone Note

1. Date: May 27, 2007

2. Time: 4:15 PM

3. Patient is calling from home.

4. Prescription: Viagra refill.

5. Sent electronic task to the physician.

6. Medical Assistant: Fauna Stout.

7. Print and label it Task 4-11.

Competency Checklists

Student Name: _____   Date: _____   Score: _____

Competency Checklist
PROCEDURE 2-1   Performing Routine Maintenance on Clinical Equipment

Task: To perform routine maintenance on clinical equipment

Condition: Given an equipment maintenance log, a writing pen, a telephone that can be used to simulate calling the supplier or manufacturer, and a classmate to play the part of the technician, the student will determine which pieces of clinical equipment are ready for maintenance and follow the proper criteria for setting up an equipment maintenance appointment by following the steps listed below.

Standards: The student will have 15 minutes to complete the procedure and will need to score an 85% or above to pass the competency. Automatic failure results if any essential steps are omitted or performed incorrectly.

STEPS START TIME: END TIME:	Points Possible	First Attempt	Second Attempt	Third Attempt
1. Read the equipment maintenance journal and correctly identified which items were ready for routine maintenance. (This may be simulated or provided in an explanation by the student.)	10			
2. Called supplier or manufacturer to set up service call to perform routine maintenance.	10			
3. Checked to make certain equipment was functioning properly and obtained any special instructions once it was returned or before technician left the premises.	10			
4. Correctly documented procedure into the maintenance log book *(Work Product, Procedure 2-1)* and placed maintenance sticker on the equipment if technician failed to do so.	10			
5. Completed the procedure within the appropriate time limit.	10			
Points Earned / Points Possible:	___ / 50			

Points possible reflect importance of step in meeting the task: Important = (5) Essential = (10).
Determine score by dividing points earned by total points possible, and multiplying results by 100.

EVALUATION
Evaluator Signature: _____   Date: _____

Evaluator Comments:

Key Competencies		
ABHES	VI.A.1.a.6.b	Operate and maintain facilities and perform routine maintenance of administrative and clinical equipment safely
CAAHEP	III.C.3.c.4.b	Perform routine maintenance of administrative and clinical equipment

Student Name: _____   Date: _____   Score: _____

DOCUMENTATION

Instructor Note: Retain work products with competency checklist.

Work Product, Procedure 2-1 (Maintenance Log Book)

Today's Date	Equipment Name, Manufacturer and Serial Number	Technician's Name	Any Repairs Needed or Special Instructions	Next Service Date	Initials of Employee

Key Competencies		
ABHES	VI.A.1.a.6.b	Operate and maintain facilities and perform routine maintenance of administrative and clinical equipment safely
CAAHEP	III.C.3.c.4.b	Perform routine maintenance of administrative and clinical equipment

Student Name: _____   Date: _____   Score: _____

Competency Checklist
PROCEDURE 3-1   Create and Maintain the EMR Using SynapseEHR 1.1 Software

Task: To create and maintain an electronic medical record

Condition: Given a computer, printer, paper, Synapse Software CD, and the competency exercises found in the Synapse modules at the rear of the workbook, the student will create and maintain an electronic record by correctly performing all of the steps in the competency exercises. ***(Students should not perform this competency until they have finished Modules 1–3 found in the Synapse exercises at the rear of the workbook.)***

Standards: The student will have 2 hours to complete the procedure and will need to score an 85% or above to pass the competency. Automatic failure results if any essential steps are omitted or performed incorrectly.

STEPS START TIME: END TIME:	Points Possible	First Attempt	Second Attempt	Third Attempt
1. Task 4-1: Accurately created the chart by properly completing all of the tabs in the Patient Information Screen.	10			
2. Task 4-1: Accurately created and printed a progress note, closing the EMR properly using the correct technique. *(Note to instructor: retain Task 4-1 printout)*	10			
3. Task 4-2: Accurately created and printed the assigned prescriptions. *(Note to instructor: retain Task 4-2 printout)*	10			
4. Task 4-3: Accurately created and printed the assigned lab requisition forms. *(Note to instructor: retain Task 4-3 printout)*	10			
5. Task 4-4: Accurately entered the assigned lab result in the patient's EMR and printed the completed lab log. *(Note to instructor: retain Task 4-4 printout)*	10			
6. Task 4-5: Accurately located and printed the assigned educational and VIS forms. *(Note to instructor: retain Task 4-5 printout)*	10			
7. Task 4-6: Accurately created and printed an immunization consent form to go with Task 4-5. *(Note to instructor: retain Task 4-6 printout)*	10			
8. Task 4-7: Accurately entered an immunization into the patient's EMR and printed a copy of the completed log. *(Note to instructor: retain Task 4-7 printout)*	10			
9. Task 4-8: Accurately entered an immunization within the global immunization log. *(Note to instructor: retain Task 4-8 printout)*	10			
10. Task 4-9: Accurately created a Proof of Appointment letter for the patient. *(Note to instructor: retain Task 4-9 printout)*	10			
11. Task 4-10: Accurately recorded a phone call in the patient's EMR. *(Note to instructor: retain Task 4-10 printout)*	10			
12. Completed the procedure within the appropriate time limit.	10			
Points Earned / Points Possible:	___ / 120			

Points possible reflect importance of step in meeting the task: Important = (5) Essential = (10).
Determine score by dividing points earned by total points possible, and multiplying results by 100.

Key Competencies		
ABHES	VI.A.1.a.2.n	Application of electronic technology
	VI.A.1.a.3.b	Prepare and maintain medical records
CAAHEP	III.C.3.c.2.c	Establish and maintain the medical record
	III.C.3 c.4.c	Utilize computer software to maintain office systems

Student Name: _____   Date: _____   Score: _____

EVALUATION
Evaluator Signature: _____   Date: _____

Evaluator Comments:

DOCUMENTATION
Instructor Note: Retain work products with competency checklist (all Task printouts).

Key Competencies			
ABHES	VI.A.1.a.2.n	Application of electronic technology	
	VI.A.1.a.3.b	Prepare and maintain medical records	
CAAHEP	III.C.3.c.2.c	Establish and maintain the medical record	
	III.C.3 c.4.c	Utilize computer software to maintain office systems	

Student Name: _____   Date: _____   Score: _____

Competency Checklist
PROCEDURE 5-1   Conducting a Patient Interview and Completing a Patient History Form

Task: To conduct a patient interview and complete a patient history

Condition: Given a patient chart, history form, blank progress note, pen, and a classmate on whom to perform the history, the student will conduct and record a comprehensive patient history while promoting good therapeutic communication.

Standards: The student will have 20 minutes to complete the procedure and will need to score an 85% or above to pass the competency. Automatic failure results if any essential steps are omitted or performed incorrectly.

STEPS START TIME: END TIME:	Points Possible	First Attempt	Second Attempt	Third Attempt
1. Assembled necessary supplies and prepared the interview area; patient's chair should be 4–12 inches away from your chair, when not using the examination table.	10			
2. Identified the patient using at least two identifiers.	10			
3. Identified self and explained the procedure; reassured patient information would remain confidential.	10			
4. If history form is completed prior to office visit, appropriately reviewed information with patient, or completed history form if completing form for the patient.	10			
5. Developed "YES" responses from the "Past History" section by recording the appropriate data on a separate progress note.	10			
6. Developed "YES" responses in "Family History" and "Social History" sections.	10			
7. Reviewed or recorded current prescribed and OTC medications; listed strength and how often the patient takes the medication.	10			
8. Reviewed or recorded allergy information; recorded drug allergies in red.	10			
9. Reviewed or recorded patient hospitalizations and surgeries.	10			
10. Correctly recorded the patient's chief complaint.	10			
11. Summarized and reviewed the information with the patient; made any necessary adjustments.	10			
12. Maintained good eye contact with patient throughout the procedure.	5			
13. Thanked patient for cooperation.	5			
14. Explained how to properly disrobe for the exam and what to expect for the remainder of the visit.	10			
15. Gave patient reading materials, if time permitted.	5			
16. Placed the completed history form *(Work Product, Procedure 5-1)* in the patient's chart for the doctor to review.	5			
17. Completed the procedure within the appropriate time limit.	10			
Points Earned / Points Possible:	___ / 150			

Points possible reflect importance of step in meeting the task: Important = (5) Essential = (10).
Determine score by dividing points earned by total points possible, and multiplying results by 100.

Key Competencies		
ABHES	VI.A.1.a.2.f	Interview effectively
	VI.A.1.a.4.a	Interview and record patient history
CAAHEP	III.C.3.b.4.c	Obtain and record patient history

Student Name: _____   Date: _____   Score: _____

EVALUATION
Evaluator Signature: _____   Date: _____

Evaluator Comments:

DOCUMENTATION
Instructor Note: Retain work products with competency checklist.
Work Product, Procedure 5-1 (Progress Note)

Progress Note for Patient: Date:	**DOUGLASVILLE MEDICINE ASSOCIATES** **5076 BRAND BLVD** **DOUGLASVILLE, NY 01234** **(123) 456-7890**

Work Product, Procedure 5-1 (Patient History Form)

Form located on following pages.

Key Competencies		
ABHES	VI.A.1.a.2.f	Interview effectively
	VI.A.1.a.4.a	Interview and record patient history
CAAHEP	III.C.3.b.4.c	Obtain and record patient history

CONFIDENTIAL HEALTH HISTORY

Name: _____ Date: _____

Birthdate: _____ Age: _____ Date of last physical examination: _____

Occupation: _____

Reason for visit today: _____

MEDICATIONS List all medications you are currently taking	**ALLERGIES** List all allergies

SYMPTOMS Check (✓) symptoms you currently have or have had in the past year.

GENERAL
- ☐ Chills
- ☐ Depression
- ☐ Dizziness
- ☐ Fainting
- ☐ Fever
- ☐ Forgetfulness
- ☐ Headache
- ☐ Loss of sleep
- ☐ Loss of weight
- ☐ Nervousness
- ☐ Numbness
- ☐ Sweats

MUSCLE/JOINT/BONE
Pain, weakness, numbness in:
- ☐ Arms
- ☐ Back
- ☐ Feet
- ☐ Hands
- ☐ Hips
- ☐ Legs
- ☐ Neck
- ☐ Shoulders

GENITO-URINARY
- ☐ Blood in urine
- ☐ Frequent urination
- ☐ Lack of bladder control
- ☐ Painful urination

GASTROINTESTINAL
- ☐ Appetite poor
- ☐ Bloating
- ☐ Bowel changes
- ☐ Constipation
- ☐ Diarrhea
- ☐ Excessive hunger
- ☐ Excessive thirst
- ☐ Gas
- ☐ Hemorrhoids
- ☐ Indigestion
- ☐ Nausea
- ☐ Rectal bleeding
- ☐ Stomach pain
- ☐ Vomiting
- ☐ Vomiting blood

CARDIOVASCULAR
- ☐ Chest pain
- ☐ High blood pressure
- ☐ Irregular heart beat
- ☐ Low blood pressure
- ☐ Poor circulation
- ☐ Rapid heart beat
- ☐ Swelling of ankles
- ☐ Varicose veins

EYE, EAR, NOSE, THROAT
- ☐ Bleeding gums
- ☐ Blurred vision
- ☐ Crossed eyes
- ☐ Difficulty swallowing
- ☐ Double vision
- ☐ Earache
- ☐ Ear discharge
- ☐ Hay fever
- ☐ Hoarseness
- ☐ Loss of hearing
- ☐ Nosebleeds
- ☐ Persistent cough
- ☐ Ringing in ears
- ☐ Sinus problems
- ☐ Vision - Flashes
- ☐ Vision - Halos

SKIN
- ☐ Bruise easily
- ☐ Hives
- ☐ Itching
- ☐ Change in moles
- ☐ Rash
- ☐ Scars
- ☐ Sores that won't heal

MEN only
- ☐ Breast lump
- ☐ Erection difficulties
- ☐ Lump in testicles
- ☐ Penis discharge
- ☐ Sore on penis
- ☐ Other

WOMEN only
- ☐ Abnormal Pap Smear
- ☐ Bleeding between periods
- ☐ Breast lump
- ☐ Extreme menstrual pain
- ☐ Hot flashes
- ☐ Nipple discharge
- ☐ Painful intercourse
- ☐ Vaginal discharge
- ☐ Other

Date of last
menstrual period _____

Date of last
Pap Smear _____

Have you had
a mammogram? _____

Are you pregnant? _____

Number of children _____

MEDICAL HISTORY Check (✓) the medical conditions you have or have had in the past.

- ☐ AIDS
- ☐ Alcoholism
- ☐ Anemia
- ☐ Anorexia
- ☐ Appendicitis
- ☐ Arthritis
- ☐ Asthma
- ☐ Bleeding Disorders
- ☐ Breast Lump
- ☐ Bronchitis
- ☐ Bulimia
- ☐ Cancer
- ☐ Cataracts

- ☐ Chemical Dependency
- ☐ Chicken Pox
- ☐ Diabetes
- ☐ Emphysema
- ☐ Epilepsy
- ☐ Gall Bladder Disease
- ☐ Glaucoma
- ☐ Goiter
- ☐ Gonorrhea
- ☐ Gout
- ☐ Heart Disease
- ☐ Hepatitis
- ☐ Hernia

- ☐ Herpes
- ☐ High Cholesterol
- ☐ HIV Positive
- ☐ Kidney Disease
- ☐ Liver Disease
- ☐ Measles
- ☐ Migraine Headaches
- ☐ Miscarriage
- ☐ Mononucleosis
- ☐ Multiple Sclerosis
- ☐ Mumps
- ☐ Pacemaker
- ☐ Pneumonia

- ☐ Polio
- ☐ Prostate Problem
- ☐ Psychiatric Care
- ☐ Rheumatic Fever
- ☐ Scarlet Fever
- ☐ Stroke
- ☐ Suicide Attempt
- ☐ Thyroid Problems
- ☐ Tonsillitis
- ☐ Tuberculosis
- ☐ Typhoid Fever
- ☐ Ulcers
- ☐ Vaginal Infections
- ☐ Venereal Disease

CONFIDENTIAL HEALTH HISTORY

HOSPITALIZATIONS

Year	Hospital	Reason for Hospitalization and Outcome

Have you ever had a blood transfusion? ☐ Yes ☐ No

If yes, please give approximate dates: _____

OCCUPATIONAL CONCERNS Check (✓) if your work exposes you to the following:	**HEALTH HABITS** Check (✓) which substances you use and indicate how much you use per day/week.	**PREGNANCY HISTORY**		
		Year of Birth	Sex of Birth	Complications if any
☐ Stress	☐ Caffeine			
☐ Hazardous Substances	☐ Tobacco			
☐ Heavy Lifting	☐ Drugs			
☐ Other	☐ Alcohol			

SERIOUS ILLNESS/INJURIES	DATE	OUTCOME

FAMILY HISTORY Fill in health information about your family.

Relation	Age	State of Health	Age at Death	Cause of Death	Check (✓) if your blood relatives had any of the following Disease	Relationship to you
Father					☐ Arthritis, Gout	
Mother					☐ Asthma, Hay Fever	
Brothers					☐ Cancer	
					☐ Chemical Dependency	
					☐ Diabetes	
					☐ Heart Disease, Strokes	
Sisters					☐ High Blood Pressure	
					☐ Kidney Disease	
					☐ Tuberculosis	
					☐ Other	

I certify that the above information is correct to the best of my knowledge. I will not hold my doctor or any members of his/her staff responsible for any errors or ommisions that I may have made in the completion of this form.

_____   _____
Signature   Date

_____   _____
Reviewed By   Date

Student Name: _____   Date: _____   Score: _____

Competency Checklist
PROCEDURE 6-1   Conduct and Record Results from an In-Office Screening

Task: To conduct an in-office screening and document a chief complaint

Condition: Given a patient chart, progress note, pen, and a patient with a pre-assigned complaint by the teacher, the student will conduct and record an in-office screening while promoting good therapeutic communication.

Standards: The student will have 15 minutes to complete the procedure and will need to score an 85% or above to pass the competency. Automatic failure results if any essential steps are omitted or performed incorrectly.

STEPS START TIME: END TIME:	Points Possible	First Attempt	Second Attempt	Third Attempt
1. Checked the reason for the visit with the appointment list and gathered necessary supplies before bringing back patient.	5			
2. Greeted and escorted patient back to the examination room.	5			
3. Checked patient's name again with the name on the chart and asked another identifier to verify that the chart belonged to the patient.	10			
4. Seated the patient in a comfortable manner; patient was able to easily view the student.	5			
5. Asked patient the reason for the visit (chief complaint) if not clear from the appointment list, or otherwise confirmed the reason for the visit. Demonstrated a caring attitude during the questioning phase.	10			
6. Performed a brief HPI to determine how to proceed with setting up the room and patient.	10			
7. Updated any prescribed or OTC medications, including vitamins or minerals being taken by the patient.	10			
8. Updated allergy listings.	10			
9. Reviewed information for accuracy.	10			
10. Properly set up the room and any trays according to patient's complaint and gave patient appropriate disrobing instructions.	10			
11. Student dismissed him/herself in a professional manner.	5			
12. Alerted provider patient was ready for examination. (This could be through a light or flag system, or by mouth or computer.)	10			
13. *Entry Information (Work Product, Procedure 6-1):* The entry was properly organized and legible and included today's date and time, reason for visit, related symptoms, updated medication list and drug allergies listed in red.	10			
14. Student signed the entry using an appropriate closing signature.	10			
15. Entry had no spelling errors.	10			
16. Completed the procedure within the appropriate time limit.	10			
Points Earned / Points Possible:	___ / 140			

Points possible reflect importance of step in meeting the task: Important = (5) Essential = (10).
Determine score by dividing points earned by total points possible, and multiplying results by 100.

Key Competencies		
ABHES	VI.A.1.a.2.f	Interview effectively
	VI. A.1.a.4.ff	Perform telephone and in-person screening
CAAHEP	III.C.3.b.4.a	Perform telephone and in-person screening

Student Name: _____   Date: _____   Score: _____

EVALUATION

Evaluator Signature: _____   Date: _____

Evaluator Comments:

DOCUMENTATION

Instructor Note: Retain work products with competency checklist.
Work Product, Procedure 6-1 (Progress Note)

Progress Note for	**DOUGLASVILLE MEDICINE ASSOCIATES**
	5076 BRAND BLVD
Patient:	**DOUGLASVILLE, NY 01234**
Date:	**(123) 456-7890**

Key Competencies		
ABHES	VI.A.1.a.2.f	Interview effectively
	VI. A.1.a.4.ff	Perform telephone and in-person screening
CAAHEP	III.C.3.b.4.a	Perform telephone and in-person screening

Student Name: _____   Date: _____   Score: _____

Competency Checklist
PROCEDURE 6-2   Conduct a Follow-Up Interview and Develop a Progress Note

Task: To conduct a follow-up interview and develop and document a progress note

Condition: Given a patient chart, progress note, pen, and a patient with a pre-assigned follow-up complaint by the instructor, the student will conduct a follow-up interview and document the findings onto a progress note.

Standards: The student will have 10 minutes to complete the procedure and will need to score an 85% or above to pass the competency. Automatic failure results if any essential steps are omitted or performed incorrectly.

STEPS START TIME: END TIME:	Points Possible	First Attempt	Second Attempt	Third Attempt
1. Assembled equipment and supplies.	10			
2. Properly identified the patient using at least two identifiers and explained the procedure.	10			
3. Seated the patient in a comfortable manner; patient was able to easily view the student.	5			
4. Asked patient about current health status (symptoms better or worse?).	10			
5. Asked patient about compliance with homecare instructions (taking medication as prescribed, any problems with dressing changes, etc.).	10			
6. Made any observations that the provider will not be able to make (such as the appearance of the bandage after being removed, any difficulty walking, confusion, etc.).	10			
7. Gave patient disrobing instructions and set up any necessary supplies or equipment.	10			
8. Gave patient indication on how the long wait will be and what they could expect the remainder of the visit.	5			
9. Excused self in a professional manner.	5			
10. Gathered all of the lab or diagnostic test results from last visit and placed the information in the front of the chart.	10			
11. Alerted provider patient was ready for examination.	10			
12. *Entry Information (Work Product, Procedure 6-2):* The entry was properly organized and included the following information: today's date, time, reason for visit, current health status, compliance of patient to follow home care instructions, and any observations made by the medical assistant.	10			
13. Signed the entry using an appropriate closing signature.	10			
14. Completed the procedure within the appropriate time limit.	10			
Points Earned / Points Possible:	___ / 125			

Points possible reflect importance of step in meeting the task: Important = (5) Essential = (10).
Determine score by dividing points earned by total points possible, and multiplying results by 100.

Key Competencies		
ABHES	VI.A.1.a.2.f	Interview effectively
	VI.A.1.a.4.ff	Perform telephone and in-office screenings
CAAHEP	III.C.3.b.4.a	Perform telephone and in-person screening

Student Name: _____   Date: _____   Score: _____

EVALUATION
Evaluator Signature: _____   Date: _____

Evaluator Comments:

DOCUMENTATION
Instructor Note: Retain work products with competency checklist.
Work Product, Procedure 6-2 (Progress Note)

Progress Note for Patient: Date:	**DOUGLASVILLE MEDICINE ASSOCIATES** **5076 BRAND BLVD** **DOUGLASVILLE, NY 01234** **(123) 456-7890**

Key Competencies			
ABHES	VI.A.1.a.2.f	Interview effectively	
	VI.A.1.a.4.ff	Perform telephone and in-office screenings	
CAAHEP	III.C.3.b.4.a	Perform telephone and in-person screening	

Student Name: _____   Date: _____   Score: _____

Competency Checklist
PROCEDURE 7-1   Perform a Telephone Screening

Task: To perform a telephone screening

Condition: Given a patient chart, progress note, pen, telephone screening book, and a classmate with a preassigned complaint to play the patient on the other end of the phone, the student will perform a telephone screening, following the steps listed below.

Standards: The student will have 10 minutes to complete the procedure and will need to score an 85% or above to pass the competency. Automatic failure results if any essential steps are omitted or performed incorrectly.

STEPS START TIME: END TIME:	Points Possible	First Attempt	Second Attempt	Third Attempt
1. Properly identified self and stated title.	10			
2. Properly identified the patient using at least two identifiers.	10			
3. Asked the patient if call was an emergency; if call was an emergency proceeded to step 5; if not, placed the caller on hold and pulled the patient's chart.	10			
4. Thanked the patient for waiting.	5			
5. Asked patient for a brief description of the complaint.	10			
6. Opened telephone screening manual and turned to the appropriate complaint.	10			
7. Proceeded down the list of questions until the patient gave a "yes" response. Gave patient instructions listed in the action column beside the "yes" response.	10			
8. If patient refused to follow instructions, stated the importance of following the instructions and the possible consequences of not following instructions.	10			
9. If patient still refused to follow instructions, referred call to supervisor or provider.	10			
10. Thanked the patient for calling and let patient hang up first.	5			
11. *Entry Information (Work Product, Procedure 7-1):* The entry was properly organized and legible and included today's date and time, the reason for the call, instructions given to the patient, where the instructions came from (telephone screening manual, page XX, provider, etc.), and the patient's confirmation or refusal to follow instructions.	10			
12. Signed the entry using an appropriate closing signature.	10			
13. Entry had no spelling errors.	10			
14. Completed the procedure within the appropriate time limit.	10			
Points Earned / Points Possible:	___ / 130			

Points possible reflect importance of step in meeting the task: Important = (5) Essential = (10).
Determine score by dividing points earned by total points possible, and multiplying results by 100.

Key Competencies		
ABHES	VI.A.1.a.4.ff	Perform telephone and in-person screening
	VI.A.1.a.2.e	Use proper telephone techniques
	VI.A.1.a.4.l	Screen and follow up patient test results
CAAHEP	III.C.3.b.4.a	Perform telephone and in-person screening
	III.C.3.c.1.d	Demonstrate telephone techniques
	III.C.3.c.4.i	Screen and follow up test results

Student Name: _____   Date: _____   Score: _____

EVALUATION
Evaluator Signature: _____   Date: _____

Evaluator Comments:

DOCUMENTATION
Instructor Note: Retain work products with competency checklist.
Work Product, Procedure 7-1 (Progress Note)

Progress Note for Patient: Date:	**DOUGLASVILLE MEDICINE ASSOCIATES** **5076 BRAND BLVD** **DOUGLASVILLE, NY 01234** **(123) 456-7890**

Key Competencies		
ABHES	VI.A.1.a.4.ff	Perform telephone and in-person screening
	VI.A.1.a.2.e	Use proper telephone techniques
	VI.A.1.a.4.l	Screen and follow up patient test results
CAAHEP	III.C.3.b.4.a	Perform telephone and in-person screening
	III.C.3.c.1.d	Demonstrate telephone techniques
	III.C.3.c.4.i	Screen and follow up test results

Student Name: _____   Date: _____   Score: _____

Competency Checklist
PROCEDURE 7-2   Screen and Follow Up on Test Results (Determine the Order of Prioritization)

Task: To screen a few lab reports and place in order of priority, to simulate calling a patient back with lab results, and to provide the patient with any special instructions to follow as a result of the lab findings

Condition: Given a few patient charts, some abnormal lab reports, a telephone, a writing utensil, and a classmate to play the part of the patient, the student will prioritize labs (by placing the labs in order from most critical to least critical). The instructor will then pull one of the labs from the pile and attach instructions that are to be given to the patient. The student will simulate calling the patient and provide the results of the tests and instructions that are to be given to the patient.

Standards: The student will have 10 minutes to complete the procedure and will need to score an 85% or above to pass the competency. Automatic failure results if any essential steps are omitted or performed incorrectly.

STEPS START TIME: END TIME:	Points Possible	First Attempt	Second Attempt	Third Attempt
1. Retrieved completed lab reports from the lab printer.	10			
2. Divided the labs according to their ranking in priority, with critical labs on top.	10			
3. Attached the lab reports to the charts and placed them on provider's desk for review.	10			
4. Reviewed charts once placed back on desk from provider and placed in order of importance.	10			
5. Gathered necessary supplies to telephone patient.	10			
6. Checked the patient's privacy information to determine how test results were to be handled in the event the patient was unavailable.	10			
7. Called patient's phone number and asked to speak to the patient. Identified self, stated title, and stated the name of the office.	10			
8. Gave the patient test results and listed any instructions given by the provider.	10			
9. Had patient repeat results/instructions back for accuracy.	10			
10. Encouraged the patient to contact the office if he or she had any further questions regarding the test results or instructions.	5			
11. Thanked the patient for his or her time.	5			
12. Let patient hang up first.	5			
13. *Entry Information (Work Product, Procedure 7-2):* The entry was properly organized and included: the date and time of the call, the information given to the patient, instructions given to patient, and a confirmation that the patient understood the directions.	10			
14. Signed the entry using an appropriate closing signature.	10			
15. Entry had no spelling errors.	10			
16. Completed the procedure within the appropriate time limit.	10			
Points Earned / Points Possible:	___ /145			

Points possible reflect importance of step in meeting the task: Important = (5) Essential = (10).
Determine score by dividing points earned by total points possible, and multiplying results by 100.

Key Competencies		
ABHES	VI.A.1.a.4.l	Screen and follow up patient test results
	VI.A.1.a.2.e	Use proper telephone techniques
	VI.A.1.a.4.ff	Perform telephone and in-person screenings
CAAHEP	III.C.3.b.4.i	Screen and follow-up test results
	III.C.3.b.4.a	Perform telephone and in-person screenings
	III.C.3.c.1.d	Demonstrate telephone techniques

Student Name: _____   Date: _____   Score: _____

EVALUATION
Evaluator Signature: _____   Date: _____

Evaluator Comments:

DOCUMENTATION
Instructor Note: Retain work products with competency checklist.
Work Product, Procedure 7-2 (Progress Note)

Progress Note for Patient: Date:	**DOUGLASVILLE MEDICINE ASSOCIATES** **5076 BRAND BLVD** **DOUGLASVILLE, NY 01234** **(123) 456-7890**

Key Competencies		
ABHES	VI.A.1.a.4.l	Screen and follow up patient test results
	VI.A.1.a.2.e	Use proper telephone techniques
	VI.A.1.a.4.ff	Perform telephone and in-person screenings
CAAHEP	III.C.3.b.4.i	Screen and follow-up test results
	III.C.3.b.4.a	Perform telephone and in-person screenings
	III.C.3.c.1.d	Demonstrate telephone techniques

Student Name: _____   Date: _____   Score: _____

Competency Checklist
PROCEDURE 8-1   Effectively Communicate with Patients from Different Cultures

Task: To effectively communicate with patients from different cultures

Condition: Given a chart, pen, necessary brochures, any supplies or equipment necessary for the screening, a classmate to play the part of the culturally diverse patient and another classmate to play the role of the interpreter, the student will interview the patient, following the steps listed below.

Standards: The student will have 15 minutes to complete the procedure and will need to score an 85% or above to pass the competency. Automatic failure results if any essential steps are omitted or performed incorrectly.

STEPS START TIME: END TIME:	Points Possible	First Attempt	Second Attempt	Third Attempt
1. Prepared interview area. (If interpreter was used, the interpreter's chair was placed beside the patient's chair and angled slightly toward the patient for easy viewing of the interpreter. The medical assistant's chair was placed directly across from the patient's and interpreter's chairs.)	10			
2. Identified self and stated title and identified the patient; asked for correct pronunciation if unable to pronounce name correctly and wrote the phonetic spelling in the appropriate section of the chart.	10			
3. If patient was not the same gender, asked patient if he or she would like someone of the same gender to assist during the interview process.	10			
4. Asked patient to introduce any family members present and state their relationship.	5			
5. Assessed patient's language skills by asking some questions about the patient's career or family.	10			
6. If limited English, gave patient brochures in native language that expressed the patient's right to have an interpreter present.	10			
7. Contacted interpreting company if necessary and waited until an interpreter was available before proceeding with the questioning.	10			
8. Asked patient to explain goals for today's visit or the reason for the visit.	10			
9. Spoke clearly, avoiding the use of slang or medical jargon, and talked directly to the patient instead of the interpreter.	10			
10. Had patient repeat back any instructions to ensure that the patient understood the information. Listened to interpreter to ascertain the patient understood the information.	10			
11. Gave patient disrobing instructions. Provided patient with gown, sheets or drapes and explained what the patient could expect for the remainder of the visit.	10			
12. Thanked the patient, family members, or interpreter for cooperating.	5			
13. Documented the visit *(Work Product, Procedure 8-1)* and stated if an interpreter was present.	10			
14. Completed the procedure within the appropriate time limit.	10			
Points Earned / Points Possible:	___ / 130			

Points possible reflect importance of step in meeting the task: Important = (5) Essential = (10).
Determine score by dividing points earned by total points possible, and multiplying results by 100.

Key Competencies		
ABHES	VI.A.1.a.2.m	Adaptation for individualized needs
	VI.A.1.a.7.b	Instruct patients with special needs
CAAHEP	III.C.3.c.3.b	Instruct individuals according to their needs

Student Name: _____ Date: _____ Score: _____

EVALUATION

Evaluator Signature: _____ Date: _____

Evaluator Comments:

DOCUMENTATION

Instructor Note: Retain work products with competency checklist.

Work Product, Procedure 8-1 (Progress Note)

Progress Note for Patient: Date:	**DOUGLASVILLE MEDICINE ASSOCIATES** **5076 BRAND BLVD** **DOUGLASVILLE, NY 01234** **(123) 456-7890**

Key Competencies			
ABHES	VI.A.1.a.2.m	Adaptation for individualized needs	
	VI.A.1.a.7.b	Instruct patients with special needs	
CAAHEP	III.C.3.c.3.b	Instruct individuals according to their needs	

Student Name: _____   Date: _____   Score: _____

Competency Checklist
PROCEDURE 8-2   Effectively Communicate with Sight Impaired or Blind Patients

Task: To provide sighted guide assistance

Condition: Given a chart, supplies and equipment necessary for the screening, and a classmate to play the part of a blind patient, the student will simulate assisting a blind patient during an office visit, by acting as a sighted guide.

Standards: The student will have 20 minutes to complete the procedure and will need to score an 85% or above to pass the competency. Automatic failure results if any essential steps are omitted or performed incorrectly.

STEPS START TIME: END TIME:	Points Possible	First Attempt	Second Attempt	Third Attempt
1. Prepared patient's room and walkway from reception room to examination room by clearing objects that could cause the patient to trip or fall.	10			
2. Approached patient in the reception room and gently called out the patient's name; didn't startle patient.	5			
3. Identified self and stated title.	10			
4. Asked patient if he or she would like to have sighted guide assistance; asked patient if he or she wanted to be on a particular side.	10			
5. Positioned self on the side that patient indicated and allowed patient to grasp his or her arm just above the elbow.	10			
6. Walked a half step in front of patient; patient's shoulder should be lined up behind the opposite shoulder of the guide.	10			
7. Warned patient when coming to stairs, doorway or elevator, or about any obstacles that could not be moved.	10			
8. Once inside examination room, described the type of seating (chair with/without arms, approximate height of the seating, etc).	10			
9. Escorted patient to the front of the chair, allowing the patient's knees or feet to just slightly touch the front of the chair.	10			
10. Placed patient's hand that was being guided on the arm of the chair and allowed patient to finish seating herself.	10			
11. Interviewed patient in a normal fashion.	5			
12. When performing any procedures (vitals, etc) explained the procedure and gave patient warning before touching the patient.	10			
13. Explained how to disrobe and placed any gowns or drapes directly beside the patient—describing the exact location of the drapes.	10			
14. Asked patient if he or she needed any assistance disrobing.	10			
15. Notified the patient when exiting the room and explained that the provider will knock before entering.	10			
16. Completed the procedure within the appropriate time limit.	10			
Points Earned / Points Possible:	___ / 150			

Points possible reflect importance of step in meeting the task: Important = (5) Essential = (10).
Determine score by dividing points earned by total points possible, and multiplying results by 100.

Key Competencies		
ABHES	VI.A.1.a.2.m	Adaptation for individualized needs
	VI.A.1.a.7.b	Instruct patients with special needs
CAAHEP	III.C.3.c.3.b	Instruct individuals according to their needs

Student Name: _____   Date: _____   Score: _____

EVALUATION

Evaluator Signature: _____   Date: _____

Evaluator Comments:

Key Competencies			
ABHES	VI.A.1.a.2.m	Adaptation for individualized needs	
	VI.A.1.a.7.b	Instruct patients with special needs	
CAAHEP	III.C.3.c.3.b	Instruct individuals according to their needs	

Student Name: _____   Date: _____   Score: _____

Competency Checklist
PROCEDURE 8-3   Effectively Communicate with Hearing Impaired or Deaf Patients when an Interpreter is Present

Task: To effectively communicate with a deaf patient when an interpreter is present

Condition: Given a chart, pen, equipment and supplies necessary for the screening, a classmate to play the part of a deaf patient, and a classmate to play the role of the interpreter, the student will effectively communicate with a deaf patient with the aid of an interpreter, following the steps listed below.

Standards: The student will have 20 minutes to complete the procedure and will need to score an 85% or above to pass the competency. Automatic failure results if any essential steps are omitted or performed incorrectly.

STEPS START TIME: END TIME:	Points Possible	First Attempt	Second Attempt	Third Attempt
1. Set the room up correctly by placing chairs in a triangular pattern; placed patient at the point of triangle and centered the other two chairs directly across from the patient's chair.	10			
2. Identified self and stated title to the patient; asked the interpreter to introduce him/herself to the patient.	10			
3. Asked patient to introduce him/herself and state any signing preferences.	10			
4. Looked directly at the patient during the communication encounter and talked at a normal rate of speed (for lip reading).	10			
5. Asked the patient to repeat back instructions (via the interpreter); listened to the patient's response through the interpreter while looking at the patient.	10			
6. Gave patient written instructions to take home.	5			
7. Thanked both the patient and the interpreter for their participation. (If the patient indicated he/she felt particularly comfortable with this particular interpreter, made a note in the patient's chart.)	5			
8. Correctly documented visit and stated that an interpreter was present for the visit (*Work Product, Procedure 8-3*).	10			
9. Completed the procedure within the appropriate time limit.	10			
Points Earned / Points Possible:	___ / 80			

Points possible reflect importance of step in meeting the task: Important = (5) Essential = (10).
Determine score by dividing points earned by total points possible, and multiplying results by 100.

EVALUATION
Evaluator Signature: _____   Date: _____

Evaluator Comments:

Key Competencies		
ABHES	VI.A.1.a.2.m	Adaptation for individualized needs
	VI.A.1.a.7.b	Instruct patients with special needs
CAAHEP	III.C.3.c.3.b	Instruct individuals according to their needs

Student Name: _____   Date: _____   Score: _____

DOCUMENTATION

Instructor Note: Retain work products with competency checklist.
Work Product, Procedure 8-3 (Progress Note)

Progress Note for	DOUGLASVILLE MEDICINE ASSOCIATES
	5076 BRAND BLVD
Patient:	DOUGLASVILLE, NY 01234
Date:	(123) 456-7890

Key Competencies		
ABHES	VI.A.1.a.2.m	Adaptation for individualized needs
	VI.A.1.a.7.b	Instruct patients with special needs
CAAHEP	III.C.3.c.3.b	Instruct individuals according to their needs

Student Name: _____   Date: _____   Score: _____

Competency Checklist
PROCEDURE 8-4   Effectively Communicate with a Hearing Impaired or Deaf Patient Who Speech Reads

Task: To effectively communicate with a hearing impaired or deaf patient who speech reads

Condition: Given a patient chart, pen, any supplies or equipment needed for the screening, and a classmate to play the part of the hearing impaired patient, the student will provide effective communication for a hearing impaired patient who can read lips by following the steps listed below.

Standards: The student will have 20 minutes to complete the procedure and will need to score an 85% or above to pass the competency. Automatic failure results if any essential steps are omitted or performed incorrectly.

STEPS START TIME: END TIME:	Points Possible	First Attempt	Second Attempt	Third Attempt
1. Selected an exam room that was quiet and had good lighting. (If possible, positioned light source so that it would shine on the medical assistant.)	10			
2. Positioned self directly across from the patient, at the same eye level.	10			
3. Spoke at a normal talking rate throughout the entire encounter.	5			
4. Used gestures, hand cues and written materials to assist in the communication process.	5			
5. Rephrased statements or questions that were confusing to the patient.	10			
6. Asked patient to repeat any homecare instructions to verify comprehension (may be through writing, gestures or speaking).	10			
7. Completed the procedure within the appropriate time limit.	10			
Points Earned / Points Possible:	___ / 60			

Points possible reflect importance of step in meeting the task: Important = (5) Essential = (10).
Determine score by dividing points earned by total points possible, and multiplying results by 100.

EVALUATION
Evaluator Signature: _____   Date: _____

Evaluator Comments:

Key Competencies		
ABHES	VI.A.1.a.2.m	Adaptation for individualized needs
	VI.A.1.a.7.b	Instruct patients with special needs
CAAHEP	III.C.3.c.3.b	Instruct individuals according to their needs

Student Name: _____   Date: _____   Score: _____

Competency Checklist
PROCEDURE 9-1   Provide Instruction for Health Maintenance and Disease Prevention and Identify Community Resources That Will Assist the Patient

Task: To provide instruction for health maintenance and disease prevention and identify community resources that will assist the patient

Condition: Given a health topic to research prior to the session, equipment and supplies as listed in the procedure, and a classmate to play the part of the patient, the student will provide an educational session following the steps listed below.

Standards: The student will have 20 minutes to complete the procedure and will need to score an 85% or above to pass the competency. Automatic failure results if any essential steps are omitted or performed incorrectly.

Student will conduct patient education on _____.

STEPS START TIME: END TIME:	Points Possible	First Attempt	Second Attempt	Third Attempt
1. Read and clarified order from physician.	10			
2. Collected necessary items and supplies including educational pamphlets, lists of community resources, models, laptop computer, etc.	10			
3. Reviewed information and asked physician questions if unclear about information in any of the resources.	10			
4. Prepared the room so that everyone in the session had a seat and could see each other; room had outlets and lighting.	10			
5. Identified the patient and family members or friends of the patient and identified self.	10			
6. Stated the purpose of the session.	10			
7. Determined the patient's preferred learning style and set goals to determine what the patient and family wanted to accomplish from the session.	10			
8. Presented the information in clear manner.	10			
9. Had checkpoints along the way to determine understanding of material.	5			
10. Summarized the information at the end of session.	10			
11. Had patient repeat the information or demonstrate the procedure back.	10			
12. Praised patient and family for comprehension of material.	5			
13. Gave patient learning pamphlets, prescriptions, any necessary supplies, and provided a list of resources that can assist the patient with special needs.	10			
14. Gave patient business card with name and office phone number; encouraged the patient to contact the office with any questions.	5			
15. Correctly documented session, including date and time, who was present and if educational material was handed out *(Work Product, Procedure 9-1)*.	10			
16. Completed the procedure within the appropriate time limit.	10			
Points Earned / Points Possible:	___ / 145			

Key Competencies		
ABHES	VI.A.1.a.7.c	Teach patients methods of health promotion and disease prevention
	VI.A.1.a.3.e	Locate resources and information for patients and employers
CAAHEP	III.C.3.c.3.c	Provide instruction for health maintenance and disease prevention
	III.C.3.c.3.d	Identify community resources

Student Name: _____   Date: _____   Score: _____

Points possible reflect importance of step in meeting the task: Important = (5) Essential = (10).
Determine score by dividing points earned by total points possible, and multiplying results by 100.

EVALUATION
Evaluator Signature: _____   Date: _____

Evaluator Comments:

DOCUMENTATION
Instructor Note: Retain work products with competency checklist.
Work Product, Procedure 9-1 (Progress Note)

Progress Note for Patient: Date:	**DOUGLASVILLE MEDICINE ASSOCIATES** **5076 BRAND BLVD** **DOUGLASVILLE, NY 01234** **(123) 456-7890**

Key Competencies		
ABHES	VI.A.1.a.7.c	Teach patients methods of health promotion and disease prevention
	VI.A.1.a.3.e	Locate resources and information for patients and employers
CAAHEP	III.C.3.c.3.c	Provide instruction for health maintenance and disease prevention
	III.C.3.c.3.d	Identify community resources

Student Name: _____   Date: _____   Score: _____

Competency Checklist
PROCEDURE 10-1 Perform Medically Aseptic Handwashing

Task: To perform a medically aseptic handwashing

Condition: Given the equipment and supplies as listed in the procedure, the student will perform the task, adhering to the standards listed below.

Standards: The student will have 5 minutes to complete the procedure and will need to score an 85% or above to pass the competency. Automatic failure results if any essential steps are omitted or performed incorrectly.

STEPS START TIME: END TIME:	Points Possible	First Attempt	Second Attempt	Third Attempt
1. Assembled necessary equipment and removed all jewelry, except a plain wedding band.	5			
2. Stood at sink (did not touch rim with hands/clothing); turned on faucet with a paper towel, adjusted water temperature, discarded towel.	10			
3. Wet hands, wrists, and forearms and applied soap.	10			
4. Used a circular motion and friction to scrub backs and palms of hands, wrists, and forearms. Interlaced fingers and thumbs and rubbed back and forth to clean all surfaces. Kept hands pointed down during entire washing process.	10			
5. For first washing of the day, cleaned cuticles and nails with orange stick.	10			
6. Rinsed hands and wrists well, with hands pointed downward.	10			
7. Blotted hands, wrists, and forearms until dry with a paper towel and discarded towel.	10			
8. Turned faucet off with clean paper towel.	10			
9. Applied antibacterial lotion.	5			
Points Earned / Points Possible:	___ / 80			

Points possible reflect importance of step in meeting the task: Important = (5) Essential = (10).
Determine score by dividing points earned by total points possible, and multiplying results by 100.

EVALUATION
Evaluator Signature: _____   Date: _____

Evaluator Comments:

Key Competencies		
ABHES	VI.A.1.a.4.c	Apply principles of aseptic techniques and infection control
CAAHEP	III.C.3.b.1.a	Perform handwashing

Student Name: _____ Date: _____ Score: _____

Competency Checklist
PROCEDURE 10-2 Perform an Alcohol-Based Hand Rub

Task: To clean hands by using an alcohol-based hand rub

Condition: Given the equipment and supplies as listed in the procedure, the student will perform the task, adhering to the steps below.

Standards: The student will have 3 minutes to complete the procedure and will need to score an 85% or above to pass the competency. Automatic failure results if any essential steps are omitted or performed incorrectly.

STEPS START TIME: END TIME:	Points Possible	First Attempt	Second Attempt	Third Attempt
1. Inspected hands for any visible soil or contamination. (If present, performed a standard medically aseptic handwashing with soap and water.)	10			
2. Removed all jewelry except a plain wedding band.	5			
3. Applied recommended amount of alcohol-based hand rub and smoothed over all surfaces of hand.	10			
4. Rubbed hands together (approximately 10–15 seconds) until dry or followed procedure on label.	10			
Points Earned / Points Possible:	___ / 35			

Points possible reflect importance of step in meeting the task: Important = (5) Essential = (10).
Determine score by dividing points earned by total points possible, and multiplying results by 100.

EVALUATION
Evaluator Signature: _____ Date: _____

Evaluator Comment:

Key Competencies		
ABHES	VI.A.1.a.4.c	Apply principles of aseptic technique and infection control
CAAHEP	III.C.3.b.1.e	Practice Standard Precautions

Student Name: _____   Date: _____   Score: _____

Competency Checklist
PROCEDURE 10-3 Remove Contaminated Gloves

Task: To properly remove contaminated gloves

Condition: Given the equipment and supplies as listed in the procedure, the student will perform the task, adhering to the standards listed below.

Standards: The student will have 5 minutes to complete the procedure and will need to score an 85% or above to pass the competency. Automatic failure results if any essential steps are omitted or performed incorrectly.

STEPS START TIME: END TIME:	Points Possible	First Attempt	Second Attempt	Third Attempt
1. With hands pointed downward and away from the body, grabbed the palm of the left glove with the right hand, turned glove inside out, and crumpled into a ball in right hand.	10			
2. Grasped contaminated glove that had been removed in gloved right hand and inserted two fingers of ungloved left hand between wrist and under cuff of other contaminated glove.	10			
3. Turned right glove inside out over the other glove.	10			
4. Disposed of contaminated gloves in biohazard waste container.	10			
5. Washed hands.	5			
Points Earned / Points Possible:	___ / 45			

Points possible reflect importance of step in meeting the task: Important = (5) Essential = (10).
Determine score by dividing points earned by total points possible, and multiplying results by 100.

EVALUATION
Evaluator Signature: _____   Date: _____

Evaluator Comments:

Key Competencies		
ABHES	VI.A.1.a.4.p	Dispose of biohazardous materials
	VI.A.1.a.4.q	Practice Standard Precautions
CAAHEP	III.C.3.b.1.d	Dispose of biohazardous materials
	III.C.3.b.1.e	Practice Standard Precautions

Student Name: _____   Date: _____   Score: _____

Competency Checklist
PROCEDURE 11-1 Obtain the Height and Weight of an Adult Patient

Task: To obtain and document an adult patient's height and weight

Condition: Given the equipment and supplies as listed in the procedure and a classmate to play the part of the patient, the student will perform and document an adult height and weight, adhering to the steps listed below.

Standards: The student will have 5 minutes to complete the procedure and will need to score an 85% or above to pass the competency. Automatic failure results if any essential steps are omitted or performed incorrectly.

STEPS START TIME: END TIME:	Points Possible	First Attempt	Second Attempt	Third Attempt
1. Washed hands, placed upper and lower scale weights at zero and checked to be sure the scale was properly balanced.	10			
2. Identified the patient using at least two identifiers, identified self, and explained the procedure.	10			
3. Assessed the stability of the patient.	5			
4. Instructed patient to remove any unnecessary clothing, including shoes.	10			
5. Placed paper towel on the platform of the scales.	10			
6. Assisted the patient onto the center of the scale platform, facing the weights, and asked patient to stand completely still.	10			
7. Slowly moved the lower weight first, into the appropriate notched groove and then adjusted the upper weight so that the indicator arrow was properly centered in the designated area.	10			
8. Recorded the measurement on a piece of paper or on the progress note, and returned the weights to zero.	5			
9. Assisted the patient off the scale, and raised the calibrated height bar to a height greater than the patient's height.	10			
10. Extended or opened the measuring bar to a horizontal position.	10			
11. Assisted the patient back onto the scale with his or her back toward the measuring bar and instructed the patient to stand totally erect and still.	10			
12. Lowered the horizontal bar (positioned at a 90-degree angle) until it touched the top of the patient's head.	10			
13. Read and recorded the height measurement on a piece of paper or progress note and returned the measurement bar back to its original position.	10			
14. Assisted patient off the scale platform and discarded paper towel.	5			
15. Washed hands and documented the results in the patient's chart if measurements were not already recorded on the patient's chart. (Converted lb to kg if necessary.) *(Work Product, Procedure 11-1)*	10			
16. Transferred information to flow chart if applicable *(Work Product, Procedure 11-1).*	10			
17. Completed the procedure within the appropriate time limit.	10			
Points Earned / Points Possible:	___ / 155			

Points possible reflect importance of step in meeting the task: Important = (5) Essential = (10).
Determine score by dividing points earned by total points possible, and multiplying results by 100.

Key Competencies		
ABHES	VI.A.1.a.4.d	Take Vital Signs
CAAHEP	III.C.3.b.4.b	Obtain Vital Signs

Student Name: _____   Date: _____   Score: _____

EVALUATION
Evaluator Signature: _____   Date: _____

Evaluator Comments:

DOCUMENTATION
Instructor Note: Retain work products with competency checklist.
Work Product, Procedure 11-1 (Progress Note)

Progress Note for Patient: Date:	**DOUGLASVILLE MEDICINE ASSOCIATES** **5076 BRAND BLVD** **DOUGLASVILLE, NY 01234** **(123) 456-7890**

Work Product, Procedure 11-1 (Flow Sheet)

HEIGHT AND WEIGHT FLOW SHEET

Patient's Name: _____   Patient's Birth Date: _____

Patient's ID #: _____   Provider's Name: _____

Today's Date	WT	HT

Key Competencies		
ABHES	VI.A.1.a.4.d	Take Vital Signs
CAAHEP	III.C.3.b.4.b	Obtain Vital Signs

Student Name: _____   Date: _____   Score: _____

Competency Checklist
PROCEDURE 11-2 Obtain an Oral Body Temperature

Task: To obtain and document an accurate oral body temperature reading

Condition: Given the equipment and supplies as listed in the procedure and a classmate to play the part of the patient, the student will perform and document an oral body temperature, adhering to the steps listed below.

Standards: The student will have 5 minutes to complete the procedure and will need to score an 85% or above to pass the competency. Automatic failure results if any essential steps are omitted or performed incorrectly.

STEPS START TIME: END TIME:	Points Possible	First Attempt	Second Attempt	Third Attempt
1. Washed hands and assembled equipment. (Applied gloves if applicable.)	10			
2. Identified the patient using at least two identifiers, identified self, and explained the procedure.	10			
3. Inquired about recent hot or cold beverages, foods and smoking; waited an appropriate amount of time if applicable before proceeding.	10			
4. Removed thermometer from base and placed a disposable probe cover on the blue/oral probe.	10			
5. Placed the probe in the patient's mouth under the tongue just to the right or left of the frenulum linguae.	10			
6. Instructed patient not to bite down on the thermometer and to keep mouth shut and lips sealed—breathing only through nose.	10			
7. Kept the thermometer in place until the signal beeped—removed probe, read the digital display, and discarded the used probe cover into the appropriate trash receptacle (following institutional guidelines).	10			
8. Placed the electronic thermometer back in the base holder for recharging.	10			
9. Washed hands and documented in progress note and in flow sheet (if applicable) *(Work Product, Procedure 11-2)*.	10			
10. Completed the procedure within the appropriate time limit.	10			
Points Earned / Points Possible:	___ / 100			

Points possible reflect importance of step in meeting the task: Important = (5) Essential = (10).
Determine score by dividing points earned by total points possible, and multiplying results by 100.

EVALUATION
Evaluator Signature: _____   Date: _____

Evaluator Comments:

Key Competencies		
ABHES	VI.A.1.a.4.d	Take Vital Signs
CAAHEP	III.C.3.b.4.b	Obtain Vital Signs

Student Name: _____   Date: _____   Score: _____

DOCUMENTATION

Instructor Note: Retain work products with competency checklist.
Work Product, Procedure 11-2 (Progress Note)

Progress Note for Patient: Date:	**DOUGLASVILLE MEDICINE ASSOCIATES** **5076 BRAND BLVD** **DOUGLASVILLE, NY 01234** **(123) 456-7890**

Work Product, Procedure 11-2 (Flow Sheet)

VITAL SIGN FLOW SHEET

Patient's Name: _____   **Patient's Birth Date:** _____

Patient's ID #: _____   **Provider's Name:** _____

Today's Date	Pain Rating	Temp	Pulse	Resp	BP	BP Med	Current Dose	Change in Dose	Provider's Initials

Key Competencies		
ABHES	VI.A.1.a.4.d	Take Vital Signs
CAAHEP	III.C.3.b.4.b	Obtain Vital Signs

Student Name: _____   Date: _____   Score: _____

Competency Checklist
PROCEDURE 11-3 Obtain an Aural Body Temperature

Task: To obtain an aural body temperature

Condition: Given the equipment and supplies as listed in the procedure and a classmate to play the part of the patient, the student will perform and document an aural temperature reading, adhering to the steps listed below.

Standards: The student will have 5 minutes to complete the procedure and will need to score an 85% or above to pass the competency. Automatic failure results if any essential steps are omitted or performed incorrectly.

STEPS START TIME: END TIME:	Points Possible	First Attempt	Second Attempt	Third Attempt
1. Washed hands and assembled equipment.	10			
2. Ensured that the thermometer was charged, cleaned, and in proper working order.	10			
3. Identified the patient using at least two identifiers, identified self, and explained the procedure.	10			
4. Placed a clean probe cover over the tympanic probe and turned the unit on, making certain that the unit was in the "ready" mode.	10			
5. Properly straightened the auditory canal by gently pulling the auricle of the ear up and back on an adult, or down and back on patients under the age of three.	10			
6. Inserted the probe into the patient's ear directing the probe towards the patient's eardrum.	10			
7. Sealed the canal properly to prevent air from entering the canal.	10			
8. Activated the thermometer and, following the beep, read the digital results.	10			
9. Disposed of the probe cover in the appropriate trash receptacle and returned thermometer to storage.	10			
10. Washed hands and documented in progress note and in flow sheet (if applicable) *(Work Product, Procedure 11-3)*.	10			
11. Completed the procedure within the appropriate time limit.	10			
Points Earned / Points Possible:	___ / 110			

Points possible reflect importance of step in meeting the task: Important = (5) Essential = (10).
Determine score by dividing points earned by total points possible, and multiplying results by 100.

EVALUATION
Evaluator Signature: _____   Date: _____

Evaluator Comments:

Key Competencies		
ABHES	VI.A.1.a.4.d	Take Vital Signs
CAAHEP	III.C.3.b.4.b	Obtain Vital Signs

Student Name: _____   Date: _____   Score: _____

DOCUMENTATION
Instructor Note: Retain work products with competency checklist.
Work Product, Procedure 11-3 (Progress Note)

Progress Note for Patient: Date:	**DOUGLASVILLE MEDICINE ASSOCIATES** **5076 BRAND BLVD** **DOUGLASVILLE, NY 01234** **(123) 456-7890**

Work Product, Procedure 11-3 (Flow Sheet)

VITAL SIGN FLOW SHEET

Patient's Name: _____   Patient's Birth Date: _____

Patient's ID #: _____   Provider's Name: _____

Today's Date	Pain Rating	Temp	Pulse	Resp	BP	BP Med	Current Dose	Change in Dose	Provider's Initials

Key Competencies		
ABHES	VI.A.1.a.4.d	Take Vital Signs
CAAHEP	III.C.3.b.4.b	Obtain Vital Signs

Student Name: _____   Date: _____   Score: _____

Competency Checklist
PROCEDURE 11-4 Obtain an Axillary Body Temperature

Task: To obtain an axillary body temperature

Condition: Given the equipment and supplies as listed in the procedure and a classmate to play the part of the patient, the student will perform and document an axillary temperature reading, adhering to the steps listed below.

Standards: The student will have 5 minutes to complete the procedure and will need to score an 85% or above to pass the competency. Automatic failure results if any essential steps are omitted or performed incorrectly.

STEPS START TIME: END TIME:	Points Possible	First Attempt	Second Attempt	Third Attempt
1. Washed hands, assembled equipment and ensured that thermometer was clean and in proper working order.	10			
2. Identified the patient using at least two identifiers, explained the procedure, and instructed patient to remove necessary clothing.	10			
3. Removed probe from base and placed a disposable probe cover over the oral/blue probe.	10			
4. If applicable, patted armpit with a paper towel or instructed patient to do so, removing any moisture from the area.	10			
5. Inserted the probe under the armpit, making a tight seal, and instructed patient to hold arm tightly against body.	10			
6. Kept thermometer in place until device emitted a beep and noted the reading.	10			
7. Discarded probe cover in appropriate container and placed the unit into the charging base.	10			
8. Washed hands and documented in progress note and in flow sheet (if applicable) (*Work Product, Procedure 11-4*).	10			
9. Completed the procedure within the appropriate time limit.	10			
Points Earned / Points Possible:	___ / 90			

Points possible reflect importance of step in meeting the task: Important = (5) Essential = (10).
Determine score by dividing points earned by total points possible, and multiplying results by 100.

EVALUATION
Evaluator Signature: _____   Date: _____

Evaluator Comments:

Key Competencies		
ABHES	VI.A.1.a.4.d	Take Vital Signs
CAAHEP	III.C.3.b.4.b	Obtain Vital Signs

Student Name: _____   Date: _____   Score: _____

DOCUMENTATION

Instructor Note: Retain work products with competency checklist.

Work Product, Procedure 11-4 (Progress Note)

Progress Note for Patient: Date:	**DOUGLASVILLE MEDICINE ASSOCIATES** **5076 BRAND BLVD** **DOUGLASVILLE, NY 01234** **(123) 456-7890**

Work Product, Procedure 11-4 (Flow Sheet)

VITAL SIGN FLOW SHEET

Patient's Name: _____   Patient's Birth Date: _____

Patient's ID #: _____   Provider's Name: _____

Today's Date	Pain Rating	Temp	Pulse	Resp	BP	BP Med	Current Dose	Change in Dose	Provider's Initials

Key Competencies		
ABHES	VI.A.1.a.4.d	Take Vital Signs
CAAHEP	III.C.3.b.4.b	Obtain Vital Signs

Student Name: _____   Date: _____   Score: _____

Competency Checklist
PROCEDURE 11-5 Obtain a Temporal Artery Body Temperature

Task: To obtain a temporal artery body temperature

Condition: Given the equipment and supplies as listed in the procedure and a classmate to play the part of the patient, the student will perform and document a temperature reading, using a temporal thermometer, adhering to the steps listed below.

Standards: The student will have 5 minutes to complete the procedure and will need to score an 85% or above to pass the competency. Automatic failure results if any essential steps are omitted or performed incorrectly.

STEPS START TIME: END TIME:	Points Possible	First Attempt	Second Attempt	Third Attempt
1. Washed hands and assembled equipment.	10			
2. Cleaned thermometer with an alcohol pad (applied probe cover if applicable), and ensured unit was working properly.	10			
3. Identified the patient using at least two identifiers and explained the procedure.	10			
4. Removed any hats or scarves and pulled back hair from the area being scanned.	10			
5. Checked forehead for perspiration and wiped dry if applicable.	10			
6. Depressed scan button and kept depressed throughout the entire procedure.	10			
7. Placed probe at midline of forehead, keeping it flush with skin. Slowly glided probe across forehead and over the temple region.	10			
8. Released scan button, lifted probe from patient's skin, and checked display for reading.	10			
9. If second reading behind the ear was necessary, left the scan button depressed when removing from over the temporal region and immediately placed the probe behind the ear, just under the mastoid process.	10			
10. Waited until scanning was finished and accurately documented the highest reading and method used in the patient's chart and in flow sheet (if applicable) (*Work Product, Procedure 11-5*).	10			
11. Completed the procedure within the appropriate time limit.	10			
Points Earned / Points Possible:	___ / 110			

Points possible reflect importance of step in meeting the task: Important = (5) Essential = (10).
Determine score by dividing points earned by total points possible, and multiplying results by 100.

EVALUATION
Evaluator Signature: _____   Date: _____

Evaluator Comments:

Key Competencies		
ABHES	VI.A.1.a.4.d	Take Vital Signs
CAAHEP	III.C.3.b.4.b	Obtain Vital Signs

Student Name: _____   Date: _____   Score: _____

DOCUMENTATION

Instructor Note: Retain work products with competency checklist.

Work Product, Procedure 11-5 (Progress Note)

Progress Note for Patient: Date:	**DOUGLASVILLE MEDICINE ASSOCIATES** **5076 BRAND BLVD** **DOUGLASVILLE, NY 01234** **(123) 456-7890**

Work Product, Procedure 11-5 (Flow Sheet)

VITAL SIGN FLOW SHEET

Patient's Name: _____   Patient's Birth Date: _____

Patient's ID #: _____   Provider's Name: _____

Today's Date	Pain Rating	Temp	Pulse	Resp	BP	BP Med	Current Dose	Change in Dose	Provider's Initials

Key Competencies			
ABHES	VI.A.1.a.4.d	Take Vital Signs
CAAHEP	III.C.3.b.4.b	Obtain Vital Signs

Student Name: _____   Date: _____   Score: _____

Competency Checklist
PROCEDURE 11-6 Obtain a Radial Pulse Rate and Respiration Rate

Task: To obtain a radial pulse rate and respiration rate

Condition: Given the equipment and supplies as listed in the procedure and a classmate to play the part of the patient, the student will perform a radial pulse and respiration, adhering to the steps listed below.

Standards: The student will have 5 minutes to complete the procedure and will need to score an 85% or above to pass the competency. Automatic failure results if any essential steps are omitted or performed incorrectly.

STEPS START TIME: END TIME:	Points Possible	First Attempt	Second Attempt	Third Attempt
1. Washed hands.	10			
2. Identified the patient using at least two identifiers, identified self, and explained the procedure.	10			
3. Allowed patient to rest for a few moments, promoting a calm environment.	5			
4. Positioned patient's wrist for easy accessibility and patient comfort.	5			
5. Placed index and middle finger over radial artery to palpate the radial pulse. Applied the correct amount of pressure so that the pulse was detectable.	10			
6. Counted the number of beats for 30 seconds, multiplying the rate by two for a full minute rate. (Note pulse rate, rhythm, and pulse.)	10			
7. Maintained fingers over the radial artery and counted the respirations for 30 seconds, multiplying the result by 2 for a full minute rate. (Note rate, volume and rhythm.)	10			
8. Washed hands and documented results in patient's progress note and in flow sheet (if applicable) (Work Product, Procedure 11-6).	10			
9. Completed the procedure within the appropriate time limit.	10			
Points Earned / Points Possible:	___ / 80			

Points possible reflect importance of step in meeting the task: Important = (5) Essential = (10).
Determine score by dividing points earned by total points possible, and multiplying results by 100.

EVALUATION
Evaluator Signature: _____   Date: _____

Evaluator Comments:

Key Competencies			
ABHES	VI.A.1.a.4.d	Take Vital Signs	
CAAHEP	III.C.3.b.4.b	Obtain Vital Signs	

Student Name: _____   Date: _____   Score: _____

DOCUMENTATION

Instructor Note: Retain work products with competency checklist.
Work Product, Procedure 11-6 (Progress Note)

Progress Note for	**DOUGLASVILLE MEDICINE ASSOCIATES**
Patient:	**5076 BRAND BLVD**
Date:	**DOUGLASVILLE, NY 01234**
	(123) 456-7890

Work Product, Procedure 11-6 (Flow Sheet)

VITAL SIGN FLOW SHEET

Patient's Name: _____   **Patient's Birth Date:** _____

Patient's ID #: _____   **Provider's Name:** _____

Today's Date	Pain Rating	Temp	Pulse	Resp	BP	BP Med	Current Dose	Change in Dose	Provider's Initials

Key Competencies			
ABHES	VI.A.1.a.4.d	Take Vital Signs
CAAHEP	III.C.3.b.4.b	Obtain Vital Signs

Student Name: _____   Date: _____   Score: _____

Competency Checklist
PROCEDURE 11-7 Obtain an Apical Pulse Rate

Task: To obtain an apical pulse reading

Condition: Given the equipment and supplies as listed in the procedure and a classmate to play the part of the patient, the student will perform an apical pulse rate, adhering to the steps listed below.

Standards: The student will have 5 minutes to complete the procedure and will need to score an 85% or above to pass the competency. Automatic failure results if any essential steps are omitted or performed incorrectly.

STEPS START TIME: END TIME:	Points Possible	First Attempt	Second Attempt	Third Attempt
1. Washed hands, sanitized stethoscope, and assembled equipment.	5			
2. Identified the patient using at least two identifiers, identified self, and explained the procedure.	10			
3. Instructed patient to expose left thoracic region by removing appropriate clothing; offered patient a gown.				
4. Located the apex of the heart (fifth intercostal space at the left midclavicular line), placed stethoscope in ears and placed chest piece of stethoscope over apex of heart.	10			
5. Counted the heartbeats for one minute, noting any irregularities.	10			
6. Removed stethoscope from patient's chest and assisted the patient with dressing, if needed.	5			
7. Washed hands and documented in progress note and in flow sheet (if applicable) *(Work Product, Procedure 11-7)*.	10			
8. Completed the procedure within the appropriate time limit.				
Points Earned / Points Possible:	___ / 50			

Points possible reflect importance of step in meeting the task: Important = (5) Essential = (10).
Determine score by dividing points earned by total points possible, and multiplying results by 100.

EVALUATION
Evaluator Signature: _____   Date: _____

Evaluator Comments:

Key Competencies		
ABHES	VI.A.1.a.4.d	Take Vital Signs
CAAHEP	III.C.3.b.4.b	Obtain Vital Signs

Student Name: _____   Date: _____   Score: _____

DOCUMENTATION

Instructor Note: Retain work products with competency checklist.

Work Product, Procedure 11-7 (Progress Note)

Progress Note for Patient: Date:	**DOUGLASVILLE MEDICINE ASSOCIATES** **5076 BRAND BLVD** **DOUGLASVILLE, NY 01234** **(123) 456-7890**

Work Product, Procedure 11-7 (Flow Sheet)

VITAL SIGN FLOW SHEET

Patient's Name: _____   **Patient's Birth Date:** _____

Patient's ID #: _____   **Provider's Name:** _____

Today's Date	Pain Rating	Temp	Pulse	Resp	BP	BP Med	Current Dose	Change in Dose	Provider's Initials

Key Competencies		
ABHES	VI.A.1.a.4.d	Take Vital Signs
CAAHEP	III.C.3.b.4.b	Obtain Vital Signs

Student Name: _____   Date: _____   Score: _____

Competency Checklist
PROCEDURE 11-8 Obtain a Blood Pressure Measurement Using the Palpatory Method

Task: To obtain a blood pressure reading

Condition: Given the equipment and supplies as listed in the procedure and a classmate to play the part of the patient, the student will perform a blood pressure reading, adhering to the steps listed below.

Standards: The student will have 5 minutes to complete the procedure and will need to score an 85% or above to pass the competency. Automatic failure results if any essential steps are omitted or performed incorrectly.

STEPS START TIME: END TIME:	Points Possible	First Attempt	Second Attempt	Third Attempt
1. Washed hands, sanitized stethoscope, and assembled equipment; checked cuff for proper working order—made certain that cuff was properly deflated and all air was removed from the cuff.	10			
2. Identified the patient using at least two identifiers, identified self, and explained the procedure.	10			
3. Assessed patient for anxiousness, if any noted, and had patient rest for a few minutes before performing the procedure.	5			
4. Instructed patient to remove any clothing that restricted access to the testing area or to pull shirt sleeve up several inches above the bend of the elbow.	10			
5. Assessed patient's arm size to make certain cuff was the appropriate size.	10			
6. Placed patient in a comfortable position and positioned arm so that it was level with the heart.	10			
7. With patient's palm upward, applied cuff to patient's arm 1–2 inches above the bend of the elbow and aligned the correct arrow over the brachial artery. Adjusted aneroid dial so that it was clearly visible.	10			
8. Tested stethoscope by gently tapping on chest piece to ascertain the correct side was in the open position for measurement.	5			
9. Palpated brachial artery for a viable pulse and noted where pulse was the strongest.	5			
10. Held bulb in dominant hand and located radial pulse with the other hand. Closed valve and squeezed bulb to inflate the cuff while palpating the radial pulse.	10			
11. Continued inflation of cuff until pulse subsided and approximately 30 mm/Hg beyond the disappearance of the pulse.	10			
12. Slowly opened valve and released air from cuff while continuing to palpate radial pulse. Noted reading when pulse returned.	10			
13. Removed all air from cuff and waited 30 seconds before continuing with the procedure.	10			
14. Placed chest piece of stethoscope over brachial artery and held in place with the index and middle fingers.	10			
15. Closed valve and pumped cuff up rapidly to 20 mm/hg above the return of the palpated pressure.	10			
16. Released pressure in cuff and observed dial carefully. Noted when first beat was heard (systolic pressure) and when the last beat was heard (diastolic pressure).	10			
17. Opened valve and completely deflated the cuff.	10			
18. Removed the stethoscope and cuff from the patient's arm and washed hands.	10			

Key Competencies		
ABHES	VI.B.1.a.4.d	Take Vital Signs
CAAHEP	III.C.3.b.4.b	Obtain Vital Signs

Student Name: _____   Date: _____   Score: _____

19. Accurately documented procedure in progress note and in flow sheet (if applicable) *(Work Product, Procedure 11-8).*	10			
20. Completed the procedure within the appropriate time limit.	10			
Points Earned / Points Possible:	___ / 185			

Points possible reflect importance of step in meeting the task: Important = (5) Essential = (10).
Determine score by dividing points earned by total points possible, and multiplying results by 100.

EVALUATION
Evaluator Signature: _____   Date: _____

Evaluator Comments:

DOCUMENTATION
Instructor Note: Retain work products with competency checklist.
Work Product, Procedure 11-8 (Progress Note)

Progress Note for Patient: Date:	**DOUGLASVILLE MEDICINE ASSOCIATES** **5076 BRAND BLVD** **DOUGLASVILLE, NY 01234** **(123) 456-7890**

Work Product, Procedure 11-8 (Flow Sheet)

VITAL SIGN FLOW SHEET

Patient's Name: _____   Patient's Birth Date: _____

Patient's ID #: _____   Provider's Name: _____

Today's Date	Pain Rating	Temp	Pulse	Resp	BP	BP Med	Current Dose	Change in Dose	Provider's Initials

Key Competencies			
ABHES	VI.B.1.a.4.d	Take Vital Signs	
CAAHEP	III.C.3.b.4.b	Obtain Vital Signs	

Student Name: _____   Date: _____   Score: _____

Competency Checklist
PROCEDURE 12-1 Prepare the Examination Room

Task: To clean an examination room and prepare it for the next patient

Condition: Given the equipment and supplies as listed in the procedure, an exam room that has been staged for cleaning by the instructor (instructor may place artificial body fluids on exam table, simulated contaminated sponges and instruments on trays, mayo stands, sharps containers, etc.), the student will prepare an examination room, adhering to the steps listed below. The student should know what type of exam or procedures were performed prior to cleaning the exam room and the reason for the next patient's visit.

Standards: The student will have 5 minutes to complete the procedure and will need to score an 85% or above to pass the competency. Automatic failure results if any essential steps are omitted or performed incorrectly.

STEPS START TIME: END TIME:	Points Possible	First Attempt	Second Attempt	Third Attempt
1. Washed hands and put on disposable gloves.	10			
2. Removed used instruments, dirty gauze, table paper, and pillow coverings and placed or discarded in appropriate trash receptacles or basins.	10			
3. Properly cleaned and disinfected exam table surfaces, countertops, and trays used during previous exam.	10			
4. Removed contaminated gloves and discarded in appropriate trash receptacle.	10			
5. Placed clean table paper on exam table and pillow covering on pillow.	10			
6. Checked exam table controls and height of exam table. Placed foot rest in proper position.	5			
7. Made certain lighting was effective.	5			
8. Restocked paper towels and other supplies used during previous exams and set up any items necessary for the next patient, including drapes, gowns, trays, etc.	10			
9. Activated room indicator (if applicable).	5			
10. Completed the procedure within the appropriate time limit.	10			
Points Earned / Points Possible:	___ / 85			

Points possible reflect importance of step in meeting the task: Important = (5) Essential = (10).
Determine score by dividing points earned by total points possible, and multiplying results by 100.

EVALUATION
Evaluator Signature: _____   Date: _____

Evaluator Comments:

Key Competencies		
ABHES	VI.A.1.a.4.g	Prepare and maintain examination and treatment area
	VI.A.1.a.4.q	Dispose of biohazardous materials
	VI.A.1.a.4.r	Practice standard precautions
CAAHEP	III.C.3.b.1.d	Dispose of Biohazardous Materials
	III.C.3.b.1.e	Practice Standard Precautions
	III.C.3.b.4.d	Prepare and maintain examination and treatment areas

Student Name: _____   Date: _____   Score: _____

Competency Checklist
PROCEDURE 12-2 Position and Drape the Patient

Task: To position and drape a patient

Condition: Given the equipment and supplies as listed in the procedure a classmate to play the part of the patient, the student will demonstrate the proper steps for placing patients in a variety of different positions (according to exam type or procedure). The instructor may use a different order for testing from the order listed below.

Standards: The student will have 15 minutes to work through the preliminary steps and each of the listed positions and will need to score an 85% or above to pass the competency. Automatic failure results if any essential steps listed in the preliminary steps are performed incorrectly or omitted. If student misses any steps for one of the listed positions, just that position will need to be repeated.

STEPS START TIME: END TIME:	Points Possible	First Attempt	Second Attempt	Third Attempt
1. Washed hands and gloved if necessary. Prepared room according to the scenario given by the instructor.	10			
2. Removed gloves, washed hands, and set out gowns and drapes necessary for each of the positions listed below.	10			
3. (Patient enters exam room.) Identified the patient using at least two identifiers, explained procedure (any procedure stated by the instructor), and provided patient with gown, drape, and disrobing instructions.	10			
4. Assisted the patient into a sitting position on the end of the exam table and placed drape over patient's lap and lower extremities. (Legs hung over the table at a 90-degree angle.)	10			
5. Starting from the sitting position, correctly placed the patient in the supine position. Placed a drape over the patient's chest and lower extremities.	10			
6. Starting from the sitting position, correctly placed the patient in the prone position. Placed a drape over the torso and lower extremities.	10			
7. Starting from the sitting position, placed patient in dorsal recumbent position. Placed diamond-shaped drape over the lower half of the body.	10			
8. Starting from the sitting position, placed patient in the Sims' position. Draped for comfort and privacy.	10			
9. Starting from the sitting position, placed patient in the full-Fowler's position (raised the head of the table to 90 degrees). Draped patient's torso and lower extremeties.	10			
10. Starting from the sitting position, placed patient in the Semi-Fowler's position (raised the head of the table to 45 degrees). Draped patient's torso and lower extremeties.	10			
11. Starting from the sitting position, placed the patient in the lithotomy position. (Made certain stirrups were at a comfortable distance.) Placed diamond shaped drape over the lower half of the body.	10			
12. Starting from a sitting position, placed the patient in the knee-chest position. Draped the buttocks region with a diamond shaped drape.	10			
13. Instituted good safety standards for each position.	5			
14. Instructed patient not to tuck drape under or around body parts.	5			

Key Competencies		
ABHES	VI.A.1.a.4.b	Prepare Patients for Procedures
	VI.A.1.a.4.h	Prepare patient for and assist physician with routine and specialty examinations and treatments and minor office surgeries
CAAHEP	III.C.3.b.4.e	Prepare Patient for and Assist with Routine and Specialty Examinations

Student Name: _____   Date: _____   Score: _____

15. Completed the procedure within the appropriate time limit.	10			
Points Earned / Points Possible:	___ / 140			

Points possible reflect importance of step in meeting the task: Important = (5) Essential = (10).
Determine score by dividing points earned by total points possible, and multiplying results by 100.

EVALUATION
Evaluator Signature: _____   Date: _____

Evaluator Comments:

Key Competencies			
ABHES	VI.A.1.a.4.b	Prepare Patients for Procedures	
	VI.A.1.a.4.h	Prepare patient for and assist physician with routine and specialty examinations and treatments and minor office surgeries	
CAAHEP	III.C.3.b.4.e	Prepare Patient for and Assist with Routine and Specialty Examinations	

Student Name: _____   Date: _____   Score: _____

Competency Checklist
PROCEDURE 12-3 Assist with the General Physical Examination

Task: To assist with the general physical examination

Condition: Given the equipment and supplies as listed in the procedure, a classmate to play the part of the patient, and a classmate to play the part of the physician, the student will demonstrate the proper steps for assisting with a general physical exam.

Standards: The student will have 10 minutes to complete the procedure and will need to score an 85% or above to pass the competency. Automatic failure results if any essential steps are omitted or performed incorrectly.

STEPS START TIME: END TIME:	Points Possible	First Attempt	Second Attempt	Third Attempt
1. Washed hands, prepared exam room, assembled supplies and necessary equipment (gloved if necessary).	10			
2. Identified the patient using at least two identifiers and explained the procedure.	10			
3. Obtained patient's vital signs, height and weight, and recorded the information in the patient's progress note *(Work Product, Procedure 12-3)*.	10			
4. Allowed patient to use restroom and collected a sample if required by physician.	10			
5. Provided patient with gown and drape and gave proper disrobing instructions.	10			
6. Asked patient to turn off cell phone/pager.	5			
7. Left the room and allowed patient time to disrobe. Knocked on door before re-entering.	10			
8. Positioned patient in sitting position and alerted physician patient was ready for exam.	10			
9. Properly positioned patient throughout the exam and assisted physician with any needs during the exam.	10			
10. Assisted patient into sitting position for reorientation.	5			
11. Instructed patient to dress, and told patient that you would follow up with homecare instructions following the exam.	10			
12. Instructed patient on any directives given by the physician and properly documented instruction in patient's chart and flow sheet *(Work Product, Procedure 12-3)*.	10			
13. Accompanied patient to check out area, as needed.	5			
14. Completed the procedure within the appropriate time limit.	10			
Points Earned / Points Possible:	___ / 125			

Points possible reflect importance of step in meeting the task: Important = (5) Essential = (10).
Determine score by dividing points earned by total points possible, and multiplying results by 100.

EVALUATION
Evaluator Signature: _____   Date: _____

Evaluator's Comments:

Key Competencies		
ABHES	VI.A.1.a.4.b	Prepare patients for procedures
	VI.A.1.a.4.h	Prepare patient for and assist physician with routine and specialty examinations and treatments and minor office surgeries
CAAHEP	III.C.3.b.4.e	Prepare patient for and assist with routine and specialty exams

Student Name: _____   Date: _____   Score: _____

DOCUMENTATION

Instructor Note: Retain work products with competency checklist.

Work Product, Procedure 12-3 (Progress Note)

Progress Note for Patient: Date:	**DOUGLASVILLE MEDICINE ASSOCIATES** **5076 BRAND BLVD** **DOUGLASVILLE, NY 01234** **(123) 456-7890**

Work Product, Procedure 12-3 (Flow Sheet)

VITAL SIGN FLOW SHEET

Patient's Name: _____   Patient's Birth Date: _____

Patient's ID #: _____   Provider's Name: _____

Today's Date	Pain Rating	Temp	Pulse	Resp	BP	BP Med	Current Dose	Change in Dose	Provider's Initials

Key Competencies		
ABHES	VI.A.1.a.4.b	Prepare patients for procedures
	VI.A.1.a.4.h	Prepare patient for and assist physician with routine and specialty examinations and treatments and minor office surgeries
CAAHEP	III.C.3.b.4.e	Prepare patient for and assist with routine and specialty exams

Student Name: _____ Date: _____ Score: _____

Competency Checklist
PROCEDURE 13-1 Snellen Chart Visual Acuity Testing

Task: To perform a Snellen chart visual acuity test

Condition: Given the equipment and supplies as listed in the procedure and a classmate to play the part of the patient, the student will perform a visual acuity test, adhering to the steps listed below.

Standards: The student will have 10 minutes to complete the procedure and will need to score an 85% or above to pass the competency. Automatic failure results if any essential steps are omitted or performed incorrectly.

STEPS START TIME: END TIME:	Points Possible	First Attempt	Second Attempt	Third Attempt
1. Washed hands, assembled equipment, cleaned occluder with alcohol and allowed occluder to air dry.	10			
2. Identified the patient using two identifiers, identified self, and explained procedure. Inquired about corrective lenses.	10			
3. If patient wore glasses, instructed patient that acuity would be tested both with and without glasses. (If patient wore contacts, instructed patient that acuity would be tested only with correction.)	10			
4. Instructed patient to stand 20 feet away from the chart and to cover the left eye with the occluder, while keeping both eyes open, and to read the letters aloud as he or she pointed to each line.	10			
5. The student started by pointing to the 20/200 line or several lines above the 20/20 line. Proceeded to the last line the patient could read without errors.	10			
6. Repeated screening on the left eye and then with both eyes.	10			
7. Pointed to the red and green color stripes and had patient identify the colors.	10			
8. Observed patient for signs of difficulty while testing such as squinting, watery eyes, or repositioning of the head.	5			
9. If patient wore glasses, tested eyes both with and without glasses.	10			
10. Cleaned the occluder with alcohol after use.	10			
11. Washed hands and documented results in the patient's chart *(Work Product, Procedure 13-1).*	10			
12. Completed the procedure within the appropriate time limit.	10			
Points Earned / Points Possible:	___ / 115			

Points possible reflect importance of step in meeting the task: Important = (5) Essential = (10).
Determine score by dividing points earned by total points possible, and multiplying results by 100.

EVALUATION
Evaluator Signature: _____ Date: _____

Evaluator Comments:

Key Competencies		
ABHES	VI.A.1.a.4.h	Prepare Patient for and Assist Physician with Routine and Specialty Examinations and Treatments and Minor Office Surgeries
CAAHEP	III.C.3.b.4.e	Prepare Patient for and Assist with Routine and Specialty Examinations

Student Name: _____   Date: _____   Score: _____

DOCUMENTATION

Instructor Note: Retain work products with competency checklist.

Work Product, Procedure 13-1 (Progress Note)

Progress Note for Patient: Date:	**DOUGLASVILLE MEDICINE ASSOCIATES** **5076 BRAND BLVD** **DOUGLASVILLE, NY 01234** **(123) 456-7890**

Key Competencies		
ABHES	VI.A.1.a.4.h	Prepare Patient for and Assist Physician with Routine and Specialty Examinations and Treatments and Minor Office Surgeries
CAAHEP	III.C.3.b.4.e	Prepare Patient for and Assist with Routine and Specialty Examinations

Student Name: _____   Date: _____   Score: _____

Competency Checklist
PROCEDURE 13-2   Screen Near Visual Acuity

Task: To screen near visual acuity

Condition: Given the equipment and supplies as listed in the procedure and a classmate to play the part of the patient, the student will perform a near visual acuity test, adhering to the steps listed below.

Standards: The student will have 10 minutes to complete the procedure and will need to score an 85% or above to pass the competency. Automatic failure results if any essential steps are omitted or performed incorrectly.

STEPS START TIME: END TIME:	Points Possible	First Attempt	Second Attempt	Third Attempt
1. Washed hands and assembled equipment.	10			
2. Cleaned occluder with alcohol and allowed the occluder to air dry.	10			
3. Identified the patient using two identifiers, identified self, and explained the procedure; inquired about corrective lenses.	10			
4. If patient wore glasses, instructed patient that acuity would be tested both with and without glasses. (If patient wore contacts, instructed patient that acuity would be tested only with correction.)	10			
5. Held acuity card or instructed patient to hold acuity card approximately 14 inches from the eyes.	10			
6. Had patient gently cover the left eye with the occluder and read each line on the card. Recorded the last line the patient could read without errors.	10			
7. Repeated procedure for the left eye (while covering the right eye) and tested both eyes without an occluder. Repeated the test with corrective lenses if applicable.	10			
8. Observed patient for squinting, watering eyes, or leaning head backward or forward.	5			
9. Cleaned occluder with alcohol wipe after use.	10			
10. Washed hands and accurately documented results in patient's chart *(Work Product, Procedure 13-2)*.	10			
11. Completed the procedure within the appropriate time limit.	10			
Points Earned / Points Possible:	___ / 105			

Points possible reflect importance of step in meeting the task: Important = (5) Essential = (10).
Determine score by dividing points earned by total points possible, and multiplying results by 100.

EVALUATION
Evaluator Signature: _____   Date: _____

Evaluator Comments:

Key Competencies		
ABHES	VI.B.1.a.4.h	Prepare Patient for and Assist Physician with Routine and Specialty Examinations and Treatments and Minor Office Surgeries
CAAHEP	III.C.3.b.4.e	Prepare Patient for and Assist with Routine and Specialty Examinations

Student Name: _____   Date: _____   Score: _____

DOCUMENTATION

Instructor Note: Retain work products with competency checklist.
Work Product, Procedure 13-2 (Progress Note)

Progress Note for Patient: Date:	**DOUGLASVILLE MEDICINE ASSOCIATES** **5076 BRAND BLVD** **DOUGLASVILLE, NY 01234** **(123) 456-7890**

Key Competencies		
ABHES	VI.B.1.a.4.h	Prepare Patient for and Assist Physician with Routine and Specialty Examinations and Treatments and Minor Office Surgeries
CAAHEP	III.C.3.b.4.e	Prepare Patient for and Assist with Routine and Specialty Examinations

Student Name: _____   Date: _____   Score: _____

Competency Checklist
PROCEDURE 13-3 Ishihara Test for Color Vision

Task: To perform a color vision screening with the Ishihara method

Condition: Given the equipment and supplies as listed in the procedure and a classmate to play the part of the patient, the student will perform an Ishihara color vision test, adhering to the steps listed below.

Standards: The student will have 10 minutes to complete the procedure and will need to score an 85% or above to pass the competency. Automatic failure results if any essential steps are omitted or performed incorrectly.

STEPS START TIME: END TIME:	Points Possible	First Attempt	Second Attempt	Third Attempt
1. Washed hands and assembled equipment.	10			
2. Identified the patient using at least two identifiers, identified self, and explained the procedure.	10			
3. Starting with the practice plate, held the plate 30 inches from the patient and at a right angle to the patient's field of vision. Instructed patient to identify the number formed by the colored dots. (Recorded results after each plate, *Work Product, Procedure 13-3.*)	10			
4. Repeated procedure with all plates, either by reading numbers aloud or tracing the winding line on the plate.	10			
5. Washed hands and correctly documented results in patient's chart (*Work Product, Procedure 13-3*).	10			
6. Stored plates or book in a dark place to protect from light.	10			
7. Completed the procedure within the appropriate time limit.	10			
Points Earned / Points Possible:	___ / 70			

Points possible reflect importance of step in meeting the task: Important = (5) Essential = (10).
Determine score by dividing points earned by total points possible, and multiplying results by 100.

EVALUATION
Evaluator Signature: _____   Date: _____

Evaluator Comments:

Key Competencies		
ABHES	VI.A.1.a.4.h	Prepare Patient for and Assist Physician with Routine and Specialty Examinations and Treatments and Minor Office Surgeries
CAAHEP	III.C.3.b.4.e	Prepare Patient for and Assist with Routine and Specialty Examinations

Student Name: _____   Date: _____   Score: _____

DOCUMENTATION

Instructor Note: Retain work products with competency checklist.

Work Product, Procedure 13-3 (Progress Note)

Progress Note for	**DOUGLASVILLE MEDICINE ASSOCIATES**
	5076 BRAND BLVD
Patient:	**DOUGLASVILLE, NY 01234**
Date:	**(123) 456-7890**

Work Product, Procedure 13-3 (Ishihara Recording Form)

Plate Number	Results
1	
2	
3	
4	
5	
6	
7	
8	
9	
10	
11	
Screener's Name	
Date of Test	
Time of Test	

Key Competencies		
ABHES	VI.A.1.a.4.h	Prepare Patient for and Assist Physician with Routine and Specialty Examinations and Treatments and Minor Office Surgeries
CAAHEP	III.C.3.b.4.e	Prepare Patient for and Assist with Routine and Specialty Examinations

Student Name: _____   Date: _____   Score: _____

Competency Checklist
PROCEDURE 13-4 Eye Instillation

Task: To perform an eye instillation

Condition: Given the equipment and supplies as listed in the procedure and a classmate to play the part of the patient, the student will perform an eye instillation using sterile saline or sterile water, or will simulate performing the procedure, adhering to the steps listed below.

Standards: The student will have 10 minutes to complete the procedure and will need to score an 85% or above to pass the competency. Automatic failure results if any essential steps are omitted or performed incorrectly.

STEPS START TIME: END TIME:	Points Possible	First Attempt	Second Attempt	Third Attempt
1. Washed hands, assembled equipment and gathered medication. If medication was refrigerated, allowed medication to come to room temperature before using.	10			
2. Checked medication against physician's orders and looked for word *ophthalmic* on label. (Checked label a total of three times to ensure the name on the label matched the physician's exact order.)	10			
3. Checked the expiration date to make certain medication was not past its expiration date.	10			
4. Identified the patient using two identifiers, identified self, and explained procedure.	10			
5. Washed hands again and applied gloves.	10			
6. Placed patient in a supine or sitting position.	10			
7. Prepared medication by inverting the medication bottle holding the drops a couple of times to mix the medication and drawing the medication into a sterile dropper. (For eye ointment, removed cap from tube without contaminating the tip or cap of the ointment.)	10			
8. Instructed patient to look up, placed gauze over cheekbone, and gently pulled down the skin under the eye with a tissue or gauze pad to expose the lower conjunctival sac.	10			
9. Instilled the correct number of drops into the center of the lower conjunctival sac or a thin line of ointment along lower surface of eyelid without touching dropper or tip of tube to the eye.	10			
10. Instructed patient to close the eye and roll eyeball around.	10			
11. Dabbed eyelid with gauze removing any excess medication that escaped from the eye.	5			
12. *For eyedrops:* discarded unused medication from the dropper and returned empty dropper to medicine bottle without contaminating the dropper. *For ointment:* wiped excess ointment from the tip of the tube with a piece of sterile gauze. Replaced cap without contaminating the ointment.	10			
13. Disposed of used equipment and supplies.	10			
14. Removed gloves, washed hands, and documented procedure in patient's chart and medication log *(Work Product, Procedure 13-4).*	10			
15. Completed the procedure within the appropriate time limit.	10			
Points Earned / Points Possible:	___ / 145			

Key Competencies		
ABHES	VI.A.1.a.4.m	Prepare and Administer Medications as Directed by the Physician
CAAHEP	III.C.3.b.4.g	Apply Pharmacology Principles to Prepare and Administer Oral and Parenteral (excluding IV) Medications

Student Name: _____   Date: _____   Score: _____

Points possible reflect importance of step in meeting the task: Important = (5) Essential = (10).
Determine score by dividing points earned by total points possible, and multiplying results by 100.

EVALUATION
Evaluator Signature: _____   Date: _____

Evaluator Comments:

DOCUMENTATION
Instructor Note: Retain work products with competency checklist.
Work Product, Procedure 13-4 (Progress Note)

Progress Note for Patient: Date:	**DOUGLASVILLE MEDICINE ASSOCIATES** **5076 BRAND BLVD** **DOUGLASVILLE, NY 01234** **(123) 456-7890**

Work Product, Procedure 13-4 (Patient Medication Log)

PATIENT MEDICATION LOG

Patient's Name: _____   **DOB:** _____

Date	Time	Medication Name	Amt Ordered	Ordering Physician	Amt Given	Location	Route	Name of Doctor	Person that Administered Medication

Key Competencies		
ABHES	VI.A.1.a.4.m	Prepare and Administer Medications as Directed by the Physician
CAAHEP	III.C.3.b.4.g	Apply Pharmacology Principles to Prepare and Administer Oral and Parenteral (excluding IV) Medications

Student Name: _____   Date: _____   Score: _____

Competency Checklist
PROCEDURE 13-5 Eye Irrigation

Task: To perform an eye irrigation using a waterpick

Condition: Given the equipment and supplies as listed in the procedure and a classmate to play the part of the patient, the student will simulate performing an eye irrigation, adhering to the steps listed below.

Standards: The student will have 15 minutes to complete the procedure and score an 85% or above to pass the competency. Automatic failure results if any essential steps are omitted or performed incorrectly.

STEPS START TIME: END TIME:	Points Possible	First Attempt	Second Attempt	Third Attempt
1. Washed hands and assembled equipment.	10			
2. Identified the patient using at least two identifiers, identified self, and explained the procedure.	10			
3. Placed patient in a supine position with head turned towards the affected eye. Placed towel on patient's shoulder and placed basin beside affected eye. Asked patient to hold basin.	10			
4. Checked expiration date of solution and checked label 3 times before use.	10			
5. Warmed solution to body temperature by placing IV bag in warm water if using IV solution, or warming solution in irrigating tank by following the directions on the unit if using a professional irrigation system. (Used bath thermometer to check temperature of solution.)	10			
6. Washed hands again and gloved.	10			
7. Cleansed eyelid from inner to outer canthus with moistened gauze. Discarded gauze after use.	10			
8. While resting the bulb of the waterpick on the bridge of the patient's nose, and holding the eye open with finger and thumb of the opposite hand, opened nozzle of waterpick and allowed to flow at a steady stream, irrigating from the inner to outer canthus directing the solution towards the basin held by the patient. (Did not touch eye or conjunctiva with tip of the waterpick.)	10			
9. Instructed patient to stare at a fixed spot throughout the procedure.	10			
10. Dried eyelid and eyelashes from inner to outer canthus with gauze pads.	10			
11. Checked return basin for any debris.	10			
12. Discarded supplies, removed gloves, and washed hands.	10			
13. Documented procedure in patient's chart *(Work Product, Procedure 13-5).*	10			
14. Completed the procedure within the appropriate time limit.	10			
Points Earned / Points Possible:	___ / 140			

Points possible reflect importance of step in meeting the task: Important = (5) Essential = (10).
Determine score by dividing points earned by total points possible, and multiplying results by 100.

Key Competencies		
ABHES	VI.A.1.a.4.b	Prepare Patients for Procedures
	VI.A.1.a.4.h	Prepare Patient for and Assist Physician with Routine and Specialty Examinations and Treatments and Minor Office Surgeries
CAAHEP	III.C.3.b.4.e	Prepare Patient for and Assist with Routine and Specialty Examinations
	III.C.3.b.4.f	Prepare Patient for and Assist with Procedures, Treatments, and Minor Office Surgeries

Student Name: _____   Date: _____   Score: _____

EVALUATION

Evaluator Signature: _____   Date: _____

Evaluator Comments:

DOCUMENTATION

Instructor Note: Retain work products with competency checklist.
Work Product, Procedure 13-5 (Progress Note)

Progress Note for Patient: Date:	**DOUGLASVILLE MEDICINE ASSOCIATES** **5076 BRAND BLVD** **DOUGLASVILLE, NY 01234** **(123) 456-7890**

Key Competencies		
ABHES	VI.A.1.a.4.b	Prepare Patients for Procedures
	VI.A.1.a.4.h	Prepare Patient for and Assist Physician with Routine and Specialty Examinations and Treatments and Minor Office Surgeries
CAAHEP	III.C.3.b.4.e	Prepare Patient for and Assist with Routine and Specialty Examinations
	III.C.3.b.4.f	Prepare Patient for and Assist with Procedures, Treatments, and Minor Office Surgeries

Student Name: _____   Date: _____   Score: _____

Competency Checklist
PROCEDURE 13-6 Ear Instillation

Task: To perform an ear instillation

Condition: Given the equipment and supplies as listed in the procedure and a classmate to play the part of the patient, the student will simulate performing an ear instillation, adhering to the steps listed below.

Standards: The student will have 5 minutes to complete the procedure and will need to score an 85% or above to pass the competency. Automatic failure results if any essential steps are omitted or performed incorrectly.

STEPS START TIME: END TIME:	Points Possible	First Attempt	Second Attempt	Third Attempt
1. Washed hands and assembled equipment.	10			
2. Identified the patient using at least two identifiers, identified self, and explained the procedure.	10			
3. Checked medication against physician's orders and verified that medication was for *otic* use. Checked expiration date and checked label 3 times before administering.	10			
4. Instructed patient to lie on unaffected side or sit with head tilted toward unaffected side. Placed towel on patient's shoulder.	10			
5. Washed hands, applied gloves, inverted medication bottle a couple of times to mix the medication, and withdrew medication from bottle using the sterile dropper, without contaminating dropper or medication.	10			
6. Grasped auricle of ear by pulling up and back on an adult or pulling down and back on a child under the age of 3. Instilled prescribed amount of medication into ear canal. Did not touch tip of dropper to ear.	10			
7. Instructed patient to remain in position for approximately 5 minutes.	10			
8. Inserted a slightly moistened cotton ball into ear canal, per physician's orders, and instructed patient to leave in place for 15 minutes.	10			
9. Disposed of used equipment and supplies.	10			
10. Removed gloves, washed hands, and documented procedure in patient's chart and medication log *(Work Product, Procedure 13-6)*.	10			
11. Completed the procedure within the appropriate time limit.	10			
Points Earned / Points Possible:	___ / 110			

Points possible reflect importance of step in meeting the task: Important = (5) Essential = (10).
Determine score by dividing points earned by total points possible, and multiplying results by 100.

EVALUATION
Evaluator Signature: _____   Date: _____

Evaluator Comments:

Key Competencies		
ABHES	VI.A.1.a.4.m	Prepare and Administer Oral and Parenteral Medications as Directed by Physician
CAAHEP	III.C.3.b.4.g	Apply Pharmacology Principles to Prepare and Administer Oral and Parenteral (excluding IV) Medications

Student Name: _____   Date: _____   Score: _____

DOCUMENTATION

Instructor Note: Retain work products with competency checklist.
Work Product, Procedure 13-6 (Progress Note)

Progress Note for Patient: Date:	**DOUGLASVILLE MEDICINE ASSOCIATES** **5076 BRAND BLVD** **DOUGLASVILLE, NY 01234** **(123) 456-7890**

Work Product, Procedure 13-6 (Patient Medication Log)

PATIENT MEDICATION LOG

Patient's Name: _____   **DOB:** _____

Date	Time	Medication Name	Amt Ordered	Ordering Physician	Amt Given	Location	Route	Name of Doctor	Person that Administered Medication

Key Competencies		
ABHES	VI.A.1.a.4.m	Prepare and Administer Oral and Parenteral Medications as Directed by Physician
CAAHEP	III.C.3.b.4.g	Apply Pharmacology Principles to Prepare and Administer Oral and Parenteral (excluding IV) Medications

Student Name: _____   Date: _____   Score: _____

Competency Checklist
PROCEDURE 13-7 Ear Irrigation

Task: To perform an ear irrigation

Condition: Given the equipment and supplies as listed in the procedure and a classmate to play the part of the patient, the student will simulate performing an ear irrigation, adhering to the steps listed below.

Standards: The student will have 15 minutes to complete the procedure and will need to score an 85% or above to pass the competency. Automatic failure results if any essential steps are omitted or performed incorrectly.

STEPS START TIME: END TIME:	Points Possible	First Attempt	Second Attempt	Third Attempt
1. Washed hands and assembled equipment.	10			
2. Identified the patient using at least two identifiers, identified self, and explained the procedure. (Informed patient there may be minimal discomfort and some dizziness due to flow of fluid against tympanic membrane.)	10			
3. Checked expiration date of irrigating solution and checked label 3 times before use. Warmed solution to body temperature following institutional guidelines.	10			
4. Placed patient in sitting position with head tilted to affected side, placed towel on patient's shoulder, and instructed patient to hold ear basin under affected ear and against neck.	10			
5. Filled ear wash sprayer bottle with the ordered amount of warmed irrigating solution and applied gloves.	10			
6. Gently pulled auricle of ear up and back on an adult or down and back on a child under the age of 3.	10			
7. Inserted the disposable tip in the ear canal, directing the solution toward the roof of the canal. Started spraying the solution at a slow, steady pace. Continued process until desired effects were achieved or solution was gone.	10			
8. Dried outer ear and checked ear with otoscope to determine if all cerumen or debris were successfully removed.	10			
9. Disposed of used equipment and supplies, removed gloves, and washed hands.	10			
10. Cleaned irrigator tubing and irrigation bottle according to institutional guidelines.	10			
11. Documented procedure in patient's chart (*Work Product, Procedure 13-7*).	10			
12. Completed the procedure within the appropriate time limit.	10			
Points Earned / Points Possible:	___ / 120			

Points possible reflect importance of step in meeting the task: Important = (5) Essential = (10).
Determine score by dividing points earned by total points possible, and multiplying results by 100.

Key Competencies		
ABHES	VI.A.1.a.4.b	Prepare Patients for Procedures
	VI.A.1.a.4.h	Prepare Patient for and Assist Physician with Routine and Specialty Examinations and Treatments and Minor Office Surgeries
CAAHEP	III.C.3.b.4.e	Prepare Patient for and Assist with Routine and Specialty Examinations
	III.C.3.b.4.f	Prepare Patient for and Assist with Procedures, Treatments, and Minor Office Surgeries

Student Name: _____   Date: _____   Score: _____

EVALUATION
Evaluator Signature: _____   Date: _____

Evaluator Comments:

DOCUMENTATION
Instructor Note: Retain work products with competency checklist.
Work Product, Procedure 13-7 (Progress Note)

Progress Note for Patient: Date:	**DOUGLASVILLE MEDICINE ASSOCIATES** **5076 BRAND BLVD** **DOUGLASVILLE, NY 01234** **(123) 456-7890**

Key Competencies		
ABHES	VI.A.1.a.4.b	Prepare Patients for Procedures
	VI.A.1.a.4.h	Prepare Patient for and Assist Physician with Routine and Specialty Examinations and Treatments and Minor Office Surgeries
CAAHEP	III.C.3.b.4.e	Prepare Patient for and Assist with Routine and Specialty Examinations
	III.C.3.b.4.f	Prepare Patient for and Assist with Procedures, Treatments, and Minor Office Surgeries

Student Name: _____ Date: _____ Score: _____

Competency Checklist
PROCEDURE 14-1 Perform a Fecal Occult Blood Test

Task: To perform a fecal occult blood test

Condition: Given the equipment and supplies as listed in the procedure and a classmate to play the part of the patient, the student will perform a fecal occult blood test, adhering to the steps listed below.

Standards: The student will have 10 minutes to complete the procedure and will need to score an 85% or above to pass the competency. Automatic failure results if any essential steps are omitted or performed incorrectly.

STEPS START TIME: END TIME:	Points Possible	First Attempt	Second Attempt	Third Attempt
Patient Instructions				
1. Washed hands and assembled supplies for testing (testing packet with cards, spatulas, directions, and collecting basin or hat).	10			
2. Identified the patient using at least two identifiers, identified self, and explained the purpose of the procedure and special dietary instructions.	10			
3. Explained the proper procedure for labeling the cards.	10			
4. Explained collection instructions, including number of collections and instructions for sending cards back to the office. Gave patient collection supplies.	10			
Testing Instructions				
5. Washed hands and applied gloves prior to testing.	10			
6. Followed developing instructions and performed a control on each test card (a blue color indicates a positive result).	10			
7. Properly disposed of test cards, cleaned work area, removed gloves, and washed hands.	10			
8. Documented procedure in patient's chart and in the lab log *(Work Product, Procedure 14-1)*.	10			
9. Completed the procedure within the appropriate time limit.	10			
Points Earned / Points Possible:	___ / 90			

Points possible reflect importance of step in meeting the task: Important = (5) Essential = (10).
Determine score by dividing points earned by total points possible, and multiplying results by 100.

EVALUATION
Evaluator Signature: _____ Date: _____

Evaluator Comments:

Key Competencies		
ABHES	VI.A.1.a.4.i	Use Quality Control
	VI.A.1.a.4.x	Instruct patient in the collection of a fecal specimen
CAAHEP	III.C.3.b.2.e	Instruct patients in the collection of fecal specimens
	III.C.3.c.4.d	Use methods of quality control

Student Name: _____   Date: _____   Score: _____

DOCUMENTATION

Instructor Note: Retain work products with competency checklist.

Work Product, Procedure 14-1 (Progress Note)

Progress Note for Patient: Date:	**DOUGLASVILLE MEDICINE ASSOCIATES** **5076 BRAND BLVD** **DOUGLASVILLE, NY 01234** **(123) 456-7890**

Work Product, Procedure 14-1 (In-House Testing Log)

IN-HOUSE TESTING LOG

Date of Testing	Date of Patient Collection	Time	Patient Name/ID	Test Name	Ordering Provider	Manufacturer	Exp Date	Lot #	Results	Initials

Key Competencies		
ABHES	VI.A.1.a.4.i	Use Quality Control
	VI.A.1.a.4.x	Instruct patient in the collection of a fecal specimen
CAAHEP	III.C.3.b.2.e	Instruct patients in the collection of fecal specimens
	III.C.3.c.4.d	Use methods of quality control

Student Name: _____   Date: _____   Score: _____

Competency Checklist
PROCEDURE 14-2 Instruct the Patient on How to Collect a Fecal Specimen

Task: To instruct the patient on how to collect a fecal specimen

Condition: Given the equipment and supplies as listed in the procedure and a classmate to play the part of the patient, the student will instruct the patient on the proper method for collecting a fecal specimen, adhering to the steps listed below.

Standards: The student will have 10 minutes to complete the procedure and will need to score an 85% or above to pass the competency. Automatic failure results if any essential steps are omitted or performed incorrectly.

STEPS START TIME: END TIME:	Points Possible	First Attempt	Second Attempt	Third Attempt
1. Washed hands and assembled all equipment.	10			
2. Identified the patient using two identifiers and identified self.	10			
3. Completed lab requisition and labeled specimen container with all pertinent patient information except time and date of specimen.	10			
4. Gave patient appropriate collection container, specimen container, spatulas, and gloves and instructed patient on how to collect the specimen and finish labeling the container. (Cautioned patient not to contaminate the specimen with urine, toilet tissue, or other foreign material.)	10			
5. Instructed patient to place lid tightly on container and return specimen to the office as soon as possible. (Told patient to place specimen in refrigerator if the specimen cannot be delivered immediately following defecation.)	10			
6. Encouraged patient to ask questions and gave written instructions.	10			
7. Correctly documented education in patient's chart *(Work Product, Procedure 14-2)*.	10			
8. Completed the education session within the appropriate time limit.	10			
Points Earned / Points Possible:	___ / 80			

Points possible reflect importance of step in meeting the task: Important = (5) Essential = (10).
Determine score by dividing points earned by total points possible, and multiplying results by 100.

EVALUATION
Evaluator Signature: _____   Date: _____

Evaluator Comments:

Key Competencies		
ABHES	VI.A.1.a.4.x	Instruct Patient in the Collection of Fecal Specimen
CAAHEP	III.C.3.b.2.e	Instruct Patients in the Collection of Fecal Specimens

Student Name: _____   Date: _____   Score: _____

DOCUMENTATION

Instructor Note: Retain work products with competency checklist.
Work Product, Procedure 14-2 (Progress Note)

Progress Note for Patient: Date:	DOUGLASVILLE MEDICINE ASSOCIATES 5076 BRAND BLVD DOUGLASVILLE, NY 01234 (123) 456-7890

Key Competencies		
ABHES	VI.A.1.a.4.x	Instruct Patient in the Collection of Fecal Specimen
CAAHEP	III.C.3.b.2.e	Instruct Patients in the Collection of Fecal Specimens

Student Name: _____   Date: _____   Score: _____

Competency Checklist
PROCEDURE 14-3 Assist with a Flexible Sigmoidoscopy

Task: To assist with a flexible sigmoidoscopy

Condition: Given the equipment and supplies as listed in the procedure and classmates to play the part of the patient and provider, the student will simulate assisting the provider with a sigmoidoscopy, adhering to the steps listed below.

Standards: The student will have 15 minutes to complete the procedure and will need to score an 85% or above to pass the competency. Automatic failure results if any essential steps are omitted or performed incorrectly.

STEPS START TIME: END TIME:	Points Possible	First Attempt	Second Attempt	Third Attempt
1. Washed hands, assembled equipment, and applied gloves.	10			
2. Identified the patient using at least two identifiers, identified self, and explained the procedure.	10			
3. Labeled sterile specimen container and instructed patient to empty bladder.	10			
4. Supplied patient with gown and drape and instructed patient to disrobe from the waist down and to put the gown on so that the opening was in the back.	10			
5. Assisted the patient into the Sims' position and placed a diamond drape over the buttocks region.	10			
6. Provided the physician with disposable gloves, placed lubricant on the first digit of the glove for the rectal exam, and lubricated the end of the sigmoidoscope.	10			
7. Assisted physician with suctioning and any other needs.	10			
8. Provided physician with biopsy forceps, if needed, and placed specimen in sterile container.	10			
9. Following completion of procedure, assisted patient into sitting position, assessed patient for good orientation, and provided patient with tissues to clean anal region.	5			
10. Prepared specimen for transport to laboratory and completed lab requisition.	10			
11. Cleaned equipment and exam room and disposed of contaminated materials properly.	10			
12. Removed gloves, washed hands, and correctly documented procedure in patient's chart *(Work Product, Procedure 14-3)*.	10			
13. Completed the procedure within the appropriate time limit.	10			
Points Earned / Points Possible:	___ / 125			

Points possible reflect importance of step in meeting the task: Important = (5) Essential = (10).
Determine score by dividing points earned by total points possible, and multiplying results by 100.

EVALUATION
Evaluator Signature: _____   Date: _____

Evaluator Comments:

Key Competencies		
ABHES	VI.A.1.a.4.h	Prepare Patients for and Assist Physician with Routine and Specialty Examinations and Treatments and Minor Office Surgeries
CAAHEP	III.C.3.b.4.e	Prepare Patient for and Assist with Routine and Specialty Examinations

Student Name: _____   Date: _____   Score: _____

DOCUMENTATION
Instructor Note: Retain work products with competency checklist.
Work Product, Procedure 14-3 (Progress Note)

Progress Note for Patient: Date:	**DOUGLASVILLE MEDICINE ASSOCIATES** **5076 BRAND BLVD** **DOUGLASVILLE, NY 01234** **(123) 456-7890**

Work Product, Procedure 14-3 (Outstanding Lab Results Tracking Report)

OUTSTANDING LAB RESULTS TRACKING REPORT

Date Sent	Patient Name/ID	Ordering Provider	Tests Ordered	Number of and Type of Specimens Sent to	Prepared By	Laboratory	Date Results Received	Results Received By

Key Competencies		
ABHES	VI.A.1.a.4.h	Prepare Patients for and Assist Physician with Routine and Specialty Examinations and Treatments and Minor Office Surgeries
CAAHEP	III.C.3.b.4.e	Prepare Patient for and Assist with Routine and Specialty Examinations

Student Name: _____   Date: _____   Score: _____

Competency Checklist
PROCEDURE 15-1   Perform a Standard 12-Lead Electrocardiogram with a Multichannel Unit

Task: To perform a standard 12-lead electrocardiogram

Condition: Given the equipment and supplies as listed in the procedure and a classmate to play the part of the patient, the student will perform a 12-lead EKG, adhering to the steps listed below.

Standards: The student will have 15 minutes to complete the procedure and will need to score an 85% or above to pass the competency. Automatic failure results if any essential steps are omitted or performed incorrectly.

STEPS START TIME: END TIME:	Points Possible	First Attempt	Second Attempt	Third Attempt
1. Washed hands and assembled equipment.	10			
2. Identified the patient using at least two identifiers, identified self, and explained the procedure. Instructed patient on what to expect throughout the procedure and to remain still during recording.	10			
3. Instructed patient to remove all clothing from the waist up and to expose lower legs. Provided patient with a gown, instructions for wearing the gown, and a drape for modesty and warmth.	10			
4. Prepped skin by scrubbing areas where electrodes are to be placed with alcohol pads or gauze pads.	10			
5. Placed electrodes on fleshy part of upper arms and the inner portion of the calf between the knee and ankle.	10			
6. Placed chest electrodes in correct positions by locating proper landmarks.	10			
7. Securely connected all lead wires to electrodes. (Cable wires were neatly placed over patient's abdomen and did not contain tangles.)	10			
8. Connected patient cable to machine, turned machine on, and correctly entered patient data.	10			
9. Pressed auto button (or equivalent) and recorded tracing.	10			
10. Observed tracing for artifacts and, if found, took steps to correct.	10			
11. Allowed provider to scan tracing before disconnecting the patient.	5			
12. Disconnected lead wires and removed electrodes from patient.	10			
13. Cleaned equipment and replaced tracing paper, as needed.	5			
14. Washed hands and documented procedure in patient's chart *(Work Product, Procedure 15-1)*.	10			
15. Placed tracing in patient's chart *(Work Product, Procedure 15-1)*.	10			
16. Completed the procedure within the appropriate time limit.	10			
Points Earned / Points Possible:	___ / 150			

Points possible reflect importance of step in meeting the task: Important = (5) Essential = (10).
Determine score by dividing points earned by total points possible, and multiplying results by 100.

Key Competencies		
ABHES	VI.A.1.a.4.dd	Perform Electrocardiograms
CAAHEP	III.C.3.b.3.a	Perform Electrocardiography

Student Name: _____   Date: _____   Score: _____

EVALUATION

Evaluator Signature: _____   Date: _____

Evaluator Comments:

DOCUMENTATION

Instructor Note: Retain work products, along with completed EKG tracing, with competency checklist.

Work Product, Procedure 15-1 (Progress Note)

Progress Note for Patient: Date:	**DOUGLASVILLE MEDICINE ASSOCIATES** **5076 BRAND BLVD** **DOUGLASVILLE, NY 01234** **(123) 456-7890**

Key Competencies		
ABHES	VI.A.1.a.4.dd	Perform Electrocardiograms
CAAHEP	III.C.3.b.3.a	Perform Electrocardiography

Student Name: _____   Date: _____   Score: _____

Competency Checklist
PROCEDURE 15-2 Apply the Holter Monitor

Task: To apply a Holter monitor

Condition: Given the equipment and supplies as listed in the procedure and a classmate to play the part of the patient, the student will apply a Holter monitor, adhering to the steps listed below.

Standards: The student will have 15 minutes to complete the procedure and will need to score an 85% or above to pass the competency. Automatic failure results if any essential steps are omitted or performed incorrectly.

STEPS START TIME: END TIME:	Points Possible	First Attempt	Second Attempt	Third Attempt
1. Washed hands and assembled equipment. (Inserted new recording device and battery in the unit.)	10			
2. Identified the patient using at least two identifiers, identified self, explained the procedure, and accurately completed information in the patient activity diary.	10			
3. Instructed patient to disrobe from the waist up and prepped patient's skin for placement of electrodes. (Dry shaved areas that were particularly hairy.)	10			
4. Attached disposable electrodes to patient's chest following manufacturer's directions and connected lead wires to electrodes— reinforcing each electrode and wire with non-allergenic tape. (Electrodes were firmly attached to skin.)	10			
5. Connected patient cable to monitor and checked recorder by running a baseline strip.	10			
6. Instructed patient to dress and placed unit in holder and draped unit around patient with shoulder or waist strap.	10			
7. Noted start time in diary and explained the importance of an accurate and complete activity diary.	10			
8. Specified exact time patient should return for removal of monitor.	10			
9. Washed hands and correctly documented procedure in patient's chart *(Work Product, Procedure 15-2).*	10			
10. Completed the procedure within the appropriate time limit.	10			
Points Earned / Points Possible:	___ / 100			

Points possible reflect importance of step in meeting the task: Important = (5) Essential = (10).
Determine score by dividing points earned by total points possible, and multiplying results by 100.

EVALUATION
Evaluator Signature: _____   Date: _____

Evaluator Comments:

Key Competencies		
ABHES	VI.A.1.a.4.k	Perform Selected Tests That Assist with Diagnosis and Treatment
	VI.A.1.a.4.b	Prepare patients for procedures
CAAHEP	III.C.3.b.4.f	Prepare Patient for and Assist with Procedures, Treatments, and Minor Office Surgeries

Student Name: _____   Date: _____   Score: _____

DOCUMENTATION
Instructor Note: Retain work products with competency checklist.
Work Product, Procedure 15-2 (Progress Note)

Progress Note for Patient: Date:	**DOUGLASVILLE MEDICINE ASSOCIATES** **5076 BRAND BLVD** **DOUGLASVILLE, NY 01234** **(123) 456-7890**

Key Competencies		
ABHES	VI.A.1.a.4.k	Perform Selected Tests That Assist with Diagnosis and Treatment
	VI.A.1.a.4.b	Prepare patients for procedures
CAAHEP	III.C.3.b.4.f	Prepare Patient for and Assist with Procedures, Treatments, and Minor Office Surgeries

Student Name: _____   Date: _____   Score: _____

Competency Checklist
PROCEDURE 16-1 Perform a Spirometry Test

Task: To perform a spirometry test

Condition: Given the equipment and supplies as listed in the procedure and a classmate to play the part of the patient, the student will perform a spirometry test, adhering to the steps listed below.

Standards: The student will have 15 minutes to complete the procedure and will need to score an 85% or above to pass the competency. Automatic failure results if any essential steps are omitted or performed incorrectly.

STEPS START TIME: END TIME:	Points Possible	First Attempt	Second Attempt	Third Attempt
1. Washed hands.	10			
2. Assembled equipment and supplies; calibrated spirometer before beginning.	10			
3. Identified the patient using at least two identifiers, identified self, and thoroughly explained and demonstrated the procedure.	10			
4. Measured patient's height and weight.	5			
5. Had patient remove restrictive clothing and placed patient in comfortable and safe environment (seated position).	10			
6. Programmed related information into the unit; inserted new mouthpiece onto hose and applied nose clip to patient's nose.	10			
7. Checked position of mouthpiece and instructed patient to take in a large deep breath; activated spirometry unit. (Coached the patient to exhale as hard and long as possible—completely emptying the lungs.)	10			
8. Reviewed the results (provided patient with ways to improve) and had patient repeat test two more times.	10			
9. Removed the nose clip from patient's nose and took mouthpiece from patient. (Properly disposed of mouthpiece.)	5			
10. Provided necessary breathing treatment and repeated procedure (if ordered).	10			
11. After dismissing patient, properly disposed of used supplies and sanitized mouthpiece tubing and area.	10			
12. Correctly documented procedure on progress note and attached results to the patient's chart.	10			
13. Completed the procedure within the appropriate time limit.	10			
Points Earned / Points Possible:	__ / 120			

Points possible reflect importance of step in meeting the task: Important = (5) Essential = (10).
Determine score by dividing points earned by total points possible, and multiplying results by 100.

EVALUATION
Evaluator Signature: _____   Date: _____

Evaluator Comments:

Key Competencies		
ABHES	VI.A.1.a.4.ee	Perform respiratory testing
CAAHEP	III.C.3.b.3.b	Perform respiratory testing

Student Name: _____   Date: _____   Score: _____

DOCUMENTATION
Instructor Note: Retain work product, along with completed PFT results, with competency checklist.
Work Product, Procedure 16-1

Progress Note for	**DOUGLASVILLE MEDICINE ASSOCIATES** **5076 BRAND BLVD** **DOUGLASVILLE, NY 01234** **(123) 456-7890**
Patient: Date:	

Key Competencies		
ABHES	VI.A.1.a.4.ee	Perform respiratory testing
CAAHEP	III.C.3.b.3.b	Perform respiratory testing

Student Name: _____   Date: _____   Score: _____

Competency Checklist
PROCEDURE 16-2 Perform Pulse Oximetry

Task: To perform pulse oximetry

Condition: Given the equipment and supplies as listed in the procedure and a classmate to play the part of the patient, the student will perform pulse oximetry, adhering to the steps listed below.

Standards: The student will have 10 minutes to complete the procedure and will need to score an 85% or above to pass the competency. Automatic failure results if any essential steps are omitted or performed incorrectly.

STEPS START TIME: END TIME:	Points Possible	First Attempt	Second Attempt	Third Attempt
1. Washed hands.	10			
2. Assembled equipment and supplies.	10			
3. Identified the patient using at least two identifiers, identified self, and explained the procedure.	10			
4. Had patient remove nail polish (if applicable) and to wash and dry hands.	10			
5. Applied pulse oximeter probe to an acceptable site and observed the perfusion indicator (perfusion strength was acceptable—observed both the heart rate and SpO2 level).	10			
6. Kept pulse oximeter probe attached to the patient and gave findings to the physician (if below 95% notified physician ASAP).	10			
7. Continued to monitor the patient according to physician's instructions.	10			
8. Correctly removed the probe and assisted patient as necessary.	5			
9. Properly disinfected equipment and returned equipment to proper location.	10			
10. Correctly documented information in patient's chart.	10			
11. Completed the procedure within the appropriate time limit.	10			
Points Earned / Points Possible:	___ / 105			

Points possible reflect importance of step in meeting the task: Important = (5) Essential = (10).
Determine score by dividing points earned by total points possible, and multiplying results by 100.

EVALUATION
Evaluator Signature: _____   Date: _____

Evaluator Comments:

Key Competencies		
ABHES	VI.A.1.a.4.h	Prepare the patient for and assist physician with routine and specialty examinations and treatments and minor office surgeries
CAAHEP	III.C.3.b.4.f	Prepare patient for and assist with procedures, treatments, and minor office surgeries

Student Name: _____   Date: _____   Score: _____

DOCUMENTATION
Instructor Note: Retain work products with competency checklist.
Work Product, Procedure 16-2 (Progress Note)

Progress Note for Patient: Date:	**DOUGLASVILLE MEDICINE ASSOCIATES** **5076 BRAND BLVD** **DOUGLASVILLE, NY 01234** **(123) 456-7890**

Key Competencies		
ABHES	VI.A.1.a.4.h	Prepare the patient for and assist physician with routine and specialty examinations and treatments and minor office surgeries
CAAHEP	III.C.3.b.4.f	Prepare patient for and assist with procedures, treatments, and minor office surgeries

Student Name: _____   Date: _____   Score: _____

Competency Checklist
PROCEDURE 16-3 Obtain a Sputum Specimen and Prepare a Smear

Task: To obtain a sputum specimen and prepare a smear

Condition: Given the equipment and supplies as listed in the procedure and a classmate to play the part of the patient, the student will instruct a patient how to obtain a sputum specimen and will prepare a smear, adhering to the steps listed below.

Standards: The student will have 10 minutes to complete the procedure and will need to score an 85% or above to pass the competency. Automatic failure results if any essential steps are omitted or performed incorrectly.

STEPS START TIME: END TIME:	Points Possible	First Attempt	Second Attempt	Third Attempt
Obtaining a Sputum Specimen				
1. Washed hands and applied PPE.	10			
2. Assembled equipment and supplies and labeled specimen container.	10			
3. Identified the patient using at least two identifiers, identified self, and explained the procedure.	10			
4. Had patient rinse out mouth with water.	10			
5. Removed lid from specimen cup and placed on counter without contaminating the lid.	10			
6. Instructed patient to take in three deep breaths and to start forcefully coughing.	10			
7. Asked patient to expectorate sputum into the center of the specimen container.	10			
8. Placed lid on the container without contaminating it and tightened it securely.	10			
9. Placed specimen in plastic transport bag with completed lab requisition form. (Refrigerated sample if sending out.)	10			
Preparing the Slide/Smear				
1. Washed hands and applied PPE.	10			
2. Labeled slides and carefully opened lid to specimen. Dipped sterile cotton-tipped applicator into the sputum and placed sample onto the slide.	10			
3. Squeezed one drop of potassium hydroxide over the smear and placed cover slip over smear.	10			
4. Placed slide under the microscope on low power for the physician to read.	10			
5. Cleaned area and removed PPE.	10			
6. Correctly documented collection on progress note and completed lab requisition/reporting form. (Results will not be documented since the student didn't perform the test.)	10			
7. Student completed the procedure within the appropriate time limit.	10			
Points Earned / Points Possible:	___ / 160			

Points possible reflect importance of step in meeting the task: Important = (5) Essential = (10).
Determine score by dividing points earned by total points possible, and multiplying results by 100.

Key Competencies		
ABHES	VI.A.1.a.4.j	Collect and process specimens
	III.C.3.b.2.c	Obtain specimens for microbiological testing

Student Name: _____   Date: _____   Score: _____

EVALUATION

Evaluator Signature: _____   Date: _____

Evaluator Comments:

DOCUMENTATION

Instructor Note: Retain work products with competency checklist

Work Product, Procedure 16-3 (Progress Note)

Progress Note for Patient: Date:	**DOUGLASVILLE MEDICINE ASSOCIATES** **5076 BRAND BLVD** **DOUGLASVILLE, NY 01234** **(123) 456-7890**

MISCELLANEOUS IN-HOUSE **LABORATORY TEST REQUISITION AND REPORT FORM**			
PHYSICIAN INFORMATION		**PATIENT INFORMATION**	
DOUGLASVILLE MEDICINE ASSOCIATES **5076 BRAND BLVD** **DOUGLASVILLE, NY 01234** **(123)456-7890** **Ordering Physician:** **Physician ID #**		Name: Address: City/State/Zip: Phone #: DOB:	
Date and Time of Collection		**Date Results Received**	
Test Ordered	**Check Test that Applies**	**Results**	**Reference Range**
Pregnancy Test			
Rapid Strep Test			
Mono Test			
Influenza Test			
H. Pylori			
Sputum (KOH)			
Name of person who prepared the specimen			

Key Competencies		
ABHES	VI.A.1.a.4.j	Collect and process specimens
	III.C.3.b.2.c	Obtain specimens for microbiological testing

Student Name: _____   Date: _____   Score: _____

Competency Checklist
PROCEDURE 16-4   Administer a Nebulizer Treatment

Task: To properly administer a nebulizer treatment

Condition: Given the equipment and supplies as listed in the procedure and a classmate to play the part of the patient, the student will correctly simulate administering a nebulizer treatment, adhering to the steps listed below.

Standards: The student will have 15 minutes to complete the procedure and will need to score an 85% or above to pass the competency. Automatic failure results if any essential steps are omitted or performed incorrectly.

Dr's Order: 2.5 mg Albluterol via Inhalation Therapy

STEPS START TIME: END TIME:	Points Possible	First Attempt	Second Attempt	Third Attempt
1. Assembled nebulizer equipment and supplies.	10			
2. Identified the patient using at least two identifiers, identified self, and explained the procedure.	10			
3. Checked medication label with medication order a minimum of three times.	10			
4. Washed hands and applied gloves.	10			
5. Poured correct amount of medication and diluent into medication dispenser, screwed lid on dispenser and gently mixed the medication.	10			
6. Connected the dispenser to the mouthpiece or mask. Connected the disposable tubing to medication dispenser and nebulizer.	10			
7. Placed patient in full-Fowler's position; turned nebulizer on and made sure there was a mist.	10			
8. Instructed patient on proper placement of mouthpiece or mask (assisted patient if necessary).	10			
9. Instructed patient to take in slow deep breaths (2–3 seconds each); continued treatment until mist disappeared.	10			
10. Turned nebulizer off and properly disposed of supplies.	10			
11. Instructed patient to take in several deep breaths and to cough up secretions that were loosened during breathing treatment.	10			
12. Removed gloves and washed hands. Gave patient home care instructions.	10			
13. Correctly documented procedure on progress note and in medication log.	10			
14. Completed the procedure within the appropriate time limit.	10			
Points Earned / Points Possible:	___ / 140			

Points possible reflect importance of step in meeting the task: Important = (5) Essential = (10).
Determine score by dividing points earned by total points possible, and multiplying results by 100.

Key Competencies		
ABHES	VI.A.1.a.4.h	Prepare patient for and assist physician with routine and specialty examinations and treatments and minor office surgeries
CAAHEP	III.C.3.b.4.g	Apply pharmacology principles to prepare and administer oral and parenteral (excluding IV) medications

Student Name: _____   Date: _____   Score: _____

EVALUATION
Evaluator Signature: _____   Date: _____

Evaluator Comments:

DOCUMENTATION
Instructor Note: Retain work products with competency checklist.
Work Product, Procedure 16-4 (Progress Note)

Progress Note for Patient: Date:	**DOUGLASVILLE MEDICINE ASSOCIATES** **5076 BRAND BLVD** **DOUGLASVILLE, NY 01234** **(123) 456-7890**

PATIENT MEDICATION LOG

Patient's Name: DOB:

Date and Time	Medication Name	Amt Ordered	Ordering Physician	Amt Given	Location	Route	Name of Doctor	Person that Administered Medication or Treatment

Key Competencies		
ABHES	VI.A.1.a.4.h	Prepare patient for and assist physician with routine and specialty examinations and treatments and minor office surgeries
CAAHEP	III.C.3.b.4.g	Apply pharmacology principles to prepare and administer oral and parenteral (excluding IV) medications

Student Name: _____   Date: _____   Score: _____

Competency Checklist
PROCEDURE 17-1 Assist with a GYN Exam and Pap Test

Task: To assist the physician with a GYN exam and Pap test

Condition: Given the equipment and supplies as listed in the procedure, a classmate to play the part of the patient, and a classmate to play the part of the provider, the student will correctly simulate assisting the physician with a GYN exam and pap test, adhering to the steps listed below.

Standards: The student will have 15 minutes to complete the simulation and will need to score an 85% or above to pass the competency. Automatic failure results if any essential steps are omitted or performed incorrectly.

STEPS START TIME: END TIME:	Points Possible	First Attempt	Second Attempt	Third Attempt
1. Washed hands, assembled necessary equipment and supplies, and warmed speculum.	10			
2. Correctly labeled slides or ThinPrep solution container.	10			
3. Identified patient using two identifiers, identified self, and instructed patient to empty her bladder and collect a specimen, if office policy.	10			
4. Obtained patient's vital signs and weight and updated patient's medical history.	10			
5. Explained procedure to patient and gave disrobing instructions.	10			
6. When physician entered the room, assisted patient into a supine position and draped for the breast exam.	10			
7. Assisted patient into lithotomy position and draped for privacy.	10			
8. Handed warmed vaginal speculum to provider and adjusted light source.	10			
9. Washed hands, applied gloves, and gave physician collection tools in the correct order. *Direct method:* Correctly held slides as physician prepared smears—immediately sprayed with fixative. *ThinPrep® method:* Held open vial so physician could place broom in vial, agitated broom in solution until all of specimen was suspended in liquid. Disposed of collection tools in biohazarous trash.	10			
10. Squeezed lubricant on physician's gloved fingers for bi-manual and rectal exam.	10			
11. Following exam—assisted patient into sitting position, provided tissues for cleansing, and instructed patient to get dressed.	10			
12. Properly disposed of used equipment and soaked vaginal speculum. (Sanitized and sterilized when convenient.)	10			
13. Prepared specimen for transport to lab and completed lab requisition form.	10			
14. Removed gloves and washed hands.	10			

Key Competencies		
ABHES	VI.A.1.a.4.h	Prepare patient for and assist physician with routine and specialty examinations and treatments and minor office surgeries
	VI.A.1.a.4.j	Collect and process specimens
	VI.A.1.a.4.q	Dispose of biohazardous wastes
	VI.A.1.a.4.r	Practice standard precautions
CAAHEP	III.C.3.b.1.d	Dispose of biohazard materials
	III.C.3.b.1.e	Practice standard precautions
	III.C.3.b.2.c	Obtain specimens for microbiological testing
	III.C.3.b.4.e	Prepare patient for and assist with routine and specialty procedures

Student Name: _____   Date: _____   Score: _____

15. Documented in patient's chart and lab log.	10			
Points Earned / Points Possible:	___ / 150			

Points possible reflect importance of step in meeting the task: Important = (5) Essential = (10).
Determine score by dividing points earned by total points possible, and multiplying results by 100.

EVALUATION
Evaluator Signature: _____   Date: _____

Evaluator Comments:

DOCUMENTATION
Instructor Note: Retain work products with competency checklist.
Work Product, Procedure 17-1

Progress Note for	**DOUGLASVILLE MEDICINE ASSOCIATES**
	5076 BRAND BLVD
Patient:	**DOUGLASVILLE, NY 01234**
Date:	**(123) 456-7890**

Work Product, Procedure 17-1 (Outstanding Lab Results Tracking Report)

OUTSTANDING LAB RESULTS TRACKING REPORT

Date Sent	Patient Name/ID	Ordering Provider	Tests Ordered	Number of and Type of Specimens Sent to	Prepared By	Laboratory	Date Results Received	Results Received By

Key Competencies		
ABHES	VI.A.1.a.4.h	Prepare patient for and assist physician with routine and specialty examinations and treatments and minor office surgeries
	VI.A.1.a.4.j	Collect and process specimens
	VI.A.1.a.4.q	Dispose of biohazardous wastes
	VI.A.1.a.4.r	Practice standard precautions
CAAHEP	III.C.3.b.1.d	Dispose of biohazard materials
	III.C.3.b.1.e	Practice standard precautions
	III.C.3.b.2.c	Obtain specimens for microbiological testing
	III.C.3.b.4.e	Prepare patient for and assist with routine and specialty procedures

Student Name: _____   Date: _____   Score: _____

Competency Checklist
PROCEDURE 17-2 Instruct the Patient in Breast Self-Examination

Task: To instruct patient on how to perform a breast self-examination

Condition: Given the equipment and supplies as listed in the procedure and a classmate to play the part of the patient, the student will correctly instruct the patient on how to perform a breast self-examination (BSE), adhering to the steps listed below.

Standards: The student will have 15 minutes to complete the education session and will need to score an 85% or above to pass the competency. Automatic failure results if any essential steps are omitted or performed incorrectly.

STEPS START TIME: END TIME:	Points Possible	First Attempt	Second Attempt	Third Attempt
1. Identified the patient using at least two identifiers, identified self, and explained the purpose of BSE.	10			
2. Gave the patient brochure on BSE and explained the procedure.	10			
3. Instructed patient to examine breasts while in shower, in front of a mirror, and while lying down—at the same time each month (preferably a few days to a week following menses).	10			
4. Instructions were as follows: *While in shower*, cover your right breast with soapy lather and place right arm over your head—gliding your hand over your breast and under your arm pit. Repeat procedure for left breast. *While in front of a mirror*, look for puckering or dimpling of the skin, redness or changes in skin texture, nipple retraction, or any change in size or shape of both breasts. Exam should be repeated with hands raised over your head, and with hands on your hips, while pressing down. *While lying down*, place a small pillow under your right shoulder, and place your right arm over your head. Applying firm pressure, rotate your fingers in a circular motion around your entire breast using the pads of your first three fingers. Repeat procedure on left side.	10 10 10			
5. Instructed patient to gently squeeze each nipple and look for discharge.	10			
6. Instructed patient to repeat the steps for each procedure and to perform an exam on the breast model.	10			
7. Patient was instructed to report any changes immediately.	10			
8. Correctly documented education session in patient's chart.	10			
9. Completed the procedure within the appropriate time limit.	10			
Points Earned / Points Possible:	___ / 110			

Points possible reflect importance of step in meeting the task: Important = (5) Essential = (10).
Determine score by dividing points earned by total points possible, and multiplying results by 100.

Key Competencies		
ABHES	VI.A.1.a.7.c	Teach Patients Methods of Health Promotion and Disease Prevention
CAAHEP	III.C.3.c.3.c	Provide Instruction for Health Maintenance and Disease Prevention

Student Name: _____   Date: _____   Score: _____

EVALUATION

Evaluator Signature: _____   Date: _____

Evaluator Comments:

DOCUMENTATION

Instructor Note: Retain work products with competency checklist.

Work Product, Procedure 17-2 (Progress Note)

Progress Note for Patient: Date:	**DOUGLASVILLE MEDICINE ASSOCIATES** **5076 BRAND BLVD** **DOUGLASVILLE, NY 01234** **(123) 456-7890**

Key Competencies		
ABHES	VI.A.1.a.7.c	Teach Patients Methods of Health Promotion and Disease Prevention
CAAHEP	III.C.3.c.3.c	Provide Instruction for Health Maintenance and Disease Prevention

Student Name: _____   Date: _____   Score: _____

Competency Checklist
PROCEDURE 17-3 Assist With the Prenatal Exam

Task: To assist with a prenatal exam

Condition: Given the equipment and supplies as listed in the procedure, a classmate to play the part of the patient, and a classmate to play the part of the provider, the student will correctly simulate assisting the provider with a prenatal exam, adhering to the steps listed below.

Standards: The student will have 15 minutes to complete the procedure and will need to score an 85% or above to pass the competency. Automatic failure results if any essential steps are omitted or performed incorrectly.

STEPS START TIME: END TIME:	Points Possible	First Attempt	Second Attempt	Third Attempt
1. Set up equipment and washed hands.	10			
2. Identified the patient using at least two identifiers, identified self, and instructed the patient to collect a urine specimen.	10			
3. Applied appropriate PPE and performed a dipstick reading for protein and glucose. Disposed of PPE and washed hands.	10			
4. Obtained patient's weight and blood pressure. If initial visit or at 36 weeks gestation or thereafter, instructed patient to disrobe completely and to put on a gown. For all other visits, instructed patient to expose belly.	10			
5. Supplied physician with equipment for fundal height measurement and a fetal monitor and gel for assessment of fetal heart tones.	10			
6. After completion of exam, assisted patient into sitting position to evaluate stability.	10			
7. Provided patient with educational materials and/or prescription for prenatal vitamins, if needed.	10			
8. Applied gloves, cleaned exam room, and properly disposed of used supplies—disinfected or sterilized used equipment. Washed hands and restocked room if necessary.	10			
9. Documented visit in patient's chart.	10			
10. Completed the procedure within the appropriate time limit.	10			
Points Earned / Points Possible:	___ / 100			

Points possible reflect importance of step in meeting the task: Important = (5) Essential = (10)
Determine score by dividing points earned by total points possible, and multiplying results by 100.

EVALUATION
Evaluator Signature: _____   Date: _____

Evaluator Comments:

Key Competencies		
ABHES	VI.A.1.a.4.h	Prepare Patients for and Assist Physician with Routine and Specialty Examinations and Treatments and Minor Office Surgeries
CAAHEP	III.C.3.b.4.e	Prepare Patient for and Assist with Routine and Specialty Examinations

Student Name: _____   Date: _____   Score: _____

DOCUMENTATION
Instructor Note: Retain work products with competency checklist.
Work Product, Procedure 17-3 (Progress Note)

Progress Note for	**DOUGLASVILLE MEDICINE ASSOCIATES**
Patient: Date:	**5076 BRAND BLVD** **DOUGLASVILLE, NY 01234** **(123) 456-7890**

Key Competencies		
ABHES	VI.A.1.a.4.h	Prepare Patients for and Assist Physician with Routine and Specialty Examinations and Treatments and Minor Office Surgeries
CAAHEP	III.C.3.b.4.e	Prepare Patient for and Assist with Routine and Specialty Examinations

Student Name: _____   Date: _____   Score: _____

Competency Checklist
PROCEDURE 18-1 Urinary Catheterization

Task: To perform a catheterization

Condition: Given the equipment and supplies as listed in the procedure and a classmate or anatomical model to play the part of the patient, the student will correctly simulate performing a catheterization, adhering to the steps listed below.

Standards: The student will have 15 minutes to complete the procedure and will need to score an 85% or above to pass the competency. Automatic failure results if any essential steps are omitted or performed incorrectly. The doctor would like a complete urinalysis and culture and sensitivity performed on the specimen.

STEPS START TIME: END TIME:	Points Possible	First Attempt	Second Attempt	Third Attempt
1. Identified the patient using at least two identifiers, identified self, and explained the procedure.	10			
2. Washed hands and assembled supplies. Placed the catheter kit on a Mayo stand or nearby counter top.	10			
3. Instructed patient to remove clothing from the waist down and provided patient with drape.	10			
4. Positioned the patient in the dorsal recumbent position. Draped with a sheet, exposing only the external genitalia.	10			
5. Placed catheter kit near working area and opened external covering of the kit.	10			
6. Carefully reached inside of the kit without contaminating the field and placed waterproof sterile drape underneath the penis for male patient and underneath buttocks for female patient. (Did not contaminate drape.)	10			
7. Washed hands and put on sterile gloves.	10			
8. Removed and opened fenestrated drape and placed over the external genitalia.	10			
9. Prepared cleaning solution, either sterile wipes or sterile cotton balls with antiseptic cleaner and squirted some of the lubricant onto a gauze pad.	10			
10. Removed catheter from container, inserted the tip of the catheter into sterile lubricant, and placed catheter on the sterile field until ready for use. Opened specimen container and placed within reach.	10			
11. For *female*, spread the labia with one hand and cleansed the genital areas from front to back with the other hand. (Right side, left side, and middle.) Used a different antiseptic wipe for each section.	10			
12. For *male*, cleansed the urinary meatus in circular motion working from the center outward. Repeated this procedure two times using a new antiseptic wipe each time.	10			
13. Inserted lubricated tip of catheter slowly into the urethral meatus.	10			
14. Progressed the catheter into the bladder until urine started to flow freely. Collected initial stream in basin and transferred the catheter to the specimen container.	10			
15. After adequate collection, emptied the remainder of the urine in the bladder into the basin.	10			
16. Slowly removed the catheter from the meatus and placed on table.	10			

Key Competencies		
ABHES	VI.A.1.a.4.h	Prepare patient for and assist physician with routine and specialty examinations and treatments and minor office surgeries
CAAHEP	III.C.3.b.4.e	Prepare patient for and assist with routine and specialty examinations

Student Name: _____   Date: _____   Score: _____

17. Removed gloves and washed hands. Assisted patient into sitting position.	10			
18. Discarded materials in the appropriate waste containers.	10			
19. Labeled container and attached completed lab requisition form.	10			
20. Correctly documented procedure on progress note, including any adverse reactions, and correctly completed requisition form.	10			
21. Completed the procedure within the appropriate time limit.	10			
Points Earned / Points Possible:	___ / 210			

Points possible reflect importance of step in meeting the task: Important = (5) Essential = (10).
Determine score by dividing points earned by total points possible, and multiplying results by 100.

EVALUATION
Evaluator Signature: _____   Date: _____

Evaluator Comments:

DOCUMENTATION
Instructor Note: Retain work products with competency checklist.
Work Product, Procedure 18-1 (Progress Note)

Progress Note for Patient: Date:	**DOUGLASVILLE MEDICINE ASSOCIATES** **5076 BRAND BLVD** **DOUGLASVILLE, NY 01234** **(123) 456-7890**

Work Product, Procedure 18-1 (Lab Requisition Form)

Form located on following page.

Key Competencies		
ABHES	VI.A.1.a.4.h	Prepare patient for and assist physician with routine and specialty examinations and treatments and minor office surgeries
CAAHEP	III.C.3.b.4.e	Prepare patient for and assist with routine and specialty examinations

LABORATORY REQUISITION

I.D. #	PATIENT LAST NAME		FIRST		M.I.	REFERRING PHYSICIAN

REFERRED BY	S.S.#		BILL: ☐ PHYSICIAN ☐ MEDICAL ☐ HMO ☐ CHDP		D.O.B	AGE	SEX
			☐ MEDICARE ☐ INSURANCE ☐ PATIENT				

PLEASE COMPLETE BILLING INFORMATION AT BOTTOM

ADDRESS		PHONE NUMBER ( )	DATE COLLECTED	TIME COLLECTED
CITY	STATE	ZIPCODE	FASTING YES NO	STAT	CALL RESULT
MEDICARE #	MEDICAL #		INFO. BELOW WILL APPEAR ON REPORT	

CUSTOM PROFILES & ADDITIONAL TESTS

173   [ ] CHEMISTRY PANEL, COMPLETE BLOOD COUNT (ZPP), LIPID PROFILE, T4

05050 [ ] CHOL, TRIG, HDL CHOL, VLDL CHOL, LDL CHOL, RISK FACTOR

PROFILES

00011 ☐	SPECIAL COMPREHENSIVE	2 SS,L	03536 ☐	HYPERTHYROID PROFILE		SS
00001 ☐	COMPREHENSIVE HEALTH SURVEY	SS,L	05037 ☐	HYPOTHYROID PROFILE		SS
00002 ☐	GENERAL SURVEY	SS,L	05051 ☐	LIPID PROFILE		SS
00003 ☐	CHEMISTRY PANEL	SS,L	05021 ☐	LIVER PROFILE		SS
CH7 ☐	CHEM 7 PANEL	SS	03359 ☐	LUPUS PROFILE		SS
03280 ☐	ANEMIA PROFILE	SS,L	03959 ☐	MENOPAUSAL PROFILE	SS /03960☐ POST MENOPAUSAL	SS
06016 ☐	ARTHRITIS PROFILE	SS,L	02280 ☐	OVARIAN FUNCTION PROFILE	SS /02281☐ TESTICULAR FUNC. PROF.	SS
05725 ☐	COMPREHENSIVE THYROID SURVEY	SS	02808 ☐	PRENATAL PROFILE		L,R
02691 ☐	EPSTEIN BARR PROFILE	SS	05006 ☐	THYROID PROFILE		SS
05010 ☐	ELECTROLYTES	SS	03191 ☐	TORCH PANEL		SS
06826 ☐	HEPATITIS PROFILE	SS	5756 ☐	URINE DRUG SCREEN	U / ☐ VENIPUNCTURE	

TESTS

0361 ☐	ABO & Rh TYPE	R,L	0141 ☐	C-REACTIVE PROTEIN	SS	0673 ☐	HEPATITIS B SURFACE ANTIGEN	SS	0237 ☐	PTT	B
0302 ☐	ALKALINE PHOSPHATASE	SS	1341 ☐	DHEA-S	SS	0245 ☐	HEPATITIS C ANTIBODY	SS	0317 ☐	RA FACTOR	SS
0109 ☐	AMYLASE	SS	0119 ☐	DIGOXIN	SS	0257 ☐	IRON	SS	0321 ☐	RUBELLA	SS
0613 ☐	ANA	SS	0224 ☐	DILANTIN	SS	LDL-A ☐	LDL CHOLESTEROL	SS	0331 ☐	RPR	SS
0366 ☐	ANTIBODY SCREEN	R	0835 ☐	ESTRADIOL	SS	0283 ☐	LEAD BLOOD	RB	0335 ☐	SEMEN ANALYSIS	SEMEN
0110 ☐	ASO (STREPTOZYME)	SS	0833 ☐	FERRITIN	SS	0281 ☐	LIPASE	SS	0328 ☐	SEDIMENTATION RATE (ESR)	L
0126 ☐	BILIRUBIN TOTAL	SS	0003 ☐	FOLIC ACID & VITAMIN B12	SS	8225 ☐	LH	SS	0349 ☐	SGOT (AST)	SS
0132 ☐	BUN	SS	0651 ☐	FSH	SS	0247 ☐	MONONUCLEOSIS	SS	0348 ☐	SGPT (ALT)	SS
8726 ☐	CA125	SS	0140 ☐	FTA-ABS	SS	0778 ☐	PHENOBARBITAL	SS	0330 ☐	SICKLE CELL SCREEN	L
0142 ☐	CALCIUM	SS	0210 ☐	GGTP	SS	0307 ☐	POTASSIUM	SS	0354 ☐	T4 (THYROXINE)	SS
0130 ☐	CBC	L	0536 ☐	GLUCOSE, FASTING	GY	0557 ☐	PREGNANCY (SERUM)	SS	1358 ☐	T4 FREE	SS
0388 ☐	CEA-ROCHE	SS	☐	GLUCOSE, ____ HR PP	GY	0308 ☐	PREGNANCY (URINE)	U	8456 ☐	TESTOSTERONE	SS
0152 ☐	CHOLESTEROL	SS	0771 ☐	GLYCOHEMOGLOBIN	L	0359 ☐	PROGESTERONE	SS	0824 ☐	THEOPHYLLINE	SS
0788 ☐	CORTISOL	SS	0534 ☐	H. PYLORI	SS	8041 ☐	PROLACTIN	SS	0360 ☐	TRIGLYCERIDE	SS
0162 ☐	CPK	SS	0823 ☐	HGG QUANTITATIVE	SS	0103 ☐	PROTEIN, TOTAL	SS	0672 ☐	TSH	SS
0445 ☐	CKMB ISOENZYME	SS	1856 ☐	HIV (ANTIBODY)	SS	2000 ☐	PROSTATE SPECIFIC ANTIGEN (PSA)	SS	0373 ☐	URIC ACID	SS
0161 ☐	CREATININE	SS	0558 ☐	HDL CHOLESTEROL	SS	0310 ☐	PT (PROTHROMBIN TIME)	B	0219 ☐	URINALYSIS	U

CYTOPATHOLOGY

☐ PREGNANT   ☐ ABORTION   ☐ POST-PARTUM   ☐ POST-MENOPAUSE
HISTORY _____

PREV. ABNORMAL CYTOL FINDINGS _____
☐ CONTRACEPTIVES   DATE _____
☐ HYSTERECTOMY   ☐ HORMONES   ☐ IUD
☐ COPHORECTOMY   ☐ TOTAL   ☐ SUPRA CX
☐ RADIATION Rx   DATE _____
☐ OTHER _____   ☐ HORMONES Rx   ☐ CHEMO Rx

LMP _____ DATE COLLECTED _____
SOURCE ☐ CERVIX   ☐ ENDOCERVIX   ☐ VAGINA
        ☐ CYTOBRUSH   ☐ OTHER SITE _____

MICROBIOLOGY

THCUL ☐ THROAT	URTHC ☐ URETHRAL	9391 ☐ CHLAMYDIA DNA
EACUL ☐ EAR	VACUL ☐ VAGINAL	9390 ☐ GONORRHEA DNA
EYCUL ☐ EYE	WOCUL ☐ WOUND	9391 ☐ OCCULT BLOOD
GOCUL ☐ GC	ROCUL ☐ CULTURE (Routine)	0293 ☐ OVA & PARASITE
SPCUL ☐ SPUTUM	URCUL ☐ URINE	WTM ☐ WET MOUNT
STCUL ☐ STOOL	GSP ☐ GRAM STAIN	
SOURCE _____	OTHER _____	

DIAGNOSIS OR COMMENTS

LAB USE ONLY (DO NOT WRITE BELOW THIS SPACE)

DATE RECEIVED	DATE REPORTED

STATEMENT OF SPECIMEN ADEQUACY

GENERAL CATEGORIZATION

DESCRIPTIVE DIAGNOSIS

HORMONAL EVALUATION

ADDITIONAL COMMENT

CYTOTECHNOLOGIST	PATHOLOGIST

BILLING INFORMATION

PRIMARY INSURED	INSURANCE COMPANY
ADDRESS	
POLICY NO. & I.D. NO.	ICD9 CODE

LEGEND

SS	Serum Separator	GY	Grey	B	Blue	U	Urine
R	Red	L	Lavender	RB	Royal Blue	G	Green

Student Name: _____   Date: _____   Score: _____

Competency Checklist
PROCEDURE 19-1 Obtain the Height/Length and Weight of an Infant

Task: To obtain the height/length and weight of an infant

Condition: Given the equipment and supplies as listed in the procedure, a classmate to play the part of the parent, and a doll or model for the role of the infant, the student will correctly simulate performing an infant height and weight measurement, adhering to the steps listed below.

Standards: The student will have 10 minutes to complete the procedure and will need to score an 85% or above to pass the competency. Automatic failure results if any essential steps are omitted or performed incorrectly.

STEPS START TIME: END TIME:	Points Possible	First Attempt	Second Attempt	Third Attempt
1. Washed hands and assembled equipment.	10			
2. Identified the patient using at least two identifiers, identified self, and asked parent to remove all clothing from the infant, except the diaper.	10			
3. Placed the infant face up on the exam table with the top of the infant's head flush with the top measuring bar of the caliper.	10			
4. Stretched infant's legs to full length and placed sole of foot flush with bottom measuring bar of caliper.	10			
5. Read the measurement and documented immediately in the infant's chart and on growth chart.	10			
6. After completing the height measurement, lined the scale with a paper towel or exam paper, balanced the scale at zero, and placed infant on scale.	10			
7. Instructed parent to comfort and support infant but not to exert any pressure.	10			
8. Obtained the weight reading, removed the infant from the scale, and instructed parent to remove the infant's diaper. Weighed the diaper and subtracted the weight of the diaper from the weight of the infant.	10			
9. Correctly documented results on progress note and on growth chart *(Work Product, Procedure 19-1)*.	10			
10. Completed the procedure within the appropriate time limit.	10			
Points Earned / Points Possible:	___ / 100			

Points possible reflect importance of step in meeting the task: Important = (5) Essential = (10).
Determine score by dividing points earned by total points possible, and multiplying results by 100.

EVALUATION
Evaluator Signature: _____   Date: _____

Evaluator Comments:

Key Competencies		
ABHES	VI.A.1.a.4.d	Take Vital Signs
CAAHEP	III.C.3.b.4.b	Obtain Vital Signs

Student Name: _____   Date: _____   Score: _____

DOCUMENTATION

Instructor Note: Retain work products with competency checklist.
Work Product, 19-1 (Progress Note)

Progress Note for	**DOUGLASVILLE MEDICINE ASSOCIATES**
	5076 BRAND BLVD
Patient:	**DOUGLASVILLE, NY 01234**
Date:	**(123) 456-7890**

Work Product, Procedure 19-1 (Infant Growth Chart)

Charts for boys and girls located on following pages.

Key Competencies			
ABHES	VI.A.1.a.4.d	Take Vital Signs	
CAAHEP	III.C.3.b.4.b	Obtain Vital Signs	

Birth to 36 months: Girls
Length-for-age and Weight-for-age percentiles

NAME _____

RECORD # _____

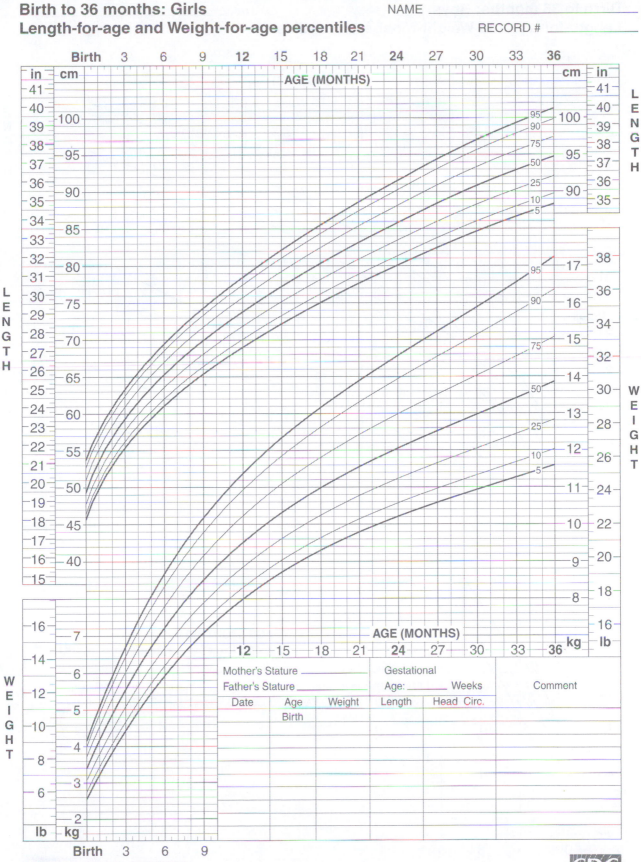

Published May 30, 2000 (modified 4/20/01).
SOURCE: Developed by the National Center for Health Statistics in collaboration with
the National Center for Chronic Disease Prevention and Health Promotion (2000).
http://www.cdc.gov/growthcharts

SAFER • HEALTHIER • PEOPLE™

Birth to 36 months: Boys
Length-for-age and Weight-for-age percentiles

NAME _____

RECORD # _____

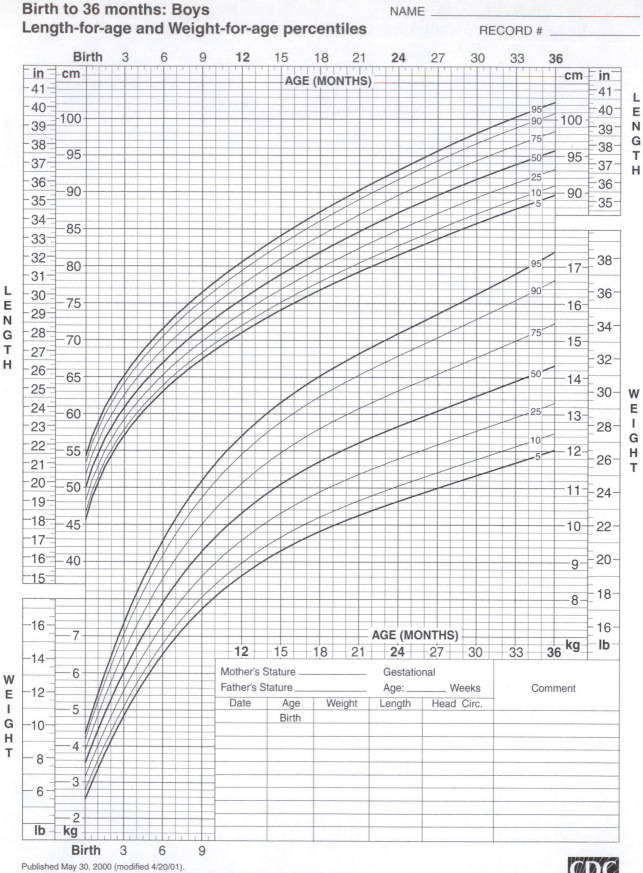

Published May 30, 2000 (modified 4/20/01).
SOURCE: Developed by the National Center for Health Statistics in collaboration with
the National Center for Chronic Disease Prevention and Health Promotion (2000).
http://www.cdc.gov/growthcharts

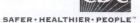

SAFER • HEALTHIER • PEOPLE™

Student Name: _____   Date: _____   Score: _____

Competency Checklist
PROCEDURE 19-2 Obtain the Temperature of an Infant or Young Child

Task: To obtain a rectal, aural and temporal temperature on an infant

Condition: Given the equipment and supplies as listed in the procedure, a classmate to play the part of the parent, and a doll or model for the role of the infant, the student will correctly simulate performing a rectal, aural, and temporal temperature on an infant, adhering to the steps listed below.

Standards: The student will have 15 minutes to complete the procedure and will need to score an 85% or above to pass the competency. Automatic failure results if any essential steps are omitted or performed incorrectly.

STEPS START TIME: END TIME:	Points Possible	First Attempt	Second Attempt	Third Attempt
1. Washed hands, assembled equipment. (Applied gloves if policy of office right before insertion of thermometer.)	10			
2. Identified the patient using at least two identifiers, explained the procedure to the parent, and had parent remove appropriate clothing from infant.	10			
Rectal temperature:				
3. Correctly positioned patient. Applied a clean probe cover over the thermometer probe and lubricated probe.	10			
4. Gently inserted probe into infant's rectum, approximately 1 inch, and held securely in place until the thermometer beeped.	10			
5. Observed reading and removed probe. Discarded sheath in appropriate trash receptacle, disinfected probe, and placed probe back in unit.	10			
6. Removed excess lubricant from infant's anal area and instructed parent to dress child.	5			
Aural Temperature:				
7. Placed a probe cover on the probe, pulled down and back on the infant's earlobe, and gently inserted thermometer into ear canal.	10			
8. Pressed activation button, waited for signal, removed probe, and obtained reading.	10			
9. Discarded probe cover in appropriate trash receptacle.	10			
Temporal Temperature:				
10. Cleaned thermometer with alcohol swab or placed a sheath over the probe. Checked infant's forehead for any moisture—dried if moisture was present.	10			
11. Placed probe at midline of forehead and kept probe flush with skin. Pressed and held scan button while gliding thermometer across forehead—over to the side of the head over the temporal artery. Took reading behind ear if necessary.	10			
12. Read reading and discarded probe in proper trash receptacle.	10			
13. Washed hands and documented information in infant's chart, indicating method performed *(Work Product, Procedure 19-2).*	10			
14. Completed the procedure within the appropriate time limit.	10			
Points Earned / Points Possible:	___ / 135			

Points possible reflect importance of step in meeting the task: Important = (5) Essential = (10).
Determine score by dividing points earned by total points possible, and multiplying results by 100.

Key Competencies		
ABHES	VI.A.1.a.4.d	Take Vital Signs
CAAHEP	III.C.3.b.4.b	Obtain Vital Signs

Student Name: _____   Date: _____   Score: _____

EVALUATION
Evaluator Signature: _____   Date: _____

Evaluator Comments:

DOCUMENTATION
Instructor Note: Retain work products with competency checklist.
Work Product, Procedure 19-2 (Progress Note)

Progress Note for Patient: Date:	**DOUGLASVILLE MEDICINE ASSOCIATES** **5076 BRAND BLVD** **DOUGLASVILLE, NY 01234** **(123) 456-7890**

Key Competencies		
ABHES	VI.A.1.a.4.d	Take Vital Signs
CAAHEP	III.C.3.b.4.b	Obtain Vital Signs

Student Name: _____   Date: _____   Score: _____

Competency Checklist
PROCEDURE 19-3 Perform a PKU on a Newborn

Task: To perform a PKU on a newborn

Condition: Given the equipment and supplies as listed in the procedure, a classmate to play the part of the parent, and a doll or model for the role of the infant, the student will correctly simulate performing a heel capillary stick to obtain blood for a PKU, adhering to the steps listed below.

Standards: The student will have 15 minutes to complete the procedure and will need to score an 85% or above to pass the competency. Automatic failure results if any essential steps are omitted or performed incorrectly.

STEPS START TIME: END TIME:	Points Possible	First Attempt	Second Attempt	Third Attempt
1. Washed hands and assembled equipment. Completed required patient information on test card and applied gloves.	10			
2. Identified the patient using at least two identifiers, identified self, and explained procedure to parent or caregiver.	10			
3. Applied gloves, exposed infant's heel. Located puncture site and warmed area with warm compresses.	10			
4. Cleansed site with alcohol wipe and allowed to air dry.	10			
5. Securely grasped foot, punctured heel perpendicular to lines on sole, and wiped away first drop of blood.	10			
6. Gently squeezed heel, placed test card on drop of blood, and allowed circle to fill until saturated. Filled all circles correctly and allowed card to dry. (Color in the circles of the card with a red marker to represent the blood.) *(Work Product, Procedure 19-3)*	10			
7. Covered puncture site with gauze and applied pressure until bleeding stopped. Applied small adhesive bandage to area.	10			
8. Discarded used materials in appropriate containers, removed gloves, and washed hands.	10			
9. Documented results of procedure in patient's chart. *(Work Product, Procedure 19-3)*	10			
Two hours later (student will simulate waiting two hours)				
10. Placed PKU card in envelope for transport to lab.	10			
11. Correctly documented procedure in chart.	10			
12. Completed the procedure within the appropriate time limit.	10			
Points Earned / Points Possible:	___ / 120			

Points possible reflect importance of step in meeting the task: Important = (5) Essential = (10).
Determine score by dividing points earned by total points possible, and multiplying results by 100.

EVALUATION
Evaluator Signature: _____   Date: _____

Evaluator Comments:

Key Competencies		
ABHES	VI.A.1.a.4.t	Perform Capillary Puncture
CAAHEP	III.C.3.b.2.b	Perform Capillary Puncture

Student Name: _____   Date: _____   Score: _____

DOCUMENTATION
Instructor Note: Retain work products with competency checklist.
Work Product, Procedure 19-3 (Progress Note)

Progress Note for Patient: Date:	**DOUGLASVILLE MEDICINE ASSOCIATES** **5076 BRAND BLVD** **DOUGLASVILLE, NY 01234** **(123) 456-7890**

Work Product, Procedure 19-3 (PKU Card)

Key Competencies		
ABHES	VI.A.1.a.4.t	Perform Capillary Puncture
CAAHEP	III.C.3.b.2.b	Perform Capillary Puncture

Student Name: _____   Date: _____   Score: _____

Competency Checklist
PROCEDURE 19-4 Perform a Pediatric Injection

Task: To perform a pediatric injection

Condition: Given the equipment and supplies as listed in the procedure, a classmate to play the part of the parent, and a doll or model to play the role of the infant, the student will correctly simulate performing a pediatric injection, adhering to the steps listed below.

Standards: The student will have 10 minutes to complete the procedure and will need to score an 85% or above to pass the competency. Automatic failure results if any essential steps are omitted or performed incorrectly.

STEPS START TIME: END TIME:	Points Possible	First Attempt	Second Attempt	Third Attempt
1. Washed hands, assembled equipment, and prepared medication.	10			
2. Identified the patient using at least two identifiers, identified self and explained procedure to parent, and child—if age appropriate.	10			
3. Washed hands again and applied gloves.	10			
4. Located site for injection, cleansed site with antiseptic, and allowed site to dry.	10			
5. Pulled the skin taut and inserted needle at a 90-degree angle.	10			
6. Aspirated to make certain not in a blood vessel and slowly injected medication.	10			
7. Removed needle quickly, at same angle of insertion, placed gauze sponge over injection site, gently massaged, and applied adhesive bandage to site.	10			
8. Engaged safety device on needle and disposed of in sharps container.	10			
9. Removed gloves, washed hands, and correctly documented procedure in patient's chart and in immunization log *(Work Product, Procedure 19-4)*.	10			
10. Completed the procedure within the appropriate time limit.	10			
Points Earned / Points Possible:	___ / 100			

Points possible reflect importance of step in meeting the task: Important = (5) Essential = (10).
Determine score by dividing points earned by total points possible, and multiplying results by 100.

EVALUATION
Evaluator Signature: _____   Date: _____

Evaluator Comments:

Key Competencies		
ABHES	VI.A.1.a.4.m	Prepare and Administer Oral and Parenteral Medications as Directed by Physician
CAAHEP	III.C.3.b.4.g	Apply Pharmacology Principles to Prepare and Administer Oral and Parenteral (excluding IV) Medications

Student Name: _____   Date: _____   Score: _____

DOCUMENTATION
Instructor Note: Retain work products with competency checklist.
Work Product, Procedure 19-4 (Progress Note)

Progress Note for Patient: Date:	**DOUGLASVILLE MEDICINE ASSOCIATES** **5076 BRAND BLVD** **DOUGLASVILLE, NY 01234** **(123) 456-7890**

Work Product, Procedure 19-4 (Immunization Tracking Log)

IMMUNIZATION TRACKING LOG

Date Admin.	Patient's Name	Name of Immunization	Drug Form	Amt. Given	Ordering Physician	Manufacturer's Name	Lot Number	Exp. Date	Who Admin.

Key Competencies		
ABHES	VI.A.1.a.4.m	Prepare and Administer Oral and Parenteral Medications as Directed by Physician
CAAHEP	III.C.3.b.4.g	Apply Pharmacology Principles to Prepare and Administer Oral and Parenteral (excluding IV) Medications

Student Name: _____   Date: _____   Score: _____

Competency Checklist
PROCEDURE 21-1 Administer Heat Therapy Treatments

Task: To administer a heat therapy treatment

Condition: Given the equipment and supplies as listed in the procedure and a classmate to play the part of the patient, the student will simulate administering heat therapy to a patient, adhering to the steps listed below.

Standards: The student will have 15 minutes to complete the procedure and will need to score an 85% or above to pass the competency. Automatic failure results if any essential steps are omitted or performed incorrectly.

STEPS START TIME: END TIME:	Points Possible	First Attempt	Second Attempt	Third Attempt
1. Washed hands and assembled equipment and supplies.	10			
2. Identified the patient using at least two identifiers, identified self and explained procedure.	10			
3. Instructed patient to remove clothing and put on a gown, if necessary, exposing area to be treated. Properly positioned patient for treatment.	10			
Heating pad:				
4. Placed protective covering on heating pad, connected cord to outlet and set temperature control—as indicated by physician.	10			
5. Placed heating pad on affected area (*did not* allow patient to lie on heating pad). Checked with patient about temperature tolerance.	10			
Hot water bottle:				
6. Filled hot water bottle approximately ½ full with water. (Temperature was between 105–110°F or 40.5–43°C.)	10			
7. Compressed air from bottle, closed lid tightly, and covered water bottle with cloth or towel.	10			
8. Applied water bottle to the affected area and left in place for prescribed amount of time.	10			
Hot compress:				
9. Filled basin with water. (Temperature ranged between 105–110°F or 40.5–43°C.) Soaked gauze or cloth in water, wrung out excess moisture, placed compress on affected area, and covered with plastic covering.	10			
10. Re-wet compress every few minutes to maintain correct temperature for amount of time prescribed by physician.	10			
Hot pack:				
11. Placed pack in hot water (105–110°F), removed from water and drained a few moments. A pad was wrapped around the pack and the pack was placed over the affected area.	10			
Hot soak:				
12. Filled appropriate-size container with water approximately 110°F (43°C). Added medication to water as directed by physician.	10			
13. Placed affected body part in water for prescribed amount of time. When finished, removed body part from soaking container, dried with towel, and inspected for any redness or damage.	10			
Paraffin bath:				
14. Heated bath to approximately 127°F (53°C) and dipped affected body part in paraffin until thick coating of wax built up.	10			
15. Wrapped part in foil, plastic wrap, or cloth for 30 minutes, took covering off and peeled away wax.	10			

Key Competencies		
ABHES	VI.A.1.a.4.h	Prepare Patients for and Assist Physician with Routine and Specialty Examinations and Treatments and Minor Office Surgeries
CAAHEP	III.C.3.b.4.f	Prepare Patient for and Assist with Procedures, Treatments, and Minor Office Surgeries

Student Name: _____   Date: _____   Score: _____

For all heat treatments:				
16. Periodically checked with patient for tolerance and comfort.	10			
17. Periodically checked treatment area for redness, swelling, or other signs of irritation to the skin. Cleaned treatment area and washed hands.	10			
18. Dismissed patient and cleaned area and washed hands.	10			
19. Documented treatment in patient's chart *(Work Product, Procedure 21-1)*.	10			
20. Completed the procedure within the appropriate time limit.	10			
Points Earned / Points Possible:	___ / 200			

Points possible reflect importance of step in meeting the task: Important = (5) Essential = (10).
Determine score by dividing points earned by total points possible, and multiplying results by 100.

EVALUATION
Evaluator Signature: _____   Date: _____

Evaluator Comments:

DOCUMENTATION
Instructor Note: Retain work products with competency checklist
Work Product, Procedure 21-1 (Progress Note)

Progress Note for Patient: Date:	**DOUGLASVILLE MEDICINE ASSOCIATES** **5076 BRAND BLVD** **DOUGLASVILLE, NY 01234** **(123) 456-7890**

Key Competencies		
ABHES	VI.A.1.a.4.h	Prepare Patients for and Assist Physician with Routine and Specialty Examinations and Treatments and Minor Office Surgeries
CAAHEP	III.C.3.b.4.f	Prepare Patient for and Assist with Procedures, Treatments, and Minor Office Surgeries

Student Name: _____   Date: _____   Score: _____

Competency Checklist
PROCEDURE 21-2 Administer Cold Therapy Treatments

Task: To administer a cold therapy treatment

Condition: Given the equipment and supplies as listed in the procedure and a classmate to play the part of the patient, the student will simulate administering cold therapy to a patient, adhering to the steps listed below.

Standards: The student will have 15 minutes to complete the procedure and will need to score an 85% or above to pass the competency. Automatic failure results if any essential steps are omitted or performed incorrectly.

STEPS START TIME: END TIME:	Points Possible	First Attempt	Second Attempt	Third Attempt
1. Washed hands and assembled supplies.	10			
2. Identified the patient using at least two identifiers, identified self, and explained procedure.	10			
3. Instructed patient to put on a gown if necessary—exposing area to be treated—and placed patient in the proper position.	10			
Ice bag:				
4. Checked bag for damage or leaks and filled approximately two-thirds full with small ice chips or cubes. Squeezed bag to expel air and screwed top in place.	10			
5. Covered pack with towel, placed on affected area, and kept in place for amount of time prescribed by physician.	10			
Commercial ice pack:				
6. Placed gel pack in freezer for amount of time recommended by manufacturer.	10			
7. Covered with protective covering, placed on affected area, and left in place for amount of time prescribed by physician.	10			
8. Placed pack back in freezer after use.	10			
Chemical ice pack:				
9. Inspected pack for leaks, squeezed bag and shook, covered pack with protective covering, and applied to affected area.	10			
10. Left in place for amount of time prescribed by physician and discarded pack after use.	10			
Cold compress:				
11. Placed small volume of cold water in basin and added ice cubes.	10			
12. Soaked gauze pad or cloth in water, squeezed out excess moisture, applied to affected area. Placed an ice pack over the compress.	10			
13. Re-wet, as needed, and repeated application every 2–3 minutes for amount of time prescribed by physician.	10			
Ice massage:				
14. Filled paper cup three-fourths full with water and placed in freezer.	10			
15. Exposed area to be treated, squeezed paper cup so ice was exposed, moved ice cube in circular motion over affected area for amount of time prescribed by physician, or until patient reported numbness or burning in the area.	10			
For all treatments:				
16. Periodically checked treatment area for signs of paleness, redness, or a bluish discoloration. Stopped treatment immediately if any problems.	10			

Key Competencies		
ABHES	VI.A.1.a.4.h	Prepare Patients for and Assist Physician with Routine and Specialty Examinations and Treatments and Minor Office Surgeries
CAAHEP	III.C.3.b.4.f	Prepare Patient for and Assist with Routine and Specialty Examinations

Student Name: _____   Date: _____   Score: _____

17. Cleaned work area and washed hands.	5			
18. Documented treatment in patient's chart *(Work Product, Procedure 21-2).*	10			
19. Completed the procedure within the appropriate time limit.	10			
Points Earned / Points Possible:	___ / 185			

Points possible reflect importance of step in meeting the task: Important = (5) Essential = (10).
Determine score by dividing points earned by total points possible, and multiplying results by 100.

EVALUATION
Evaluator Signature: _____   Date: _____

Evaluator Comments:

DOCUMENTATION
Instructor Note: Retain work products with competency checklist.
Work Product, Procedure 21-2 (Progress Note).

Progress Note for Patient: Date:	**DOUGLASVILLE MEDICINE ASSOCIATES** **5076 BRAND BLVD** **DOUGLASVILLE, NY 01234** **(123) 456-7890**

Key Competencies		
ABHES	VI.A.1.a.4.h	Prepare Patients for and Assist Physician with Routine and Specialty Examinations and Treatments and Minor Office Surgeries
CAAHEP	III.C.3.b.4.f	Prepare Patient for and Assist with Routine and Specialty Examinations

Student Name: _____   Date: _____   Score: _____

Competency Checklist
PROCEDURE 21-3 Instruct a Patient to Use a Cane

Task: To instruct a patient to use a cane

Condition: Given the equipment and supplies as listed in the procedure and a classmate to play the part of the patient, the student will demonstrate how to use a cane, adhering to the steps listed below.

Standards: The student will have 10 minutes to complete the procedure and will need to score an 85% or above to pass the competency. Automatic failure results if any essential steps are omitted or performed incorrectly.

STEPS START TIME: END TIME:	Points Possible	First Attempt	Second Attempt	Third Attempt
1. Washed hands, checked physician's orders, and assembled equipment.	10			
2. Identified the patient using at least two identifiers, identified self, and explained the procedure.	10			
3. Inspected cane for rubber tip and adjusted the height of the cane so that the handle of the cane was even with the patient's hip joint. Instructed patient to flex elbow at a 25- to 30-degree angle.	10			
4. Demonstrated correct usage by holding cane on strong side, moved cane and affected leg forward at the same time, and then moved strong leg forward slightly in front of cane.	10			
5. Applied gait belt to patient and allowed patient to practice.	10			
6. Washed hands and documented procedure in patient's chart *(Work Product, Procedure 21-3)*.	10			
7. Completed the procedure within the appropriate time limit.	10			
Points Earned / Points Possible:	___ / 70			

Points possible reflect importance of step in meeting the task: Important = (5) Essential = (10).
Determine score by dividing points earned by total points possible, and multiplying results by 100.

EVALUATION
Evaluator Signature: _____   Date: _____

Evaluator Comments:

Key Competencies		
ABHES	VI.A.1.a.7.b	Instruct Patient with Special Needs
CAAHEP	III.C.3.b.3.b	Instruct Individuals According to Their Needs

Student Name: _____   Date: _____   Score: _____

DOCUMENTATION

Instructor Note: Retain work products with competency checklist.

Work Product, Procedure 21-3 (Progress Note)

Progress Note for	**DOUGLASVILLE MEDICINE ASSOCIATES**
Patient:	**5076 BRAND BLVD**
Date:	**DOUGLASVILLE, NY 01234**
	(123) 456-7890

Key Competencies		
ABHES	VI.A.1.a.7.b	Instruct Patient with Special Needs
CAAHEP	III.C.3.b.3.b	Instruct Individuals According to Their Needs

Student Name: _____   Date: _____   Score: _____

Competency Checklist
PROCEDURE 21-4   Instruct a Patient to Use Axillary Crutches

Task: To instruct a patient on the proper use of axillary crutches

Condition: Given the equipment and supplies as listed in the procedure and a classmate to play the part of the patient, the student will demonstrate how to use crutches, adhering to the steps listed below.

Standards: The student will have 10 minutes to complete the procedure and will need to score an 85% or above to pass the competency. Automatic failure results if any essential steps are omitted or performed incorrectly.

STEPS START TIME: END TIME:	Points Possible	First Attempt	Second Attempt	Third Attempt
1. Washed hands, checked physician's orders, and assembled equipment.	10			
2. Identified the patient using at least two identifiers, identified self, and explained the procedure.	10			
3. Inspected pads on hand grips and axillary bar and rubber suction tips on the bottom of each crutch. Made any necessary adjustments.	10			
4. Tightened wing nuts.	10			
5. Instructed patient to stand erect and to place crutches underneath the armpits and to place the tips of each crutch 4–6 inches to the side of each foot.	10			
6. Adjusted height of crutches 2 finger-width spaces below the armpits and instructed patient to flex elbows at a 25- to 30-degree angle.	10			
7. Demonstrated proper gait—instructing the patient not to move crutches more than 6 inches ahead at a time.	10			
8. Allowed patient to practice and made sure that the patient was supporting his or her weight on the hand grips and not the axillary bar.	10			
9. Gave patient written instructions.	10			
10. Washed hands and correctly documented the educational session in patient's chart *(Work Product, Procedure 21-4)*.	10			
11. Completed the procedure within the appropriate time limit.	10			
Points Earned / Points Possible:	___ / 110			

Points possible reflect importance of step in meeting the task: Important = (5) Essential = (10).
Determine score by dividing points earned by total points possible, and multiplying results by 100.

EVALUATION
Evaluator Signature: _____   Date: _____

Evaluator Comments:

Key Competencies		
ABHES	VI.A.1.a.7.b	Instruct Patients with Special Needs
CAAHEP	III.C.3.b.3.b	Instruct Individuals According to Their Needs

Student Name: _____   Date: _____   Score: _____

DOCUMENTATION

Instructor Note: Retain work products with competency checklist.

Work Product, Procedure 21-4 (Progress Note)

Progress Note for	**DOUGLASVILLE MEDICINE ASSOCIATES**
	5076 BRAND BLVD
Patient:	**DOUGLASVILLE, NY 01234**
Date:	**(123) 456-7890**

Key Competencies		
ABHES	VI.A.1.a.7.b	Instruct Patients with Special Needs
CAAHEP	III.C.3.b.3.b	Instruct Individuals According to Their Needs

Student Name: _____   Date: _____   Score: _____

Competency Checklist
PROCEDURE 21-5 Instruct a Patient to Use a Walker

Task: To instruct a patient to use a walker

Condition: Given the equipment and supplies as listed in the procedure and a classmate to play the part of the patient, the student will demonstrate how to use a walker, adhering to the steps listed below.

Standards: The student will have 10 minutes to complete the procedure and will need to score an 85% or above to pass the competency. Automatic failure results if any essential steps are omitted or performed incorrectly.

STEPS START TIME: END TIME:	Points Possible	First Attempt	Second Attempt	Third Attempt
1. Washed hands and assembled equipment.	10			
2. Identified the patient using at least two identifiers, identified self, explained procedure, and applied a gait belt to the patient.	10			
3. Inspected tips and hand grips of walker and adjusted the height of the walker so that the hand grips were level with the top of the patient's hips.	10			
4. Performed a demonstration for patient, then had patient demonstrate the procedure. (Checked to make certain that the patient's arms were flexed at a 25- to 30-degree angle, that all four legs of the walker were securely on the ground before moving forward, and that the patient only moved the walker about 6 inches in front of his or her body when moving the walker forward.)	10			
5. Made any necessary adjustments following patient's demonstration and gave patient educational materials to take home.	10			
6. Washed hands and documented procedure in patient's chart *(Work Product, Procedure 21-5)*.	10			
7. Completed the procedure within the appropriate time limit.	10			
Points Earned / Points Possible:	___ / 70			

Points possible reflect importance of step in meeting the task: Important = (5) Essential = (10).
Determine score by dividing points earned by total points possible, and multiplying results by 100.

EVALUATION
Evaluator Signature: _____   Date: _____

Evaluator Comments:

Key Competencies		
ABHES	VI.A.1.a.7.b	Instruct Patients with Special Needs
CAAHEP	III.C.3.b.3.b	Instruct Individuals According to Their Needs

Student Name: _____   Date: _____   Score: _____

DOCUMENTATION

Instructor Note: Retain work products with competency checklist.
Work Product, Procedure 21-5 (Progress Note)

Progress Note for Patient: Date:	**DOUGLASVILLE MEDICINE ASSOCIATES** **5076 BRAND BLVD** **DOUGLASVILLE, NY 01234** **(123) 456-7890**

Key Competencies		
ABHES	VI.A.1.a.7.b	Instruct Patients with Special Needs
CAAHEP	III.C.3.b.3.b	Instruct Individuals According to Their Needs

Student Name: _____   Date: _____   Score: _____

Competency Checklist
PROCEDURE 22-1 Sanitization and Lubrication of Instruments

Task: To sanitize and lubricate instruments

Condition: Given the equipment and supplies as listed in the procedure, the student will demonstrate the procedure for sanitizing and lubricating instruments, adhering to the steps listed below.

Standards: The student will have 10 minutes to complete the procedure and will need to score an 85% or above to pass the competency. Automatic failure results if any essential steps are omitted or performed incorrectly.

Student will sanitize and lubricate a(n) _____.

STEPS START TIME: END TIME:	Points Possible	First Attempt	Second Attempt	Third Attempt
1. Washed hands and applied PPE.	10			
2. Assembled equipment and supplies.	10			
3. Soaked items in lined metal basin or plastic basin with deionized or distilled water, or according to institutional policy.	10			
4. Poured water out of the first basin—being careful to protect the instruments. Placed instruments in new basin filled with *warm water* and a neutral cleanser.	10			
5. Thoroughly scrubbed each part of each instrument (paying particular attention to crevices, teeth and serrations).	10			
6. Thoroughly rinsed each instrument in distilled water or approved rinsing solution.	10			
7. Placed each instrument on waterproof drape and dried each instrument with muslin cloth or comparable material.	10			
8. Inspected each instrument for defects—checked blades on cutting instruments by cutting through a piece of material or piece of rubber. Removed instruments that were damaged.	10			
9. Sprayed instruments with box locks with an approved lubricant.	10			
10. Allowed the lubricated instruments to dry by adhering to the instructions on lubricant label.	10			
11. Prepared instruments for disinfection or wrapping.	5			
12. Cleaned area using disinfectant; removed PPE and washed hands.	10			
13. Completed the procedure within the appropriate time limit.	10			
Points Earned / Points Possible:	___ / 125			

Points possible reflect importance of step in meeting the task: Important = (5) Essential = (10).
Determine score by dividing points earned by total points possible, and multiplying results by 100.

EVALUATION
Evaluator Signature: _____   Date: _____

Evaluator Comments:

Key Competencies		
ABHES	VI.A.1.a.4.c	Apply principles of aseptic techniques and infection control
CAAHEP	III.C.3.b.1.e	Practice standard precautions

Student Name: _____   Date: _____   Score: _____

Competency Checklist
PROCEDURE 22-2   Chemical Disinfection of Instruments

Task: To cleanse and disinfect instruments

Condition: Given the equipment and supplies as listed in the procedure, the student will demonstrate the procedure for disinfecting surgical instruments, adhering to the steps listed below.

Standards: Timing will vary on this competency according to submersion times on the disinfecting bottle. The instructor will set the time limit for this competency. The student will need to score an 85% or above to pass the competency. Automatic failure results if any essential steps are omitted or performed incorrectly.

STEPS START TIME: END TIME:	Points Possible	First Attempt	Second Attempt	Third Attempt
1. Selected a room that was well ventilated and clean.	10			
2. Washed hands and applied PPE.	10			
3. Assembled equipment and supplies (checked expiration date on disinfectant and indicator strips).	10			
4. Poured solution into disinfecting container following manufacturer's instructions.	10			
5. Recorded date that solution was opened on the bottle of the disinfectant and recorded date the solution was prepared on the disinfecting container. Placed initials on label of prepared solution.	10			
6. Placed chemical indicator strip into solution following manufacturer's instructions. Read indicator strip (if it didn't meet MEC guidelines, repeated test).	10			
7. Placed sanitized instrument to be disinfected onto the disinfecting tray and lowered tray so instrument was completely submerged in the solution; closed lid on solution.	10			
8. Set timer for the amount of time listed on the solution bottle. (Wait time may be simulated for the competency.)	10			
9. Recorded date and time that instrument was submerged into disinfecting log with initials.	10			
10. Once bell on timer rang, lifted tray out of disinfecting solution and rinsed the items according to manufacturer's instructions.	10			
11. *Drying Instruments*: For *critical devices*, used a sterile non-lent producing cloth to dry items. Transferred device using sterile transfer forceps or washed hands and applied sterile gloves to transfer the item. For *non-critical devices*, dried items with a clean non-lent producing cloth and handled with clean gloved hands when moving to airtight container.	10			
12. Cleaned area and replaced items; removed PPE and washed hands.	10			
13. Correctly documented procedure in instrument disinfection log book *(Work Product, Procedure 22-2)*.	10			
14. Completed the procedure within the appropriate time limit.	10			
Points Earned / Points Possible:	___ / 140			

Points possible reflect importance of step in meeting the task: Important = (5) Essential = (10).
Determine score by dividing points earned by total points possible, and multiplying results by 100.

Key Competencies		
ABHES	VI.A.1.a.4.c	Apply principles of aseptic techniques and infection control
	VI.A.1.a.4.p	Perform sterilization techniques
CAAHEP	III.C.3.b.1.c	Perform sterilization techniques

Student Name: _____   Date: _____   Score: _____

EVALUATION
Evaluator Signature: _____   Date: _____

Evaluator Comments:

DOCUMENTATION
Instructor Note: Retain work products with competency checklist.
Work Product 22-2 (Instrument Disinfection Log)

INSTRUMENT DISINFECTION LOG

Date of Disinfection	Name of Instrument	MEC Control Result	Name and Strength of Solution	Start Time	End Time	Initials
01/12/XX	Nasal Speculum	Acceptable	Cidex Plus	9:30 a.m.	10:00 a.m.	MH, CMA (AAMA)

Key Competencies		
ABHES	VI.A.1.a.4.c	Apply principles of aseptic techniques and infection control
	VI.A.1.a.4.p	Perform sterilization techniques
CAAHEP	III.C.3.b.1.c	Perform sterilization techniques

Student Name: _____   Date: _____   Score: _____

Competency Checklist

PROCEDURE 22-3 Wrap Instruments for Sterilization and Operate an Automated Autoclave

Task: To wrap instruments for sterilization and operate an automated autoclave

Condition: Given the equipment and supplies as listed in the procedure, the student will demonstrate the procedure for wrapping surgical instruments and sterilizing them in a fully automated autoclave, adhering to the steps listed below.

Standards: The student will have 1 hour to complete the procedure and will need to score an 85% or above to pass the competency. Automatic failure results if any essential steps are omitted or performed incorrectly.

STEPS START TIME: END TIME:	Points Possible	First Attempt	Second Attempt	Third Attempt
1. Washed hands.	10			
2. Assembled equipment and supplies and applied gloves.	10			
3. Checked integrity of wrapping materials for flaws, checked expiration date on sterilization indicators, placed items on a clean, dry surface.	10			
Items Wrapped in Paper or Muslin:				
4. Placed one or two sheets of paper/cloth facing diagonally resembling a diamond (one corner pointing towards the student and the other corner pointing the opposite direction).	10			
5. Placed sanitized instrument in center of paper; hinged instruments were either completely opened or taken apart. The tips of sharp instruments were shielded with gauze. Placed sterilization indicator beside the instrument.	10			
6. Correctly wrapped instrument using the fan-fold method. (If double wrapping, wrapped the instrument again with a second piece of wrapping material, using the fan-fold method.)	10			
7. Correctly secured the pack with autoclave tape. (Wrote the name of the instrument, date of sterilization and initials on the tape.)	10			
Items in Plastic Peel-Apart Wrap:				
8. Wrote the name of the item, date of sterilization and initials on the envelope.	10			
9. Placed instrument or supply in the peel apart envelope so that the handle of the instrument was facing the end that will be peeled back during the opening procedure.	10			
10. Removed the backing off of the adhesive strip and folded the adhesive flap, sealing the envelope.	10			
Autoclaving:				
11. Arranged items on autoclave trays so that steam could penetrate all surfaces of each instrument. (Packets were placed vertically on the tray and separated 1–3 inches; jars were placed on their sides with lids ajar or removed.)	10			
12. Checked gauge of water reservoir and added distilled water to fill line.	10			
13. Placed trays into the autoclave; made necessary adjustments to accommodate proper positioning, closed and latched door.	10			
14. Selected the appropriate sterilization cycle according to the load's contents and pressed start button.	10			

Key Competencies		
ABHES	VI.A.1.a.4.o	Wrap items for autoclaving
	VI.A.1.a.4.p	Perform sterilization techniques
CAAHEP	III.C.3.b.1.b	Wrap items for autoclave
	III.C.3.b.1.c	Perform sterilization techniques

Student Name: _____   Date: _____   Score: _____

15. Following the vent cycle—put on thermal gloves and opened door according to manufacturer's instructions. Let items remain in autoclave for 20–30 minutes to facilitate drying (optional).	10				
16. Pulled out trays using caution (gloves or pot holder). Removed items and checked to make certain that the strips on autoclave tape turned the appropriate color.	10				
17. Placed items in a clean covered environment (plastic container, cabinet, etc.).	10				
18. Correctly documented procedure in the sterilization log *(Work Product, Procedure 22-4)*.	10				
19. Completed the procedure within the appropriate time limit.	10				
Points Earned / Points Possible:	___ /190				

Points possible reflect importance of step in meeting the task: Important = (5) Essential = (10).
Determine score by dividing points earned by total points possible, and multiplying results by 100.

EVALUATION
Evaluator Signature: _____   Date: _____

Evaluator Comments:

DOCUMENTATION
Instructor Note: Retain work products with competency checklist.
Work Product, Procedure 22-3 (Sterilization Log)

STERILIZATION LOG

Date	Start Time	Finish Time	Items Autoclaved	Controls Used to Test Sterility	Results of Control	Initials
01/12/XX	*1:30 p.m.*	*2:15 p.m.*	*2 Laceration Trays & 2 Wrapped Vaginal Speculums*	*Autoclave Tape Chemical Indicator Pellet*	*Both tape and Indicator Pellet positive for sterilization*	*DE, CMA (AAMA)*

Key Competencies		
ABHES	VI.A.1.a.4.o	Wrap items for autoclaving
	VI.A.1.a.4.p	Perform sterilization techniques
CAAHEP	III.C.3.b.1.b	Wrap items for autoclave
	III.C.3.b.1.c	Perform sterilization techniques

Student Name: _____   Date: _____   Score: _____

Competency Checklist
PROCEDURE 23-1 Apply Skin Closures

Task: To apply sterile skin closures

Condition: Given the equipment and supplies as listed in the procedure, the student will demonstrate the proper steps for applying sterile skin closures, adhering to the steps listed below.

Standards: The student will have 15 minutes to complete the procedure and will need to score an 85% or above to pass the competency. Automatic failure results if any essential steps are omitted or performed incorrectly.

STEPS START TIME: END TIME:	Points Possible	First Attempt	Second Attempt	Third Attempt
1. Washed hands.	10			
2. Assembled equipment and supplies.	10			
3. Identified the patient using at least two identifiers, identified self, and explained the procedure.	10			
4. Inspected the wound and selected size of adhesive strips that best matched the patient's wound (checked to see if patient is allergic to adhesive).	10			
5. Positioned patient in comfortable position and placed tray for easy access.	5			
6. Cleaned tray and set up necessary items. (Maintained the sterility of the strips.)	10			
7. Washed hands and applied sterile gloves.	10			
8. Cleansed the skin with an approved antiseptic so that cleansing extended 2–3 inches (5–7 cm) around the wound—working from the inner periphery to the outer periphery. Repeated two more times.	10			
9. Allowed the area to completely dry; removed gloves and washed hands.	10			
10. Applied a thin coat of tincture of benzoin to the periphery of the wound using new sterile cotton tip applicators for each side (tincture of benzoin did not touch wound).	10			
11. Followed manufacturer's instructions for removing strips from the inner pack and applying them to the skin.	10			
12. Lined the first strip up with the *center of the wound*. Starting with the side furthest away from the student—or the medial edge of the wound—applied pressure to the strip (securing it to the skin) and gently stretched the strip while lining up both wound edges so that they just came together.)	10			
13. Once skin lined up even on both sides, pulled strip to the opposite side while pressing down firmly on the skin.	10			
14. Applied the next strip approximately $\frac{1}{8}$ inch from the first strip on either side of the first strip.	10			
15. Performed the same step on the opposite side of the wound; continued process until wound was completely closed.	10			
16. If needed, applied one closure approximately ½ inch away from the strip's edges running parallel to the wound on each side of the strips.	5			
17. Made certain there was good approximation of the wound; applied dressing if necessary.	10			
18. Removed gloves and washed hands; gave patient home care instructions.	10			

Key Competencies		
ABHES	VI.A.1.a.4.h	Assist physician with examination and treatments
CAAHEP	III.C.3.b.4.f	Prepare patient for and assist with procedures, treatments, and minor office surgeries

Student Name: _____   Date: _____   Score: _____

19. Correctly documented procedure on progress note.	10			
20. Completed the procedure within the appropriate time limit.	10			
Points Earned / Points Possible:	___ / 190			

Points possible reflect importance of step in meeting the task: Important = (5) Essential = (10).
Determine score by dividing points earned by total points possible, and multiplying results by 100.

EVALUATION
Evaluator Signature: _____   Date: _____

Evaluator Comments:

DOCUMENTATION
Instructor Note: Retain work product with competency checklist.
Work Product, Procedure 23-1 (Progress Note)

Progress Note for Patient: Date:	**DOUGLASVILLE MEDICINE ASSOCIATES** **5076 BRAND BLVD** **DOUGLASVILLE, NY 01234** **(123) 456-7890**

Key Competencies		
ABHES	VI.A.1.a.4.h	Assist physician with examination and treatments
CAAHEP	III.C.3.b.4.f	Prepare patient for and assist with procedures, treatments, and minor office surgeries

Student Name: _____   Date: _____   Score: _____

Competency Checklist
PROCEDURE 23-2 Suture or Staple Removal

Task: To remove sutures and staples

Condition: Given the equipment and supplies as listed in the procedure, the student will demonstrate the proper steps for removing sutures or staples, adhering to the steps listed below.

Standards: The student will have 15 minutes to complete the procedure and will need to score an 85% or above to pass the competency. Automatic failure results if any essential steps are omitted or performed incorrectly.

STEPS START TIME: END TIME:	Points Possible	First Attempt	Second Attempt	Third Attempt
1. Washed hands.	10			
2. Assembled equipment and supplies.	10			
3. Identified the patient using at least two identifiers, identified self, and explained the procedure.	10			
4. Asked patient if he/she finished all of the antibiotic and followed all other home care instructions.	10			
5. Examined the outside of the patient's bandage—making a mental note; washed hands and applied examination gloves.	10			
6. Removed dressing and observed both the inside of the dressing and wound area for any signs of infection (made mental note).	10			
7. Discarded dressing into biohazard trash and washed hands.	10			
8. Asked physician to observe wound *before* starting procedure; applied waterproof drape underneath the patient's wound.	10			
9. Set up sterile tray; poured sterile saline into sterile container. Opened sterile suture removal instrument pack and dropped items on sterile field. Placed pack of antiseptic swabs nearby for easy access. Washed hands and applied sterile gloves.	10			
Suture Removal:				
10. If sutures were adhered to the skin, irrigated the wound according to the physician's instructions. Cleansed skin with skin antiseptic, if applicable.	10			
11. Removed first suture by grasping one side of the knot with thumb forceps and gently *tugging upward*. Using the other hand, worked the suture scissors under the knot as close to the skin as possible and cut the suture.	10			
12. Pulled the knot *toward* the wound (no part of the suture that was on the outside went through the inside of the wound). Removed remainder of sutures using the same procedure.	10			
Staple Removal:				
13. Gently grasped the staple with staple remover, squeezed handle of staple remover until the staple popped up and out.	10			
14. Continued to remove all staples until all staples were removed.	10			
All Wounds:				
15. Checked to make certain the tissue was well approximated and healed following procedure. (If any problems alerted physician.)	10			
16. Applied antiseptic cream (if ordered) and dressed wound according to physician's instructions.	10			
17. Removed gloves and washed hands.	10			
18. Gave patient home care instructions and dismissed; properly cleaned area.	10			
19. Correctly documented procedure on progress note.	10			
20. Completed the procedure within the appropriate time limit.	10			

Key Competencies		
ABHES	VI.A.1.a.4.h	Assist physician with examination and treatments
CAAHEP	III.C.3.b.4.f	Prepare patient for and assist with procedures, treatments, and minor office surgeries

Student Name: _____   Date: _____   Score: _____

Points Earned / Points Possible:	___ / 200			

Points possible reflect importance of step in meeting the task: Important = (5) Essential = (10).
Determine score by dividing points earned by total points possible, and multiplying results by 100.

EVALUATION
Evaluator Signature: _____   Date: _____

Evaluator Comments:

DOCUMENTATION
Instructor Note: Retain work products with competency checklist.
Work Product, Procedure 23-2 (Progress Note)

Progress Note for Patient: Date:	**DOUGLASVILLE MEDICINE ASSOCIATES** **5076 BRAND BLVD** **DOUGLASVILLE, NY 01234** **(123) 456-7890**

Key Competencies		
ABHES	VI.A.1.a.4.h	Assist physician with examination and treatments
CAAHEP	III.C.3.b.4.f	Prepare patient for and assist with procedures, treatments, and minor office surgeries

Student Name: _____   Date: _____   Score: _____

Competency Checklist
PROCEDURE 24-1   Perform a Surgical Handwash and Apply Surgical Gloves

Task: To perform a surgical handwash and apply surgical gloves

Condition: Given the equipment and supplies as listed in the procedure, the student will demonstrate the proper steps for performing a surgical handwash and applying sterile gloves, adhering to the steps listed below.

Standards: The student will have 15 minutes to complete the procedure and will need to score an 85% or above to pass the competency. Automatic failure results if any essential steps are omitted or performed incorrectly.

STEPS START TIME: END TIME:	Points Possible	First Attempt	Second Attempt	Third Attempt
1. Assembled equipment and supplies; opened sterile towel without contaminating on clean dry surface (close to handwash area).	10			
2. Placed appropriate-size gloves beside sterile towel and removed from outer wrapper, unfolded pack to lay flat and opened each flap of the inner wrapper to expose gloves (cuffs of gloves facing you and thumbs pointing outward).	10			
3. Opened sterile scrub pack containing the impregnated scrub brush and nail cleaner; placed in the sink area.	10			
4. Removed any jewelry on hands or wrists.	10			
5. Turned water on using automatic sensor and adjusted temperature to a warm setting.	10			
6. Rinsed hands under the water keeping hands and fingers pointed upward and arms well above the waist.	10			
7. Using the nail stick, cleaned under each nail. Dropped nail stick in the sink and rinsed hands.	10			
8. Completely wet hands, wrists, and forearms, keepings hands and fingers pointed upward and positioned above the waist.	10			
9. Obtained impregnated brush and started scrub on the palm of hand—moving downward to base of the thumb—using a circular pattern. (Did not go over an area that had already been scrubbed.)	10			
10. Moved to fingers, scrubbing each surface—using several vertical strokes—moving *from the base of each finger to the nail* (scrubbed all four surfaces and skin between the thumb and index finger). (Offices may have specific instructions for timing of scrub or amount of strokes necessary—check office policy.)	10			
11. Turned hand over and scrubbed posterior portion of the hand extending to below the wrists using circular pattern (hands and fingers were positioned upward).	10			
12. Scrubbed forearm using circular pattern from the wrists to slightly above the elbow. (Scrubbed all four surfaces of the forearm.)	10			
13. Rinsed both arms with arms well above waist and fingers pointed upward. (Water ran *from fingertips down the arms* over the elbow.)	10			
14. Washed opposite arm using same steps listed above, dropped scrub brush into sink and rinsed thoroughly.	10			
15. Turned off water and picked up towel in dominant hand by holding onto the corners. Started at fingertips on non-dominant hand—patted dry all the way to the elbow using one side of towel (hands above waist and fingers pointed upward).	10			

Key Competencies		
ABHES	VI.A.1.a.4.c	Apply principles of aseptic techniques and infection control
CAAHEP	III.C.3.b.1.a	Perform handwashing

Student Name: _____   Date: _____   Score: _____

16. Repeated procedure with dominant hand using the opposite side of the sterile towel.	10			
Gloving:				
17. Picked up first glove by inside cuff using non-dominant hand. Lifted glove up and away from flat surface. Slid glove in an upward motion, over the dominant hand.	10			
18. Picked up second glove by slipping the four fingers from the gloved hand underneath the cuff of second glove—while keeping the thumb facing outward. Slid glove onto the nondominant hand without contaminating either glove.	10			
19. Leaving fingers under the cuff, unfolded the cuff so that it slid down over the wrist. Repeated procedure for other side.	10			
20. Examined both gloves for any tears or problems.	10			
21. Kept hands above waist level and did not touch anything besides sterile items.				
22. Student completed the procedure within the appropriate time limit.	10			
Points Earned / Points Possible:	___ / 210			

Points possible reflect importance of step in meeting the task: Important = (5) Essential = (10).
Determine score by dividing points earned by total points possible, and multiplying results by 100.

EVALUATION
Evaluator Signature: _____   Date: _____

Evaluator Comments:

Key Competencies		
ABHES	VI.A.1.a.4.c	Apply principles of aseptic techniques and infection control
CAAHEP	III.C.3.b.1.a	Perform handwashing

Student Name: _____   Date: _____   Score: _____

Competency Checklist
PROCEDURE 24-2   Prepare the Patient's Skin for the Surgical Procedure Using a One-Step Scrub

Task: To prepare the patient's skin for the surgical procedure using a one-step scrub

Condition: Given the equipment and supplies as listed in the procedure, the student will demonstrate the proper steps for performing a surgical scrub on the patient's skin using a one step scrub, adhering to the steps listed below. (This type of scrub is only used if the patient was sent home with special soaps and instructions for cleansing the skin prior to procedure.)

Standards: The student will have 15 minutes to complete the procedure and will need to score an 85% or above to pass the competency. Automatic failure results if any essential steps are omitted or performed incorrectly.

STEPS START TIME: END TIME:	Points Possible	First Attempt	Second Attempt	Third Attempt
1. Washed hands.	10			
2. Assembled necessary supplies and equipment.	10			
3. Identified the patient using at least two identifiers, identified self, and explained the procedure. Verified that patient followed home care cleansing instructions.	10			
4. Asked patient to remove necessary clothing. Exposed the surgical site and draped patient for modesty.	10			
5. Positioned patient for comfort and placed absorbent drapes under area to be cleansed.	10			
6. Adjusted the light over surgical site. Inspected skin for any gross contamination (if so, cleansed the skin with antiseptic cleanser).	10			
7. Opened skin prep kit without contaminating the swab or sponge applicator.	10			
8. Washed hands and applied sterile gloves.	10			
9. Removed swab/sponge, touching only the applicator.	10			
10. Applied antiseptic by painting concentric circles over the site for 30 seconds to 2 minutes or three separate applications with three separate applicators.	10			
11. Only shaved if physician ordered for area to be shaved (pulled skin taut and shaved in the direction that the hair grows). Re-cleansed the skin according to office policy.	10			
12. Removed absorbent pads and discarded.	10			
13. Placed sterile pad under the surgical site.	10			
14. Applied fenestrated drape and other surgical drapes according to physician's preference.	10			
15. Instructed patient to keep hands below the drapes.	10			
16. Completed the procedure within the appropriate time limit.	10			
Points Earned / Points Possible:	___ / 160			

Points possible reflect importance of step in meeting the task: Important = (5) Essential = (10).
Determine score by dividing points earned by total points possible, and multiplying results by 100.

Key Competencies		
ABHES	VI.B.1.a.4.b	Prepare patients for procedures
	VI.B.1.a.4.c	Apply principles of aseptic techniques and infection control
CAAHEP	III.C.3.b.4.f	Prepare patient for and assist with procedures, treatments, and minor office surgeries

Student Name: _____   Date: _____   Score: _____

EVALUATION
Evaluator Signature: _____   Date: _____

Evaluator Comments:

Key Competencies		
ABHES	VI.B.1.a.4.b	Prepare patients for procedures
	VI.B.1.a.4.c	Apply principles of aseptic techniques and infection control
CAAHEP	III.C.3.b.4.f	Prepare patient for and assist with procedures, treatments, and minor office surgeries

Student Name: _____   Date: _____   Score: _____

Competency Checklist
PROCEDURE 24-3 Disinfect a Surgical Tray and Place a Sterile Barrier on the Tray

Task: To disinfect a surgical tray and place a sterile barrier on the tray

Condition: Given the equipment and supplies as listed in the procedure, and a student to play the part of the patient, the student will demonstrate the proper steps for disinfecting a surgical tray and placing a sterile barrier on the tray, adhering to the steps listed below.

Standards: The student will have 10 minutes to complete the procedure and will need to score an 85% or above to pass the competency. Automatic failure results if any essential steps are omitted or performed incorrectly.

STEPS START TIME: END TIME:	Points Possible	First Attempt	Second Attempt	Third Attempt
1. Washed hands.	10			
2. Assembled necessary supplies and equipment; positioned Mayo tray so that it was at waist level.	10			
3. Cleaned the tray using 4x4s saturated with disinfectant (not dripping) using a circular motion until the entire tray was completely cleansed.	10			
4. Allowed the tray to air dry.	10			
5. Selected appropriate sterile barrier and placed it on a clean dry surface.	10			
6. Peeled back the top flap of the sterile barrier pack—completely exposing the drape. (Cut corners were facing the student.)	10			
7. Using thumb and forefinger, gently pulled up on one of the top corner edges of the drape without contaminating the drape.	10			
8. Grabbed opposing corner so that both corners were held along the top edge of drape (drape was well above waist and away from the body). Pulled drape over the Mayo stand without contaminating drape.	10			
9. Completed the procedure within the appropriate time limit.	10			
Points Earned / Points Possible:	___ / 90			

Points possible reflect importance of step in meeting the task: Important = (5) Essential = (10).
Determine score by dividing points earned by total points possible, and multiplying results by 100.

EVALUATION
Evaluator Signature: _____   Date: _____

Evaluator Comments:

Key Competencies		
ABHES	VI.B.1.a.4.c	Apply principles of aseptic technique and infection control
CAAHEP	III.C.3.b.4.f	Prepare patient for and assist with procedures, treatments, and minor office surgeries

Student Name: _____   Date: _____   Score: _____

Competency Checklist
PROCEDURE 24-4 Open Sterile Items and Place Them on the Sterile Field

Task: To open sterile items and place them on the sterile field

Condition: Given the equipment and supplies as listed in the procedure, the student will demonstrate the proper steps for opening sterile items and placing them on a sterile field, adhering to the steps listed below.

Standards: The student will have 15 minutes to complete the procedure and will need to score an 85% or above to pass the competency. Automatic failure results if any essential steps are omitted or performed incorrectly.

STEPS START TIME: END TIME:	Points Possible	First Attempt	Second Attempt	Third Attempt
Opening Sterile Pack and Using Sterile Transfer Forceps to Transfer a Sterile Item to the Sterile Field:				
1. Washed hands.	10			
2. Assembled necessary supplies and equipment; adjusted Mayo stand so that it was waist high. Prepared tray and placed sterile barrier on tray.	10			
3. Placed sterilized pack of transfer forceps on the side table.	10			
4. Placed unopened sterilized instrument on the side table and examined autoclave tape to make certain that the stripes turned the appropriate color. Checked expiration date and the quality of the wrapper.	10			
5. Removed tape from instrument to be transferred and placed it on the side table.	5			
6. Using thumb and index finger, grasped tip of the first flap—pulling it away from the student or to the opposite side.	10			
7. Grasped the right side flap-using just the right thumb and index finger—pulling it all the way to the right side of the pack.	10			
8. Grasped the left side flap—using just the left thumb and index finger—pulling it all the way to the left side of the pack.	10			
9. Grasped the tip of last folded flap using dominant thumb and index finger and pulled last flap toward self (student) without contaminating the wrap or instrument. (Entire instrument was visible for easy retrieval.)	10			
10. Checked sterilization indicator in pack to see if appropriate color.	10			
11. Checked tape of transfer forceps and opened in the same manner as first instrument without contaminating the forceps.	10			
12. Grasped the handles of transfer forceps using thumb and index fingers. Lifted transfer forceps straight up keeping tips facing downward but above the height of side table.	10			
13. Moved the transfer forceps to the instrument that needed to be transferred. Grasped and lifted the instrument above the height of the side table and gently transferred the instrument—lowering the sterile instrument onto the sterile tray.	10			
14. Once transfer was completed, pulled the sterile transfer forceps up and away from the field, setting them back on side table.	10			
Opening a Peel-Apart Pack:				
15. Inspected package and made certain integrity of wrap was not altered. Checked control strip and expiration date.	10			
16. Positioned self in front of tray with a few inches in between.	10			

Key Competencies		
ABHES	VI.A.1.a.4.c	Apply principles of aseptic techniques and infection control
CAAHEP	III.C.3.b.4.f	Prepare patient for and assist with procedures, treatments, and minor office surgeries

Student Name: _____   Date: _____   Score: _____

17. Grasped both top edges of the peel apart pack and carefully peeled them apart by rolling wrap downward on both sides.	10			
18. Once wrap was peeled to point of instrument transfer, turned hands inward and pushed the pack forward to the edge of the sterile field (instrument/item was well above the sterile field). Gently dropped item onto field.	10			
19. Completed the procedure within the appropriate time limit.	10			
Points Earned / Points Possible:	___ / 185			

Points possible reflect importance of step in meeting the task: Important = (5) Essential = (10).
Determine score by dividing points earned by total points possible, and multiplying results by 100.

EVALUATION
Evaluator Signature: _____   Date: _____

Evaluator Comments:

Key Competencies		
ABHES	VI.A.1.a.4.c	Apply principles of aseptic techniques and infection control
CAAHEP	III.C.3.b.4.f	Prepare patient for and assist with procedures, treatments, and minor office surgeries

Student Name: _____   Date: _____   Score: _____

Competency Checklist
PROCEDURE 24-5 Set Up a Complete Sterile Tray and
Pour a Sterile Solution

Task: To set up a complete sterile tray and pour a sterile solution

Condition: Given the equipment and supplies as listed in the procedure, the student will demonstrate the proper steps for setting up a sterile tray and pouring sterile solutions, adhering to the steps listed below.

Standards: The student will have 15 minutes to complete the procedure and will need to score an 85% or above to pass the competency. Automatic failure results if any essential steps are omitted or performed incorrectly.

STEPS START TIME: END TIME:	Points Possible	First Attempt	Second Attempt	Third Attempt
1. Performed aseptic hand wash (antibacterial soap and water).	10			
2. Assembled necessary supplies and equipment; placed Mayo stand at waist height.	10			
3. Cleaned Mayo stand with 4x4s saturated with disinfectant (but not dripping), cleaning in circular motion from the inner periphery to the outer periphery.	10			
4. Allowed stand to air dry.	10			
5. Checked instrument pack for integrity; checked tape stripes for correct color and checked expiration date on pack.	10			
6. Pulled tape off pack and placed on side table.	5			
7. Placed sterile pack on the center of Mayo stand so the flap that was taped was facing self (student).	10			
8. Using index finger and thumb of dominant hand, grasped tip of folded flap—pulling away from self (student) to the opposite side.	10			
9. Grasped the right side flap—using just the right thumb and index finger—pulling it all the way to the right side of the pack.	10			
10. Grasped the left side flap—using just the left thumb and index finger—pulling it all the way to the left side of the pack.	10			
11. Grasped the tip of last folded flap using dominant thumb and index finger and pulled last flap toward self (student) without contaminating the wrap or instrument.	10			
12. Repeated steps for second layer of wrap; moved to side table without turning back on the field.	10			
13. Opened sterile gloves and removed from wrapper; opened inner layer of wrapper without contaminating the gloves.	10			
14. Washed hands with alcohol-based hand sanitizer following manufacturer's instructions.	10			
15. Applied surgical gloves and held hands above the waist.	10			
16. Approached field facing forward, started removing items from inside of the tray—placing them on the sterile field in logical sequence. Placed basins for iodine and saline on the corner of the stand facing upward.	10			
17. Once field was organized, removed sterilization indicator and checked to see that it turned the proper color.	10			
18. Placed tray that held the instruments onto the side table; removed gloves and washed hands with dry soap.	10			
19. Picked up new bottle of iodine, read the label and checked the expiration date; palmed the label.	10			

Key Competencies		
ABHES	VI.A.1.a.4.c	Apply principles of aseptic techniques and infection control
CAAHEP	III.C.3.b.4.f	Prepare patient for and assist with procedures, treatments, and minor office surgeries

Student Name: _____   Date: _____   Score: _____

20. Removed the cap and placed to side with the lid facing upward. Removed protective seal and placed on side table.	10				
21. Moved to stand and approached the corner on which the basins were sitting; poured iodine into the container labeled as iodine—pouring at a distance of 2–6 inches above the field. (Did not splash solution.) Replaced cap.	10				
22. Repeated the steps for pouring iodine for pouring the sterile saline—pouring the solution in the basin labeled as saline.	10				
23. If not all contents were used replaced caps on sterile solutions and followed institution's policy for storing.	5				
24. Completed procedure within the appropriate time limit.	10				
Points Earned / Points Possible:	___ / 230				

Points possible reflect importance of step in meeting the task: Important = (5) Essential = (10).
Determine score by dividing points earned by total points possible, and multiplying results by 100.

EVALUATION
Evaluator Signature: _____   Date: _____

Evaluator Comments:

Key Competencies		
ABHES	VI.A.1.a.4.c	Apply principles of aseptic techniques and infection control
CAAHEP	III.C.3.b.4.f	Prepare patient for and assist with procedures, treatments, and minor office surgeries

Student Name: _____   Date: _____   Score: _____

Competency Checklist
PROCEDURE 24-6 Apply Surgical Attire

Task: To apply surgical attire

Condition: Given the equipment and supplies as listed in the procedure, and a student to play the part of the second medical assistant, the student will demonstrate the proper steps for applying surgical attire, adhering to the steps listed below.

Standards: The student will have 15 minutes to complete the procedure and will need to score an 85% or above to pass the competency. Automatic failure results if any essential steps are omitted or performed incorrectly.

STEPS START TIME: END TIME:	Points Possible	First Attempt	Second Attempt	Third Attempt
1. Assembled necessary supplies and equipment.	10			
2. Removed jewelry; performed aseptic handwash.	10			
3. Placed sterile gown pack and sterile gloves on Mayo stand or clean dry counter near the sink. Opened both sterile gown and sterile glove packages without contaminating.	10			
4. Applied cap, goggles and mask.	10			
5. Opened sterile scrub pack containing the scrub brush and nail stick; proceeded with surgical handwash as in Procedure 24-1.	10			
6. Reached down and lifted upward on the folded gown by grasping the inside of the gown below the neckline; stepped away from the table into an unobstructed area.	10			
7. Kept inside of gown toward body, allowed gown to unfold, keeping hands well above the waist. Slipped both hands into the armholes without extending beyond the cuffs of the gown.	10			
8. Had another medical assistant pull gown up over shoulders by grasping the inside shoulder and neck seams. Had medical assistant fasten at the neck and waist level only.	10			
9. Used only outside cuff of surgical gown from dominant hand to pick up the glove for non-dominant hand. Placed glove on the palm side of the outside cuff of non-dominant hand (fingers of glove pointed towards the elbow and thumb side of glove faced down).	10			
10. Used both hands (while still tucked within the inside cuffs of the sleeves) to pinch the rolled edges of the glove—stretching the glove up and over the gown cuff while working fingers out of the cuff of the gown into the glove.	10			
11. Gently slid fingers into the glove. Repeated steps again for gloving dominant hand using gloved hand to put on glove. Made certain cuffs on gloves were pulled over stockinette cuffs.	10			
12. Passed cardboard tab to second medical assistant. Grasped the string attached to the cardboard as the medical assistant pulled the cardboard toward the outside.	10			
13. Picked up other loose string attached to the front of the gown and tied both strings at the waist and secured.	10			
14. Made sure hands stayed above level of the waist at all of times.	10			
15. Completed the procedure within the appropriate time limit.	10			
Points Earned / Points Possible:	___ / 150			

Points possible reflect importance of step in meeting the task: Important = (5) Essential = (10).
Determine score by dividing points earned by total points possible, and multiplying results by 100.

Key Competencies		
ABHES	VI.A.1.a.4.c	Apply principles of aseptic techniques and infection control
CAAHEP	III.C.3.b.4.f	Prepare patient for and assist with procedures, treatments, and minor office surgeries

Student Name: _____   Date: _____   Score: _____

EVALUATION
Evaluator Signature: _____   Date: _____

Evaluator Comments:

Key Competencies		
ABHES	VI.A.1.a.4.c	Apply principles of aseptic techniques and infection control
CAAHEP	III.C.3.b.4.f	Prepare patient for and assist with procedures, treatments, and minor office surgeries

Student Name: _____   Date: _____   Score: _____

Competency Checklist
PROCEDURE 24-7   Remove an Old Dressing, Irrigate the Wound, and Apply a New Dressing

Task: To remove an old dressing, irrigate the wound, and apply a new dressing

Condition: Given the equipment and supplies as listed in the procedure, and a student to play the part of the patient, the student will demonstrate the proper steps for removing an old dressing, irrigating a wound, and applying a new dressing, adhering to the steps listed below.

Standards: The student will have 15 minutes to complete the procedure and will need to score an 85% or above to pass the competency. Automatic failure results if any essential steps are omitted or performed incorrectly.

STEPS START TIME: END TIME:	Points Possible	First Attempt	Second Attempt	Third Attempt
1. Checked patient's chart to determine type and strength of irrigating solution and the type of dressing to be used.	10			
2. Gathered supplies; checked the label on the irrigating solution three times against the physician's order; checked the expiration date on the solution.	10			
3. Identified the patient using at least two identifiers, identified self, and explained the procedure.	10			
4. Asked patient if any problems occurred since surgery and about compliance regarding home care instructions.	10			
5. Had patient expose the affected area; placed waterproof pad under the wound area and positioned the affected area for easy accessibility.	10			
6. Washed hands using aseptic technique and applied non-sterile examination gloves.	10			
7. Inspected outer covering of bandage (bandage torn, dirty, or wet?).	10			
8. Cut the bandage with bandage scissors *along side* of the wound. Removed bandage; pulling bandage corners *towards* the wound.	10			
9. Inspected inner portion of bandage for drainage or odor; discarded bandage into biohazard container.	10			
10. Looked at the wound area and inspected for signs of infection (edema, erythema, or drainage).	10			
11. Removed gloves and washed hands; notified doctor to examine wound (following office policy).	10			
12. Positioned Mayo tray and cleaned tray with 4x4s containing disinfectant; allowed to air dry. Applied sterile drape.	10			
13. Used sterile technique and placed one of the wrapped sterile basins on the Mayo stand.	10			
14. Opened the peel-apart package containing 4x4s and dropped contents from packet onto the sterile field.	10			
15. Opened sterile dressing and placed on sterile field, opened sterile bandage and placed on the field.	10			
16. Dropped sterile 20 mL syringe onto the field.	10			
17. Poured small amount of sterile saline into the sterile basin.	10			
18. Placed waterproof drape under the wound using sterile technique. Placed second sterile basin from side table on the waterproof drape for irrigating solution to run off in. Opened in a sterile manner. Instructed patient not to touch basin or drape.	10			

Key Competencies		
ABHES	VI.A.1.a.4.c	Apply principles of aseptic techniques and infection control
	VI.A.1.a.4.r	Practice standard precautions
CAAHEP	III.C.3.b.1d	Dispose of biohazardous materials
	III.C.3.b.1e	Practice standard precautions

Student Name: _____   Date: _____   Score: _____

19. Thoroughly washed hands using alcohol-dry soap on the side table and donned sterile gloves.	10			
20. Arranged items on tray for easy access.	5			
21. Drew up irrigating solution from basin with sterile syringe. Irrigated the patient's wound so water ran into the basin on the sterile field.	10			
22. Dried wound with sterile gauze; opened sterile dressing and placed over wound.	10			
23. Selected bandage technique that best suited the patient's wound.	10			
24. Threw away all trash into trash receptacle and gave patient home care instructions and prescriptions.	10			
25. Dismissed patient and correctly documented the procedure (*Work Product, Procedure 24-7*).	10			
26. Completed the procedure within the appropriate time limit.	10			
Points Earned / Points Possible:	___ / 255			

Points possible reflect importance of step in meeting the task: Important = (5) Essential = (10).
Determine score by dividing points earned by total points possible, and multiplying results by 100.

EVALUATION
Evaluator Signature: _____   Date: _____

Evaluator Comments:

DOCUMENTATION
Instructor Note: Retain work products with competency checklist.
Work Product, Procedure 24-7 (Progress Note)

Progress Note for Patient: Date:	**DOUGLASVILLE MEDICINE ASSOCIATES** **5076 BRAND BLVD** **DOUGLASVILLE, NY 01234** **(123) 456-7890**

Key Competencies			
ABHES	VI.A.1.a.4.c	Apply principles of aseptic techniques and infection control	
	VI.A.1.a.4.r	Practice standard precautions	
CAAHEP	III.C.3.b.1d	Dispose of biohazardous materials	
	III.C.3.b.1e	Practice standard precautions	

Student Name: _____   Date: _____   Score: _____

Competency Checklist
PROCEDURE 25-1 Review and Report Laboratory Results

Task: To review and report laboratory results

Condition: Given the equipment and supplies as listed in the procedure, and a student to play the part of the physician, the student will review a laboratory reporting form and will handle the results in an appropriate manner, adhering to the steps listed below.

Standards: The student will have 15 minutes to complete the procedure and will need to score an 85% or above to pass the competency. Automatic failure results if any essential steps are omitted or performed incorrectly.

STEPS START TIME: END TIME:	Points Possible	First Attempt	Second Attempt	Third Attempt
1. Reviewed laboratory report form, verified all patient and physician information.	10			
2. Verified all tests ordered were performed and checked results with laboratory reference ranges. Marked any abnormal results if office policy to do so.	10			
3. Immediately reported panic or critical values to the physician.	10			
4. Attached report form to patient's chart and placed on physician's desk for review.	10			
5. Following physician's review, filed report form in patient's chart and reported results to patient according to office protocol.	10			
6. Documented results in lab log as though the student both processed and received the specimen. (Used information on lab report to determine date of draw and name of test.) Documented instructions from physician on what to do with results in patient's chart *(Work Product, Procedure 25-1)*.	10			
7. Completed the procedure within the appropriate time limit.	10			
Points Earned / Points Possible:	___ / 70			

Points possible reflect importance of step in meeting the task: Important = (5) Essential = (10).
Determine score by dividing points earned by total points possible, and multiplying results by 100.

EVALUATION
Evaluator Signature: _____   Date: _____

Evaluator Comments:

DOCUMENTATION
Instructor Note: Retain work products with competency checklist.
Work Product, Procedure 25-1 (Progress Note)

Progress Note for Patient: Date:	**DOUGLASVILLE MEDICINE ASSOCIATES** **5076 BRAND BLVD** **DOUGLASVILLE, NY 01234** **(123) 456-7890**

Key Competencies		
ABHES	VI.A.1.a.4.l	Screen and Follow up Patient Test Results
CAAHEP	III.C.3.b.4.i	Screen and Follow-up Test Results

Student Name: _____   Date: _____   Score: _____

Work Product, Procedure 25-1 (Outstanding Lab Results Tracking Report)

OUTSTANDING LAB RESULTS TRACKING REPORT

Date Sent	Patient Name/ ID	Ordering Provider	Tests Ordered	Number and Type of Specimens Sent to (include tube colors)	Prepared By	Laboratory	Date Results Received	Results Received By

Work Product, Procedure 25-1 (Hematology Report Form)

ABC Laboratory
Hematology Report Form

PHYSICIAN INFORMATION	PATIENT INFORMATION		
DOUGLASVILLE MEDICINE ASSOCIATES **5076 BRAND BLVD** **DOUGLASVILLE, NY 01234** **(123) 456-7890** Ordering Physician: Wm. Green, M.D. Physician ID # 1563524	Name: **Susan Hampton** Address: **2020 Maple Grove Blvd.** City/State/Zip: **Douglasville NY, 01234** Phone #: **(123)456-9988** ID #: **77850**		

Date and Time of Collection	Date and Time of Testing		
10/10/2011 1400	10/10/2011 1830		

Test Ordered	Results	Reference Range	Abnormal Results
Complete Blood Count (CBC):			
White Blood Cell Count		4,500-11,000/cu mm	20,000/cu mm
Red Blood Cell Count	5.0 million/cu mm	M: 4.5-6.0 million/cu mm F: 4.0-5.5/ cu mm	
Hemoglobin	15 gm/dL	M: 13-18 gm/dL F: 12-16 gm/dL	
Hematocrit	45%	M: 42-52% F: 36-45%	
MCV	89 fL	82-98 fL	
MCH	32 pG	26-34 pG	
MCHC	34 g/dL	32-36 g/dL	
Platelet Count	75,000/cu mm	150,000-400,000/ cu mm	
Differential White Blood Cell Count:			
Neutrophilic Bands		0-2%	5%
Neutrophils		40-65%	75%
Eosinophils	0%	1-3%	
Basophils	1%	0-1%	
Lymphocytes		25-40%	10%
Monocytes	9%	3-9%	
RBC Morphology:	normochromic/normocytic		
ID of Technician Conducting the Testing:	**Office Information Received Report on:**	**Received by:**	**Doctor Reviewed and Released for Reporting on:**
20365			

Key Competencies		
ABHES	VI.A.1.a.4.l	Screen and Follow up Patient Test Results
CAAHEP	III.C.3.b.4.i	Screen and Follow-up Test Results

Student Name: _____   Date: _____   Score: _____

Competency Checklist
PROCEDURE 25-2 Specimen Collection for Off-Site Testing

Task: To collect a specimen for off-site testing.

Condition: Given the equipment and supplies as listed in the procedure and a student to play the part of the patient, the student will simulate collecting and processing a lab specimen and will complete a lab requisition form using the student's information, adhering to the steps listed below. The instructor will provide the student with the name(s) of tests to be performed.

Standards: The student will have 15 minutes to complete the procedure and will need to score an 85% or above to pass the competency. Automatic failure results if any essential steps are omitted or performed incorrectly.

Test(s) to be performed: _____

STEPS START TIME: END TIME:	Points Possible	First Attempt	Second Attempt	Third Attempt
1. Verified physician's order in patient's chart and reviewed laboratory guidelines for specimen collection and transport.	10			
2. Assembled the proper equipment and labeled all specimen tubes and containers with the patient's name, date and time of collection, student initials and any other required information from the lab.	10			
3. Washed hands and applied appropriate PPE.	10			
4. Identified the patient using at least two identifiers, identified self, and explained the procedure.	10			
5. Verified compliance of fasting instructions and any medication restrictions with the patient.	10			
6. Properly collected specimen according to laboratory guidelines.	10			
7. Processed and prepared specimen for transport to off-site lab. Completed lab requisition form and included with specimen (*Work Product, Procedure 25-2*).	10			
8. Stored specimen according to the lab's specifications.	10			
9. Documented procedure in patient's chart and lab log (*Work Product, Procedure 25-2*).	10			
10. Completed the procedure within the appropriate time limit.	10			
Points Earned / Points Possible:	___ / 100			

Points possible reflect importance of step in meeting the task: Important = (5) Essential = (10).
Determine score by dividing points earned by total points possible, and multiplying results by 100.

EVALUATION
Evaluator Signature: _____   Date: _____

Evaluator Comments:

Key Competencies			
ABHES	VI.A.1.a.4.j	Collect and Process Specimens	
CAAHEP	III.C.3.b.2	Specimen Collection	

Student Name: _____   Date: _____   Score: _____

DOCUMENTATION

Instructor Note: Retain work products (progress note, lab requisition form, and lab log) with competency checklist.
Work Product, Procedure 25-2 (Progress Note)

Progress Note for Patient: Date:	**DOUGLASVILLE MEDICINE ASSOCIATES** **5076 BRAND BLVD** **DOUGLASVILLE, NY 01234** **(123) 456-7890**

Work Product, Procedure 25-2 (Outside Lab Tracking Log)

OUTSIDE LAB TRACKING LOG

Date Sent	Patient Name/ID	Ordering Provider	Tests Ordered	Number of and Type of Specimens Sent to	Prepared By	Laboratory	Date Results Received	Results Received By

Work Product, Procedure 25-2 (Lab Requisition Form)

Form located on following page.

Key Competencies		
ABHES	VI.A.1.a.4.j	Collect and Process Specimens
CAAHEP	III.C.3.b.2	Specimen Collection

LAB REQUISITION FORM

DILL	PLEASE LEAVE BLANK	C-3 REQUEST FORM	USA Biomedical Labs
☐ ACCOUNT	AREA _____	INSTRUCTIONS ① FOR PATIENT BILLING, COMPLETE BOX A.	957 Central Avenue
☐ PATIENT SEE ①	DEPT. _____	② FOR 3RD PARTY BILLING, COMPLETE BOX A	Heartland, NY 11112
☐ 3RD PARTY SEE ②	BILL CD _____	AND FILL IN DIAGNOSIS, THEN EITHER B, C, or D.	

PATIENT NAME (LAST)   (FIRST)   SPECIES   SEX   AGE YRS. MOS.   DATE COLLECTED MO. DAY YR.   TIME COLLECTED

PATIENT ADDRESS   STREET   MISC. INFORMATION   DR. I.D.   MEDICARE: #

CITY   STATE   ZIP   DIAGNOSIS

PHYSICIAN   WELFARE: #   CASE NAME:

PROGRAM: PATIENT 1ST NAME: DATE OF BIRTH MO. DAY YR.   ALL CLAIMS

INSURANCE GR. #   I.D.   SERVICE CODE:

SUBSCRIBER NAME: RELATION: PHONE

N7708

STANDARD PROFILES

2987 ( )	Diagnostic (Multi-Chem) Profile
2804 ( )	Health Survey (SMA-12)
2824 ( )	Executive Profile A
2825 ( )	Executive Profile B
2826 ( )	Executive Profile C
2858 ( )	Amenorrhea Profile
7330 ( )	Anticonvulsant Group
2927 ( )	Autoimmune Profile
2801 ( )	Calcium Metabolism Profile
2859 ( )	Diabetes Management Profile
7701 ( )	Drug Abuse Screen
( )	Drug Analysis Comprehensive (S & U or G)
( )	Drug Analysis, Qual (U/G)
7340 ( )	Drug Analysis, Quant. (S)
2022 ( )	Electrolyte Profile
( )	Exanthem Group
( )	Glucose/Insulin Response
2871 ( )	Hepatitis Profile I
2872 ( )	Hepatitis Profile II
2873 ( )	Hepatitis Profile III
2874 ( )	Hepatitis Profile IV
2875 ( )	Hepatitis Profile V
2876 ( )	Hepatitis Profile VI
2879 ( )	Hepatitis Profile VII
2864 ( )	Hirsutism Profile
2865 ( )	Hypertension Screen

8350 ( )	Immunologic Evaluation*
2814 ( )	Lipid Profile A
2817 ( )	Lipid Profile B
2003 ( )	Lipid Profile C
2805 ( )	Liver Profile A
2867 ( )	Liver Profile B
2868 ( )	MMR Immunity Panel
2869 ( )	Myocardial Infarction Profile
2585 ( )	Parathyroid Panel A (Mid-Molecule)
2586 ( )	Parathyroid Panel B (Dialysis)
2587 ( )	Parathyroid Panel C (Adenoma)
2818 ( )	Prenatal Profile A
2819 ( )	Prenatal Profile B
2820 ( )	Prenatal Profile C
2877 ( )	Prenatal Profile D
( )	Respiratory Infection Profile A
( )	Respiratory Infection Profile B
( )	Respiratory Infection Profile C
( )	Respiratory Infection Profile D
2821 ( )	Rheumatoid Profile A
2878 ( )	Rheumatoid Profile B
2882 ( )	T & B Lymphocyte Differential Panel
2883 ( )	Testicular Function Profile
2832 ( )	Thyroid Panel A
2032 ( )	Thyroid Panel B
2833 ( )	Thyroid Panel C

SINGLE TESTS

5165 ( )	ABO and Rho (B) (S)
6555 ( )	Alpha-Fetoprotein RIA (S)
3015 ( )	Alk. Phosphatase (S)
3041 ( )	Amylase (S)
5163 ( )	Antibody Screen ( ) If pos. ID & Titer (S) (B)
5166 ( )	Antibody ID (B&S)
5164 ( )	Antibody Titer (B&S) (Previous Pat. # _____)
5208 ( )	ANA. Fluorescent (S)
5169 ( )	ASO Titer (B) (S)
3147 ( )	Bilirubin, Direct (S)
3010 ( )	BUN (S)
3018 ( )	Calcium (S)
6472 ( )	CEA (RIA) (Plasma Only)
2995 ( )	CBC with Automated Diff. (Abnormal Follow-Up Studies) (B) (SL)
2996 ( )	CBC less Diff. (B)
3022 ( )	Cholesterol (S)
3042 ( )	CPK (S)
6500 ( )	Digoxin (S)
6501 ( )	Digitoxin (S)
3606 ( )	GGT (S)
3006 ( )	Glucose (S) Fasting
3009 ( )	Glucose (P) Fasting
3023 ( )	Glucose P.P. (P) Hrs. _____
3650 ( )	HDL Cholesterol (S)
5180 ( )	Heterophile Screen (Mono) (S)
5179 ( )	Heterophile Absorption (S)
3342 ( )	Hemoglobin A_{1C} (B)
6416 ( )	IgE (S)
3078 ( )	Iron and T.I.B.C. (S)

6526 ( )	Neonatal T_4 (S)
6525 ( )	Neonatal TSH (S)
7941 ( )	Neonatal T_4 Blood Spot
3019 ( )	Phosphorus (S)
4132 ( )	Platelet Count (B) (S)
3026 ( )	Potassium (S)
( )	Pregnancy Test, (S or U)
5187 ( )	Premarital RPR (S)
6505 ( )	Prostatic Acid Phosphatase (RIA) (S)*
2992 ( )	Protein Electrophoresis (S) IEP If Abnormal ( ) 9085
4149 ( )	Prothrombin Time (P)*
4144 ( )	Reticulocyte Count (B)
5207 ( )	RA Latex Fixation (S)
5194 ( )	RPR
5195 ( )	Rubella H.I. (S)
3016 ( )	SGOT (S)
3045 ( )	SGPT (S)
3031 ( )	T-3 Uptake (S)
3032 ( )	T-4 (S)
2832 ( )	Thyroxine Index, Free (T_7) (S)
3036 ( )	Triglycerides (S)
4111 ( )	Urinalysis (U)
5277 ( )	Urogenital GC Assay

UNLISTED TESTS OR PROFILES

_____

_____

_____

_____

★ FROZEN   (B) BLOOD   (P) PLASMA   (U) URINE   (S) SERUM   (SL) SLIDES   (Rev. 1-84)

FOLD THIS FORM IN HALF SO TEST(S) ORDERED IS CLEARLY VISIBLE

Student Name: _____   Date: _____   Score: _____

Competency Checklist
PROCEDURE 25-3 Use the Microscope

Task: To properly use the microscope

Condition: Given the equipment and supplies as listed in the procedure, the student will demonstrate the steps that are necessary to properly use and care for a microscope.

Standards: The student will have 15 minutes to complete the procedure and will need to score an 85% or above to pass the competency. Automatic failure results if any essential steps are omitted or performed incorrectly.

STEPS START TIME: END TIME:	Points Possible	First Attempt	Second Attempt	Third Attempt
1. Washed hands, assembled supplies, and applied gloves.	10			
2. Cleaned oculars and objectives with lens paper.	10			
3. Turned on light source and adjusted light to low level.	10			
4. Rotated objectives to the low power objective (10x) and clicked into place.	10			
5. Placed slide on stage, moved stage upward until objective was in its lowest position. (Observed stage movement so objective did not come into contact with slide.)	10			
6. Adjusted oculars to a comfortable width. Viewed slide through oculars and brought specimen into focus using the coarse adjustment knob.	10			
7. Adjusted light intensity, as needed.	10			
8. Brought specimen into sharp, clear focus using fine adjustment knob.	10			
9. Adjusted the stage and rotated to high power objective (40x) and clicked into place. Used course and fine adjustment knobs to bring slide into focus.	10			
10. Adjusted the stage and rotated oil immersion objective (100x) off to the side. Placed a drop of oil onto slide. Rotated objective until it locked in place.	10			
11. Brought specimen into sharp focus using the course and fine adjustment knobs and adjusted light to bright intensity.	10			
12. Following observation, rotated objective to the side and removed slide from stage.	10			
13. Cleaned objectives with lens paper and wiped stage clean with tissue or gauze.	10			
14. Turned off light source and covered scope with dust cover.	10			
15. Completed the procedure within the appropriate time limit.	10			
Points Earned / Points Possible:	___ / 150			

Points possible reflect importance of step in meeting the task: Important = (5) Essential = (10).
Determine score by dividing points earned by total points possible, and multiplying results by 100.

EVALUATION
Evaluator Signature: _____   Date: _____

Evaluator Comments:

Key Competencies		
ABHES		
CAAHEP		

Student Name: _____ Date: _____ Score: _____

Competency Checklist
PROCEDURE 26-1 Venipuncture (Syringe Method)

Task: To perform a venipuncture using the syringe method

Condition: Given the equipment and supplies as listed in the procedure, and a student to play the part of the patient, the student will demonstrate the proper steps for performing a venipuncture using the syringe method, adhering to the steps listed below. Instructor will inform student what tests are to be drawn.

Standards: The student will have 15 minutes to complete the procedure and will need to score an 85% or above to pass the competency. Automatic failure results if any essential steps are omitted or performed incorrectly.

STEPS START TIME: END TIME:	Points Possible	First Attempt	Second Attempt	Third Attempt
1. Verified provider's order and completed lab requisition form.	10			
2. Washed hands and applied PPE.				
3. Assembled equipment, loosened plunger, and labeled tubes.	10			
4. Identified the patient using at least two identifiers, identified self, and explained procedure.	10			
5. Verified compliance of fasting instructions and any other restrictions or special instructions (such as any reason you can't draw blood from one side or the other; the patient has a history of fainting).	10			
6. Visually inspected patient's veins on both arms (asked patient for preference), selected potential site, and applied tourniquet 3–4 inches above the bend of the elbow.	10			
7. Palpated vein, moving index finger up and down the vein to check the direction of the vein.	10			
8. Instructed patient to make a fist and to place fist of other hand under the elbow of the arm being used for blood draw.	5			
9. Cleansed site with alcohol—using a circular motion. Allowed site to air dry or performed a dry wipe over area with a clean/sterile cotton ball or gauze (followed institutional guidelines).	10			
10. Pulled skin taut to anchor vein, inserted needle (bevel up) using a 15- to 30-degree angle. Observed hub for appearance of blood.	10			
11. Once blood appeared in hub, pulled back slowly and steadily on the plunger using hand that anchored the vein.	10			
12. Allowed syringe to fill to desired level and instructed patient to open fist.	10			
13. Released tourniquet, placed dry cotton ball/gauze above the site, removed the needle, and instructed patient to apply firm pressure for 2–5 minutes.	10			
14. Engaged safety device over needle and carefully removed the needle from the syringe; placed immediately in sharps container.	10			
15. Using a safety transfer device, carefully transferred blood from syringe to tubes following manufacturer's instructions and mixed tubes according to laboratory guidelines.	10			
16. Discarded equipment according to OSHA standards, checked puncture site, and applied pressure bandage.	10			
17. Dismissed patient, cleaned work area, removed PPE, and washed hands.	10			

Key Competencies		
ABHES	VI.A.1.a.4.j	Collect and Process Specimens
	VI.A.1.a.4.q	Dispose of Biohazardous Materials
	VI.A.1.a.4.r	Practice Standard Precautions
	VI.A.1.a.4.s	Perform Venipuncture
CAAHEP	III.C.3.b.1.d	Dispose of Biohazardous Materials
	III.C.3.b.1.e	Practice Standard Precautions
	III.C.3.b.2.a	Perform Venipuncture

Student Name: _____   Date: _____   Score: _____

18. Correctly documented procedure on lab requisition form, in patient's chart, and in lab log (*Work Product, Procedure 26-1*).	10			
19. Completed the procedure within the appropriate time limit.	10			
Points Earned / Points Possible:	___ / 175			

Points possible reflect importance of step in meeting the task: Important = (5) Essential = (10).
Determine score by dividing points earned by total points possible, and multiplying results by 100.

EVALUATION
Evaluator Signature: _____   Date: _____

Evaluator Comments:

DOCUMENTATION
Instructor Note: Retain work products with competency checklist.
Work Product, Procedure 26-1 (Progress Note)

Progress Note for Patient: Date:	**DOUGLASVILLE MEDICINE ASSOCIATES** **5076 BRAND BLVD** **DOUGLASVILLE, NY 01234** **(123) 456-7890**

Work Product, Procedure 26-1 (Outstanding Lab Results Tracking Report)

OUTSTANDING LAB RESULTS TRACKING REPORT								
Date Sent	Patient Name/ID	Ordering Provider	Tests Ordered	Number of and Type of Specimens Sent to (include tube colors)	Prepared By	Laboratory	Date Results Received	Results Received By

Work Product, Procedure 26-1 (Lab Requisition Form)

Form located on following page.

Key Competencies		
ABHES	VI.A.1.a.4.j	Collect and Process Specimens
	VI.A.1.a.4.q	Dispose of Biohazardous Materials
	VI.A.1.a.4.r	Practice Standard Precautions
	VI.A.1.a.4.s	Perform Venipuncture
CAAHEP	III.C.3.b.1.d	Dispose of Biohazardous Materials
	III.C.3.b.1.e	Practice Standard Precautions
	III.C.3.b.2.a	Perform Venipuncture

LAB REQUISITION FORM

BILL	PLEASE LEAVE BLANK	C-3 REQUEST FORM	USA Biomedical Labs
☐ ACCOUNT	AREA _____	INSTRUCTIONS ① FOR PATIENT BILLING, COMPLETE BOX A.	957 Central Avenue
☐ PATIENT SEE ①	DEPT. _____	② FOR 3RD PARTY BILLING, COMPLETE BOX A	Heartland, NY 11112
☐ 3RD PARTY SEE ②	BILL CD _____	AND FILL IN DIAGNOSIS, THEN EITHER B, C, or D.	

PATIENT NAME (LAST)	(FIRST)	SPECIES	SEX	AGE YRS. MOS.	DATE COLLECTED MO. DAY YR.	TIME COLLECTED

PATIENT ADDRESS STREET	MISC. INFORMATION	DR. I.D.	MEDICARE: #

CITY STATE ZIP	DIAGNOSIS	WELFARE: #

PHYSICIAN		CASE NAME:

PROGRAM:	PATIENT 1ST NAME:	DATE OF BIRTH MO. DAY YR. ALL CLAIMS

INSURANCE GR. #	I.D.	SERVICE CODE:

SUBSCRIBER NAME:	RELATION: PHONE

N7708

STANDARD PROFILES

2987 ( )	Diagnostic (Multi-Chem) Profile	
2804 ( )	Health Survey (SMA-12)	
2824 ( )	Executive Profile A	
2825 ( )	Executive Profile B	
2826 ( )	Executive Profile C	
2858 ( )	Amenorrhea Profile	
7330 ( )	Anticonvulsant Group	
2927 ( )	Autoimmune Profile	
2801 ( )	Calcium Metabolism Profile	
2859 ( )	Diabetes Management Profile	
7701 ( )	Drug Abuse Screen	
( )	Drug Analysis Comprehensive (S & U or G)	
( )	Drug Analysis, Qual (U/G)	
7340 ( )	Drug Analysis, Quant. (S)	
2022 ( )	Electrolyte Profile	
( )	Exanthem Group	
( )	Glucose/Insulin Response	
2871 ( )	Hepatitis Profile I	
2872 ( )	Hepatitis Profile II	
2873 ( )	Hepatitis Profile III	
2874 ( )	Hepatitis Profile IV	
2875 ( )	Hepatitis Profile V	
2876 ( )	Hepatitis Profile VI	
2879 ( )	Hepatitis Profile VII	
2864 ( )	Hirsutism Profile	
2865 ( )	Hypertension Screen	

8350 ( )	Immunologic Evaluation*
2814 ( )	Lipid Profile A
2817 ( )	Lipid Profile B
2003 ( )	Lipid Profile C
2805 ( )	Liver Profile A
2867 ( )	Liver Profile B
2868 ( )	MMR Immunity Panel
2869 ( )	Myocardial Infarction Profile
2585 ( )	Parathyroid Panel A (Mid-Molecule)
2586 ( )	Parathyroid Panel B (Dialysis)
2587 ( )	Parathyroid Panel C (Adenoma)
2818 ( )	Prenatal Profile A
2819 ( )	Prenatal Profile B
2820 ( )	Prenatal Profile C
2877 ( )	Prenatal Profile D
( )	Respiratory Infection Profile A
( )	Respiratory Infection Profile B
( )	Respiratory Infection Profile C
( )	Respiratory Infection Profile D
2821 ( )	Rheumatoid Profile A
2878 ( )	Rheumatoid Profile B
2882 ( )	T & B Lymphocyte Differential Panel
2883 ( )	Testicular Function Profile
2832 ( )	Thyroid Panel A
2032 ( )	Thyroid Panel B
2833 ( )	Thyroid Panel C

SINGLE TESTS

5165 ( )	ABO and Rho (B) (S)
6555 ( )	Alpha-Fetoprotein RIA (S)
3015 ( )	Alk. Phosphatase (S)
3041 ( )	Amylase (S)
5163 ( )	Antibody Screen ( ) If pos. ID & Titer (S) (B)
5166 ( )	Antibody ID (B&S)
5164 ( )	Antibody Titer (B&S) (Previous Pat. # _____)
5208 ( )	ANA, Fluorescent (S)
5169 ( )	ASO Titer (B) (S)
3147 ( )	Bilirubin, Direct (S)
3010 ( )	BUN (S)
3018 ( )	Calcium (S)
6472 ( )	CEA (RIA) (Plasma Only)
2995 ( )	CBC with Automated Diff. (Abnormal Follow-Up Studies) (B) (SL)
2996 ( )	CBC less Diff. (B)
3022 ( )	Cholesterol (S)
3042 ( )	CPK (S)
6500 ( )	Digoxin (S)
6501 ( )	Digitoxin (S)
3606 ( )	GGT (S)
3006 ( )	Glucose (S) Fasting
3009 ( )	Glucose (P) Fasting
3023 ( )	Glucose P.P. (P) Hrs. _____
3650 ( )	HDL Cholesterol (S)
5180 ( )	Heterophile Screen (Mono) (S)
5179 ( )	Heterophile Absorption (S)
3342 ( )	Hemoglobin A$_{1C}$ (B)
6416 ( )	IgE (S)
3078 ( )	Iron and T.I.B.C. (S)

6526 ( )	Neonatal T$_4$ (S)
6525 ( )	Neonatal TSH (S)
7941 ( )	Neonatal T$_4$ Blood Spot
3019 ( )	Phosphorus (S)
4132 ( )	Platelet Count (B) (S)
3026 ( )	Potassium (S)
( )	Pregnancy Test, (S or U)
5187 ( )	Premarital RPR (S)
6505 ( )	Prostatic Acid Phosphatase (RIA) (S)*
2992 ( )	Protein Electrophoresis (S) IEP if Abnormal ( ) 9085
4149 ( )	Prothrombin Time (P)*
4144 ( )	Reticulocyte Count (B)
5207 ( )	RA Latex Fixation (S)
5194 ( )	RPR
5195 ( )	Rubella H.I. (S)
3016 ( )	SGOT (S)
3045 ( )	SGPT (S)
3031 ( )	T-3 Uptake (S)
3032 ( )	T-4 (S)
2832 ( )	Thyroxine Index, Free (T$_7$) (S)
3036 ( )	Triglycerides (S)
4111 ( )	Urinalysis (U)
5277 ( )	Urogenital GC Assay

UNLISTED TESTS OR PROFILES

_____
_____
_____
_____
_____
_____

★ FROZEN	(B) BLOOD	(P) PLASMA	(U) URINE	(S) SERUM	(SL) SLIDES	(Rev. 1-84)

FOLD THIS FORM IN HALF SO TEST(S) ORDERED IS CLEARLY VISIBLE

Student Name: _____   Date: _____   Score: _____

Competency Checklist
PROCEDURE 26-2 Venipuncture (Vacuum Tube Method)

Task: To perform a venipuncture using the vacuum tube method

Condition: Given the equipment and supplies as listed in the procedure, and a student to play the part of the patient, the student will demonstrate the proper steps for performing a venipuncture using the vacuum tube method, adhering to the steps listed below. Instructor will provide the name of the test(s) to be performed.

Standards: The student will have 10 minutes to complete the procedure and will need to score an 85% or above to pass the competency. Automatic failure results if any essential steps are omitted or performed incorrectly.

STEPS START TIME: END TIME:	Points Possible	First Attempt	Second Attempt	Third Attempt
1. Checked the provider's order and completed lab requisition form.	10			
2. Washed hands and applied PPE.	10			
3. Assembled all necessary equipment and labeled specimen tubes.	10			
4. Identified the patient using at least two identifiers, identified self and explained the procedure.	10			
5. Verified compliance of fasting instructions and other restrictions or problems.	10			
6. Visually inspected patient's veins in both arms (asked patient for preference) selected potential site and applied tourniquet 3–4 inches above the elbow.	10			
7. Asked patient to make a fist and placed other fist under the elbow.	5			
8. Palpated vein and selected site.	10			
9. Cleansed site with alcohol and allowed to air dry or dry wiped area with a clean/sterile cotton ball.	10			
10. Pulled skin taut to anchor. Inserted needle bevel-up/label-down and at a 15- to 30-degree angle.	10			
11. Using hand that anchored vein, grasped flanges of holder and pushed in tube until needle punctured stopper and blood started flowing into the tube.	10			
12. Allowed tube to fill completely before removing.	10			
13. Removed tube and inverted (if tube contained an additive).	10			
14. Continued to change tubes until all tubes were collected.	10			
15. Instructed patient to open fist, released tourniquet, removed final tube, and placed a cotton ball above site before withdrawing the needle.	10			
16. Following needle removal, asked patient to apply firm pressure to site for 2–5 minutes.	10			
17. Engaged safety device; disposed entire unit in sharps container.	10			
18. Discarded equipment according to OSHA standards, checked puncture site, and applied pressure bandage.	10			
19. Dismissed patient; cleaned work area; removed gloves; washed hands.	10			
20. Correctly documented procedure on lab requisition form, in patient's chart, and in lab log (*Work Product, Procedure 26-2*).	10			
21. Completed the procedure within the appropriate time limit.				

Key Competencies			
ABHES	VI.A.1.a.4.j	Collect and Process Specimens	
	VI.A.1.a.4.q	Dispose of Biohazardous Materials	
	VI.A.1.a.4.r	Practice Standard Precautions	
	VI.A.1.a.4.s	Perform Venipuncture	
CAAHEP	III.C.3.b.1.d	Dispose of Biohazardous Materials	
	III.C.3.b.1.e	Practice Standard Precautions	
	III.C.3.b.2.a	Perform Venipuncture	

Student Name: _____   Date: _____   Score: _____

	Points Earned / Points Possible:	___/190		

Points possible reflect importance of step in meeting the task: Important = (5) Essential = (10).
Determine score by dividing points earned by total points possible, and multiplying results by 100.

EVALUATION

Evaluator Signature: _____   Date: _____

Evaluator Comments:

DOCUMENTATION

Instructor Note: Retain work products with competency checklist.
Work Product, Procedure 26-2 (Progress Note)

Progress Note for Patient: Date:	**DOUGLASVILLE MEDICINE ASSOCIATES** **5076 BRAND BLVD** **DOUGLASVILLE, NY 01234** **(123) 456-7890**

Work Product, Procedure 26-2 (Outstanding Lab Results Tracking Report)

	OUTSTANDING LAB RESULTS TRACKING REPORT							
Date Sent	Patient Name/ ID	Ordering Provider	Tests Ordered	Number and Type of Specimens Sent to (include tube colors)	Prepared By	Laboratory	Date Results Received	Results Received By

Work Product, Procedure 26-2 (Lab Requisition Form)

Form located on following page.

Key Competencies			
ABHES	VI.A.1.a.4.j	Collect and Process Specimens	
	VI.A.1.a.4.q	Dispose of Biohazardous Materials	
	VI.A.1.a.4.r	Practice Standard Precautions	
	VI.A.1.a.4.s	Perform Venipuncture	
CAAHEP	III.C.3.b.1.d	Dispose of Biohazardous Materials	
	III.C.3.b.1.e	Practice Standard Precautions	
	III.C.3.b.2.a	Perform Venipuncture	

LAB REQUISITION FORM

BILL	PLEASE LEAVE BLANK	C-3 REQUEST FORM	USA Biomedical Labs

BILL
☐ ACCOUNT
☐ PATIENT SEE ①
☐ 3RD PARTY SEE ②

PLEASE LEAVE BLANK
AREA _____
DEPT. _____
BILL CD _____

C-3 REQUEST FORM
INSTRUCTIONS ① FOR PATIENT BILLING, COMPLETE BOX A.
② FOR 3RD PARTY BILLING, COMPLETE BOX A AND FILL IN DIAGNOSIS, THEN EITHER B, C, or D.

USA Biomedical Labs
957 Central Avenue
Heartland, NY 11112

PATIENT NAME (LAST) (FIRST) SPECIES SEX AGE YRS. MOS. DATE COLLECTED MO. DAY YR. TIME COLLECTED

PATIENT ADDRESS STREET MISC. INFORMATION DR. I.D. MEDICARE: #

CITY STATE ZIP DIAGNOSIS WELFARE: # CASE NAME:

PHYSICIAN PROGRAM: PATIENT 1ST NAME: DATE OF BIRTH MO. DAY YR. ALL CLAIMS

INSURANCE I.D. SERVICE CODE:
GR. #
SUBSCRIBER NAME: RELATION: PHONE

STANDARD PROFILES

2987 ( ) Diagnostic (Multi-Chem) Profile	8350 ( ) Immunologic Evaluation*
2804 ( ) Health Survey (SMA-12)	2814 ( ) Lipid Profile A
2824 ( ) Executive Profile A	2817 ( ) Lipid Profile B
2825 ( ) Executive Profile B	2003 ( ) Lipid Profile C
2826 ( ) Executive Profile C	2805 ( ) Liver Profile A
2858 ( ) Amenorrhea Profile	2867 ( ) Liver Profile B
7330 ( ) Anticonvulsant Group	2868 ( ) MMR Immunity Panel
2927 ( ) Autoimmune Profile	2869 ( ) Myocardial Infarction Profile
2801 ( ) Calcium Metabolism Profile	2585 ( ) Parathyroid Panel A (Mid-Molecule)
2859 ( ) Diabetes Management Profile	2586 ( ) Parathyroid Panel B (Dialysis)
7701 ( ) Drug Abuse Screen	2587 ( ) Parathyroid Panel C (Adenoma)
( ) Drug Analysis Comprehensive (S & U or G)	2818 ( ) Prenatal Profile A
	2819 ( ) Prenatal Profile B
( ) Drug Analysis, Qual (U/G)	2820 ( ) Prenatal Profile C
7340 ( ) Drug Analysis, Quant. (S)	2877 ( ) Prenatal Profile D
2022 ( ) Electrolyte Profile	( ) Respiratory Infection Profile A
( ) Exanthem Group	( ) Respiratory Infection Profile B
( ) Glucose/Insulin Response	( ) Respiratory Infection Profile C
	( ) Respiratory Infection Profile D
2871 ( ) Hepatitis Profile I	2821 ( ) Rheumatoid Profile A
2872 ( ) Hepatitis Profile II	2878 ( ) Rheumatoid Profile B
2873 ( ) Hepatitis Profile III	2882 ( ) T & B Lymphocyte Differential Panel
2874 ( ) Hepatitis Profile IV	
2875 ( ) Hepatitis Profile V	2883 ( ) Testicular Function Profile
2876 ( ) Hepatitis Profile VI	2032 ( ) Thyroid Panel A
2879 ( ) Hepatitis Profile VII	2032 ( ) Thyroid Panel B
2864 ( ) Hirsutism Profile	2833 ( ) Thyroid Panel C
2865 ( ) Hypertension Screen	

SINGLE TESTS

5165 ( ) ABO and Rho (B) (S)	6526 ( ) Neonatal T4 (S)
6555 ( ) Alpha-Fetoprotein RIA (S)	6525 ( ) Neonatal TSH (S)
3015 ( ) Alk. Phosphatase (S)	7941 ( ) Neonatal T4 Blood Spot
3041 ( ) Amylase (S)	3019 ( ) Phosphorus (S)
5163 ( ) Antibody Screen ( ) If pos. ID & Titer (S) (B)	4132 ( ) Platelet Count (B) (S)
5166 ( ) Antibody ID (B&S)	3026 ( ) Potassium (S)
5164 ( ) Antibody Titer (B&S) (Previous Pat. #_____)	( ) Pregnancy Test, (S or U)
	5187 ( ) Premarital RPR (S)
5208 ( ) ANA. Fluorescent (S)	6505 ( ) Prostatic Acid Phosphatase (RIA) (S)*
5169 ( ) ASO Titer (B) (S)	2992 ( ) Protein Electrophoresis (S) IEP if Abnormal ( ) 9085
3147 ( ) Bilirubin, Direct (S)	4149 ( ) Prothrombin Time (P)*
3010 ( ) BUN (S)	4144 ( ) Reticulocyte Count (B)
3018 ( ) Calcium (S)	5207 ( ) RA Latex Fixation (S)
6472 ( ) CEA (RIA) (Plasma Only)	5194 ( ) RPR
2995 ( ) CBC with Automated Diff. (Abnormal Follow-Up Studies) (B) (SL)	5195 ( ) Rubella H.I. (S)
	3016 ( ) SGOT (S)
2996 ( ) CBC less Diff. (B)	3045 ( ) SGPT (S)
3022 ( ) Cholesterol (S)	3031 ( ) T-3 Uptake (S)
3042 ( ) CPK (S)	3032 ( ) T-4 (S)
6500 ( ) Digoxin (S)	2832 ( ) Thyroxine Index, Free (T7) (S)
6501 ( ) Digitoxin (S)	3036 ( ) Triglycerides (S)
3606 ( ) GGT (S)	4111 ( ) Urinalysis (U)
3006 ( ) Glucose (S) Fasting	5277 ( ) Urogenital GC Assay
3009 ( ) Glucose (P) Fasting	**UNLISTED TESTS OR PROFILES**
3023 ( ) Glucose P.P. (P) Hrs. _____	_____
3650 ( ) HDL Cholesterol (S)	_____
5180 ( ) Heterophile Screen (Mono) (S)	_____
5179 ( ) Heterophile Absorption (S)	_____
3342 ( ) Hemoglobin A1C (B)	_____
6416 ( ) IgE (S)	_____
3078 ( ) Iron and T.I.B.C. (S)	

★ FROZEN (B) BLOOD (P) PLASMA (U) URINE (S) SERUM (SL) SLIDES (Rev. 1-84)

FOLD THIS FORM IN HALF SO TEST(S) ORDERED IS CLEARLY VISIBLE

Student Name: _____   Date: _____   Score: _____

Competency Checklist
PROCEDURE 26-3 Venipuncture (Butterfly Method)

Task: To perform a venipuncture using the butterfly method

Condition: Given the equipment and supplies as listed in the procedure, and a student to play the part of the patient, the student will demonstrate the proper steps for performing a venipuncture using the butterfly method, adhering to the steps listed below. Instructor will provide the name of the test(s) to be performed.

Standards: The student will have 10 minutes to complete the procedure and will need to score an 85% or above to pass the competency. Automatic failure results if any essential steps are omitted or performed incorrectly.

STEPS START TIME: END TIME:	Points Possible	First Attempt	Second Attempt	Third Attempt
1. Checked provider's order and completed lab requisition form.	10			
2. Washed hands and applied PPE.	10			
3. Assembled all necessary equipment and labeled specimen tubes.	10			
4. Identified the patient using at least two identifiers, identified self, and explained procedure.	10			
5. Verified compliance of fasting instructions and other restrictions.	10			
6. Visually inspected patient's veins in both arms or hands; asked patient about preference. Selected arm/hand and applied tourniquet 3–4 inches above elbow (if arm stick) or above wrist (if hand stick).	10			
7. Had patient make a slight fist in the arm or hand being stuck, and to place other fist under the elbow (if arm stick) and under the wrist (if hand stick).	5			
8. Palpated vein—selecting final site.	10			
9. Cleansed site with alcohol and allowed to air dry or dry wiped area with clean/sterile cotton ball.	10			
10. Pulled skin taut, grasped wings of butterfly and inserted needle, bevel-up, at a 5- to 10-degree angle.	10			
Vacuum tube method:				
11. Once blood entered tubing, pushed tube onto needle inside tube adapter and allowed to fill completely. Removed tube and inverted several times if tube contained an additive.	10			
12. Inserted last tube and allowed to completely fill. Instructed patient to open fist, released tourniquet, removed tube, applied cotton ball above site, and withdrew the needle—engaged safety device.	10			
Syringe method:				
11. Once blood entered tubing, started pulling back on the plunger until syringe was completely full. Instructed patient to open fist, released tourniquet, placed a cotton ball above the site, and withdrew the needle.	10			
12. Engaged safety device and removed needle, placing it immediately into the sharps container. Filled tubes using a safety device.	10			
For both types:				
13. Asked patient to apply firm pressure over cotton ball for 2–5 minutes.	10			

Key Competencies			
ABHES	VI.A.1.a.4.j	Collect and Process Specimens	
	VI.A.1.a.4.q	Dispose of Biohazardous Materials	
	VI.A.1.a.4.r	Practice Standard Precautions	
	VI.A.1.a.4.s	Perform Venipuncture	
CAAHEP	III.C.3.b.1.d	Dispose of Biohazardous Materials	
	III.C.3.b.1.e	Practice Standard Precautions	
	III.C.3.b.2.a	Perform Venipuncture	

Student Name: _____   Date: _____   Score: _____

14. Discarded equipment according to OSHA standards, checked puncture site, and applied pressure bandage.	10				
15. Dismissed patient, cleaned work area, removed gloves, and washed hands.					
16. Correctly documented procedure on lab requisition form, in patient's chart, and in lab log.	10				
17. Completed the procedure within the appropriate time limit.	10				
Points Earned / Points Possible:	___ / 155				

Points possible reflect importance of step in meeting the task: Important = (5) Essential = (10).
Determine score by dividing points earned by total points possible, and multiplying results by 100.

EVALUATION
Evaluator Signature: _____   Date: _____

Evaluator Comments:

DOCUMENTATION
Instructor Note: Retain work products with competency checklist.
Work Product, Procedure 26-3 (Progress Note)

Progress Note for Patient: Date:	**DOUGLASVILLE MEDICINE ASSOCIATES** **5076 BRAND BLVD** **DOUGLASVILLE, NY 01234** **(123) 456-7890**

Work Product, Procedure 26-3 (Outside Lab Tracking Log)

OUTSIDE LAB TRACKING LOG								
Date Sent	Patient Name/ ID	Ordering Provider	Tests Ordered	Number and Type of Specimens Sent to (include tube colors)	Prepared By	Laboratory	Date Results Received	Results Received By

Work Product, Procedure 26-3 (Lab Requisition Form)

Form located on following page.

Key Competencies		
ABHES	VI.A.1.a.4.j	Collect and Process Specimens
	VI.A.1.a.4.q	Dispose of Biohazardous Materials
	VI.A.1.a.4.r	Practice Standard Precautions
	VI.A.1.a.4.s	Perform Venipuncture
CAAHEP	III.C.3.b.1.d	Dispose of Biohazardous Materials
	III.C.3.b.1.e	Practice Standard Precautions
	III.C.3.b.2.a	Perform Venipuncture

LAB REQUISITION FORM

BILL		PLEASE LEAVE BLANK		C-3 REQUEST FORM				

BILL
- ☐ ACCOUNT
- ☐ PATIENT   SEE ①
- ☐ 3RD PARTY SEE ②

PLEASE LEAVE BLANK
AREA _____
DEPT. _____
BILL CD _____

C-3 REQUEST FORM
INSTRUCTIONS ① FOR PATIENT BILLING, COMPLETE BOX A.
② FOR 3RD PARTY BILLING, COMPLETE BOX A AND FILL IN DIAGNOSIS, THEN EITHER B, C, or D.

USA Biomedical Labs
957 Central Avenue
Heartland, NY 11112

PATIENT NAME (LAST) _____ (FIRST) _____ SPECIES SEX AGE YRS. MOS. DATE COLLECTED MO. DAY YR. TIME COLLECTED

PATIENT ADDRESS   STREET   MISC. INFORMATION   DR. I.D.   MEDICARE: #

CITY   STATE   ZIP   DIAGNOSIS

PHYSICIAN   WELFARE: #   CASE NAME:

PROGRAM: PATIENT 1ST NAME: DATE OF BIRTH ALL CLAIMS   MO. DAY YR.

INSURANCE   I.D.   SERVICE CODE:
GR. #

SUBSCRIBER   RELATION: PHONE
NAME: ___ ___

N7708

STANDARD PROFILES

2987	( )	Diagnostic (Multi-Chem) Profile
2804	( )	Health Survey (SMA-12)
2824	( )	Executive Profile A
2825	( )	Executive Profile B
2826	( )	Executive Profile C
2858	( )	Amenorrhea Profile
7330	( )	Anticonvulsant Group
2927	( )	Autoimmune Profile
2801	( )	Calcium Metabolism Profile
2859	( )	Diabetes Management Profile
7701	( )	Drug Abuse Screen
	( )	Drug Analysis Comprehensive (S & U or G)
	( )	Drug Analysis, Qual (U/G)
7340	( )	Drug Analysis, Quant. (S)
2022	( )	Electrolyte Profile
	( )	Exanthem Group
	( )	Glucose/Insulin Response
2871	( )	Hepatitis Profile I
2872	( )	Hepatitis Profile II
2873	( )	Hepatitis Profile III
2874	( )	Hepatitis Profile IV
2875	( )	Hepatitis Profile V
2876	( )	Hepatitis Profile VI
2879	( )	Hepatitis Profile VII
2864	( )	Hirsutism Profile
2865	( )	Hypertension Screen

8350	( )	Immunologic Evaluation*
2814	( )	Lipid Profile A
2817	( )	Lipid Profile B
2003	( )	Lipid Profile C
2805	( )	Liver Profile A
2867	( )	Liver Profile B
2868	( )	MMR Immunity Panel
2869	( )	Myocardial Infarction Profile
2585	( )	Parathyroid Panel A (Mid-Molecule)
2586	( )	Parathyroid Panel B (Dialysis)
2587	( )	Parathyroid Panel C (Adenoma)
2818	( )	Prenatal Profile A
2819	( )	Prenatal Profile B
2820	( )	Prenatal Profile C
2877	( )	Prenatal Profile D
	( )	Respiratory Infection Profile A
	( )	Respiratory Infection Profile B
	( )	Respiratory Infection Profile C
	( )	Respiratory Infection Profile D
2821	( )	Rheumatoid Profile A
2878	( )	Rheumatoid Profile B
2882	( )	T & B Lymphocyte Differential Panel
2883	( )	Testicular Function Profile
2832	( )	Thyroid Panel A
2032	( )	Thyroid Panel B
2833	( )	Thyroid Panel C

SINGLE TESTS

5165	( )	ABO and Rho (B) (S)
6555	( )	Alpha-Fetoprotein RIA (S)
3015	( )	Alk. Phosphatase (S)
3041	( )	Amylase (S)
5163	( )	Antibody Screen ( ) If pos. ID & Titer (S) (B)
5166	( )	Antibody ID (B&S)
5164	( )	Antibody Titer (B&S) (Previous Pat. #_____)
5208	( )	ANA. Fluorescent (S)
5169	( )	ASO Titer (B) (S)
3147	( )	Bilirubin, Direct (S)
3010	( )	BUN (S)
3018	( )	Calcium (S)
6472	( )	CEA (RIA) (Plasma Only)
2995	( )	CBC with Automated Diff. (Abnormal Follow-Up Studies) (B) (SL)
2996	( )	CBC less Diff. (B)
3022	( )	Cholesterol (S)
3042	( )	CPK (S)
6500	( )	Digoxin (S)
6501	( )	Digitoxin (S)
3606	( )	GGT (S)
3006	( )	Glucose (S) Fasting
3009	( )	Glucose (P) Fasting
3023	( )	Glucose P.P. (P) Hrs. ____
3650	( )	HDL Cholesterol (S)
5180	( )	Heterophile Screen (Mono) (S)
5179	( )	Heterophile Absorption (S)
3342	( )	Hemoglobin A$_{1C}$ (B)
6416	( )	IgE (S)
3078	( )	Iron and T.I.B.C. (S)

6526	( )	Neonatal T$_4$ (S)
6525	( )	Neonatal TSH (S)
7941	( )	Neonatal T$_4$ Blood Spot
3019	( )	Phosphorus (S)
4132	( )	Platelet Count (B) (S)
3026	( )	Potassium (S)
	( )	Pregnancy Test, (S or U)
5187	( )	Premarital RPR (S)
6505	( )	Prostatic Acid Phosphatase (RIA) (S)*
2992	( )	Protein Electrophoresis (S) IEP if Abnormal ( ) 9085
4149	( )	Prothrombin Time (P)*
4144	( )	Reticulocyte Count (B)
5207	( )	RA Latex Fixation (S)
5194	( )	RPR
5195	( )	Rubella H.I. (S)
3016	( )	SGOT (S)
3045	( )	SGPT (S)
3031	( )	T-3 Uptake (S)
3032	( )	T-4 (S)
2832	( )	Thyroxine Index, Free (T$_7$) (S)
3036	( )	Triglycerides (S)
4111	( )	Urinalysis (U)
5277	( )	Urogenital GC Assay

UNLISTED TESTS OR PROFILES

_____
_____
_____
_____
_____

* FROZEN	(B) BLOOD	(P) PLASMA	(U) URINE	(S) SERUM	(SL) SLIDES	(Rev. 1-84)

FOLD THIS FORM IN HALF SO TEST(S) ORDERED IS CLEARLY VISIBLE

Student Name: _____   Date: _____   Score: _____

Competency Checklist
PROCEDURE 26-4 Perform a Capillary Puncture

Task: To perform a capillary puncture

Condition: Given the equipment and supplies as listed in the procedure, and a student to play the part of the patient, the student will demonstrate the proper steps for performing a capillary puncture, adhering to the steps listed below. This specimen will be sent out for testing. Instructor will provide the name of the test(s) to be performed.

Standards: The student will have 10 minutes to complete the procedure and will need to score an 85% or above to pass the competency. Automatic failure results if any essential steps are omitted or performed incorrectly.

STEPS START TIME: END TIME:	Points Possible	First Attempt	Second Attempt	Third Attempt
1. Checked provider's order to determine the test(s) to be performed. Completed lab requisition form.	10			
2. Washed hands, gloved, and applied PPE.	10			
3. Assembled necessary equipment and labeled tubes (if applicable).	10			
4. Identified the patient using at least two identifiers, identified self and explained the procedure.	10			
5. Selected the fleshy portion of the patient's distal middle or ring finger on the non-dominant hand.	10			
6. Had patient run hands under warm water or applied warm compress to the site if fingers were cold.	10			
7. Cleaned the site with alcohol (using a circular motion); allowed site to air dry.	10			
8. Grasped finger securely, and punctured fingertip at a right angle to fingerprint.	10			
9. Disposed lancet in sharps container according to OSHA guidelines.	10			
10. Wiped away first drop of blood with gauze or cotton ball. Applied gentle pressure to site by gently squeezing and releasing the fingertip.	10			
11. Collected needed samples in micro-collection tubes following the manufacturer's instructions.	10			
12. Instructed patient to apply pressure to puncture site with a clean, dry cotton ball or gauze square.	10			
13. Checked puncture site and applied adhesive bandage.	10			
14. Dismissed patient, properly disposed of all contaminated equipment, and cleaned work area.	10			
15. Removed gloves, washed hands, and documented procedure on lab requisition form, in patient's chart, and in lab log (*Work Product, Procedure 26-4*).	10			
16. Completed the procedure within the appropriate time limit.	10			
Points Earned / Points Possible:	___ / 160			

Points possible reflect importance of step in meeting the task: Important = (5) Essential = (10).
Determine score by dividing points earned by total points possible, and multiplying results by 100.

Key Competencies		
ABHES	VI.A.1.a.4.j	Collect and Process Specimens
	VI.A.1.a.4.q	Dispose of Biohazardous Materials
	VI.A.1.a.4.r	Practice Standard Precautions
	VI.A.1.a.4.t	Perform Capillary Puncture
CAAHEP	III.C.3.b.1.d	Dispose of Biohazardous Materials
	III.C.3.b.1.e	Practice Standard Precautions
	III.C.3.b.2.b	Perform Capillary Puncture

Student Name: _____   Date: _____   Score: _____

EVALUATION
Evaluator Signature: _____   Date: _____

Evaluator Comments:

DOCUMENTATION
Instructor Note: Retain work products with competency checklist.
Work Product, Procedure 26-4 (Progress Note)

Progress Note for Patient: Date:	**DOUGLASVILLE MEDICINE ASSOCIATES** **5076 BRAND BLVD** **DOUGLASVILLE, NY 01234** **(123) 456-7890**

Work Product, Procedure 26-4 (Outstanding Lab Results Tracking Report)

OUTSTANDING LAB RESULTS TRACKING REPORT

Date	Patient Name/ ID	Ordering Provider	Tests Ordered	Number and Type of Specimens Sent to (include tube colors)	Prepared By	Laboratory	Date Results Received	Results Received By

Work Product, Procedure 26-4 (Lab Requisition Form)

Form located on following page.

Key Competencies		
ABHES	VI.A.1.a.4.j	Collect and Process Specimens
	VI.A.1.a.4.q	Dispose of Biohazardous Materials
	VI.A.1.a.4.r	Practice Standard Precautions
	VI.A.1.a.4.t	Perform Capillary Puncture
CAAHEP	III.C.3.b.1.d	Dispose of Biohazardous Materials
	III.C.3.b.1.e	Practice Standard Precautions
	III.C.3.b.2.b	Perform Capillary Puncture

LAB REQUISITION FORM

BILL	PLEASE LEAVE BLANK	C-3 REQUEST FORM	USA Biomedical Labs

BILL
☐ ACCOUNT
☐ PATIENT   SEE ①
☐ 3RD PARTY SEE ②

PLEASE LEAVE BLANK
AREA _____
DEPT. _____
BILL CD _____

C-3 REQUEST FORM
INSTRUCTIONS ① FOR PATIENT BILLING, COMPLETE BOX A.
② FOR 3RD PARTY BILLING, COMPLETE BOX A AND FILL IN DIAGNOSIS, THEN EITHER B, C, or D.

USA Biomedical Labs
957 Central Avenue
Heartland, NY 11112

PATIENT NAME (LAST) .... (FIRST) .... SPECIES | SEX | AGE YRS. MOS. | DATE COLLECTED MO. DAY YR. | TIME COLLECTED

PATIENT ADDRESS .... STREET .... MISC. INFORMATION .... DR. I.D. .... MEDICARE: #

CITY .... STATE .... ZIP | DIAGNOSIS

PHYSICIAN .... WELFARE: # .... CASE NAME:

PROGRAM: .... PATIENT 1ST NAME: .... DATE OF BIRTH MO. DAY YR. ALL CLAIMS

INSURANCE .... I.D. .... SERVICE CODE:
GR. #

SUBSCRIBER NAME: .... RELATION: PHONE

N7706

STANDARD PROFILES

2987 ( ) Diagnostic (Multi-Chem) Profile	8350 ( ) Immunologic Evaluation*
2804 ( ) Health Survey (SMA-12)	2814 ( ) Lipid Profile A
2824 ( ) Executive Profile A	2817 ( ) Lipid Profile B
2825 ( ) Executive Profile B	2003 ( ) Lipid Profile C
2826 ( ) Executive Profile C	2805 ( ) Liver Profile A
2858 ( ) Amenorrhea Profile	2867 ( ) Liver Profile B
7330 ( ) Anticonvulsant Group	2868 ( ) MMR Immunity Panel
2927 ( ) Autoimmune Profile	2869 ( ) Myocardial Infarction Profile
2801 ( ) Calcium Metabolism Profile	2585 ( ) Parathyroid Panel A (Mid-Molecule)
2859 ( ) Diabetes Management Profile	2586 ( ) Parathyroid Panel B (Dialysis)
7701 ( ) Drug Abuse Screen	2587 ( ) Parathyroid Panel C (Adenoma)
( ) Drug Analysis Comprehensive (S & U or G)	2818 ( ) Prenatal Profile A
	2819 ( ) Prenatal Profile B
( ) Drug Analysis, Qual (U/G)	2820 ( ) Prenatal Profile C
7340 ( ) Drug Analysis, Quant. (S)	2877 ( ) Prenatal Profile D
2022 ( ) Electrolyte Profile	( ) Respiratory Infection Profile A
( ) Exanthem Group	( ) Respiratory Infection Profile B
( ) Glucose/Insulin Response	( ) Respiratory Infection Profile C
2871 ( ) Hepatitis Profile I	( ) Respiratory Infection Profile D
2872 ( ) Hepatitis Profile II	2821 ( ) Rheumatoid Profile A
2873 ( ) Hepatitis Profile III	2878 ( ) Rheumatoid Profile B
2874 ( ) Hepatitis Profile IV	2882 ( ) T & B Lymphocyte Differential Panel
2875 ( ) Hepatitis Profile V	
2876 ( ) Hepatitis Profile VI	2883 ( ) Testicular Function Profile
2879 ( ) Hepatitis Profile VII	2832 ( ) Thyroid Panel A
2864 ( ) Hirsutism Profile	2032 ( ) Thyroid Panel B
2865 ( ) Hypertension Screen	2833 ( ) Thyroid Panel C

SINGLE TESTS

5165 ( ) ABO and Rho (B) (S)	6526 ( ) Neonatal T_4 (S)
6555 ( ) Alpha-Fetoprotein RIA (S)	6525 ( ) Neonatal TSH (S)
3015 ( ) Alk. Phosphatase (S)	7941 ( ) Neonatal T_4 Blood Spot
3041 ( ) Amylase (S)	3019 ( ) Phosphorus (S)
5163 ( ) Antibody Screen ( ) If pos. ID & Titer (B) (B)	4132 ( ) Platelet Count (B) (S)
5166 ( ) Antibody ID (B&S)	3026 ( ) Potassium (S)
5164 ( ) Antibody Titer (B&S)	( ) Pregnancy Test, (S or U)
(Previous Pat. #_____)	5187 ( ) Premarital RPR (S)
5208 ( ) ANA. Fluorescent (S)	6505 ( ) Prostatic Acid Phosphatase (RIA) (S)*
5169 ( ) ASO Titer (B) (S)	2992 ( ) Protein Electrophoresis (S) IEP If Abnormal ( ) 9085
3147 ( ) Bilirubin, Direct (S)	4149 ( ) Prothrombin Time (P)*
3010 ( ) BUN (S)	4144 ( ) Reticulocyte Count (B)
3018 ( ) Calcium (S)	5207 ( ) RA Latex Fixation (S)
6472 ( ) CEA (RIA) (Plasma Only)	5194 ( ) RPR
2995 ( ) CBC with Automated Diff. (Abnormal Follow-Up Studies) (B) (SL)	5195 ( ) Rubella H.I. (S)
2996 ( ) CBC less Diff. (B)	3016 ( ) SGOT (S)
3022 ( ) Cholesterol (S)	3045 ( ) SGPT (S)
3042 ( ) CPK (S)	3031 ( ) T-3 Uptake (S)
6500 ( ) Digoxin (S)	3032 ( ) T-4 (S)
6501 ( ) Digitoxin (S)	2832 ( ) Thyroxine Index, Free (T_7) (S)
3606 ( ) GGT (S)	3036 ( ) Triglycerides (S)
3006 ( ) Glucose (S) Fasting	4111 ( ) Urinalysis (U)
3009 ( ) Glucose (P) Fasting	5277 ( ) Urogenital GC Assay
3023 ( ) Glucose P.P. (P) Hrs. _____	UNLISTED TESTS OR PROFILES
3650 ( ) HDL Cholesterol (S)	_____
5180 ( ) Heterophile Screen (Mono) (S)	_____
5179 ( ) Heterophile Absorption (S)	_____
3342 ( ) Hemoglobin A_{1C} (B)	_____
6416 ( ) IgE (S)	_____
3078 ( ) Iron and T.I.B.C. (S)	_____

* FROZEN   (B) BLOOD   (P) PLASMA   (U) URINE   (S) SERUM   (SL) SLIDES   (Rev. 1-84)

FOLD THIS FORM IN HALF SO TEST(S) ORDERED IS CLEARLY VISIBLE

Student Name: _____   Date: _____   Score: _____

Competency Checklist
PROCEDURE 27-1 Instruct a Patient on a Clean-Catch Midstream Urine Collection

Task: To instruct a patient on a clean-catch midstream urine collection

Condition: Given the equipment and supplies as listed in the procedure, and a student to play the part of the patient, the student will demonstrate the proper steps for instructing a patient on how to obtain a clean-catch midstream urine specimen, adhering to the steps listed below.

Standards: The student will have 10 minutes to complete the procedure and will need to score an 85% or above to pass the competency. Automatic failure results if any essential steps are omitted or performed incorrectly.

STEPS START TIME: END TIME:	Points Possible	First Attempt	Second Attempt	Third Attempt
1. Washed hands and assembled necessary equipment.	10			
2. Identified the patient using at least two identifiers, identified self, and explained collection procedure.	10			
3. Gave patient gloves, towelettes, and labeled specimen cup with lid.	10			
Instructions Given to Both Males and Females:				
4. Wash your hands, apply gloves and open towelettes. (Gloves are optional.)	10			
Instructions Given to Females:				
5. Spread labia apart with one hand to expose urinary meatus, wipe down right side from front to back with one towelette, wipe down left side from front to back with another towelette, and wipe down middle of meatus with a third towelette. Discard each towelette in toilet after use. Keep the labia folds retracted throughout the procedure.	10			
Instructions Given to Males:				
5. Retract foreskin and cleanse the tip of the urethral opening from the tip of the penis toward the ring of the glans with two separate towelettes before beginning collection. Keep foreskin retracted throughout the procedure.	10			
Instructions Given to Both Males and Females:				
6. Begin flow in the toilet and switch to specimen cup. Catch the middle portion of the urine flow in the cup, and finish urinating in the toilet.	10			
7. Place lid on specimen container, wipe the outside of container with a paper towel, and leave specimen in designated area.	10			
8. Instructed patient to remove their gloves and place them in a biohazard waste container and wash hands.	10			
9. Obtained specimen and followed physician's orders.	10			
10. Removed gloves, washed hands, and documented collection in patient's chart (*Work Product, Procedure 27-1*).	10			
11. Completed the procedure within the appropriate time limit.	10			
Points Earned / Points Possible:	___ / 110			

Points possible reflect importance of step in meeting the task: Important = (5) Essential = (10).
Determine score by dividing points earned by total points possible, and multiplying results by 100.

Key Competencies		
ABHES	VI.A.1.a.4.j	Collect and Process Specimens
	VI.A.1.a.4.r	Practice Standard Precautions
CAAHEP	III.C.3.b.1.e	Dispose of Biohazardous Materials
	III.C.3.b.1.d	Instruct Patients in the Collection of a Clean-Catch Mid-Stream Urine Specimen

Student Name: _____   Date: _____   Score: _____

EVALUATION
Evaluator Signature: _____   Date: _____

Evaluator Comments:

DOCUMENTATION
Instructor Note: Retain work products with competency checklist.
Work Product, Procedure 27-1 (Progress Note)

Progress Note for Patient: Date:	**DOUGLASVILLE MEDICINE ASSOCIATES** **5076 BRAND BLVD** **DOUGLASVILLE, NY 01234** **(123) 456-7890**

Key Competencies		
ABHES	VI.A.1.a.4.j	Collect and Process Specimens
	VI.A.1.a.4.r	Practice Standard Precautions
CAAHEP	III.C.3.b.1.e	Dispose of Biohazardous Materials
	III.C.3.b.1.d	Instruct Patients in the Collection of a Clean-Catch Mid-Stream Urine Specimen

Student Name: _____   Date: _____   Score: _____

Competency Checklist
PROCEDURE 27-2 Perform A Physical and Chemical Urinalysis and Prepare a Slide for the Provider

Task: To perform a physical and chemical urinalysis and prepare a slide for microscopic examination

Condition: Given the equipment and supplies as listed in the procedure, and a urine specimen to test, the student will demonstrate the proper steps for performing a physical and chemical urinalysis and preparing a slide for microscopic examination, adhering to the steps listed below.

Standards: The student will have 15 minutes to complete the procedure and will need to score an 85% or above to pass the competency. Automatic failure results if any essential steps are omitted or performed incorrectly.

STEPS START TIME: END TIME:	Points Possible	First Attempt	Second Attempt	Third Attempt
1. Washed hands, assembled necessary equipment and supplies and applied appropriate PPE.	10			
2. Identified the patient using at least two identifiers, identified self, and instructed patient to properly collect a urine specimen.	10			
3. Gently mixed specimen, poured specimen into clear centrifuge tube, assessed the color and clarity of the urine and noticed any unusual odors.	10			
4. Measured specific gravity with a digital refractometer, following manufacturer's instructions (if applicable).	10			
5. Dipped reagent strip in urine specimen being certain to cover entire strip. Tilted strip sideways on paper towel allowing excess urine to drain onto towel. Began timing immediately after removing strip from specimen.	10			
6. Held strip next to color chart, reading each test at the appropriate time requirement.	10			
7. Recorded results on report form and log using a pen covered with a disposable plastic sheath *(Work Product, Procedure 27-2)*. Followed office protocol for all positive results.	10			
8. Centrifuged urine for 5 minutes at 2500 rpm.	10			
9. Carefully poured off supernatant and mixed sediment well.	10			
10. Placed one drop of well mixed sediment on glass slide and placed cover slip over drop of urine. Placed slide under microscope using low power (10x) objective.	10			
11. Informed physician specimen is ready to examine.	10			
12. Following physician examination, properly disposed of all supplies and specimens.	10			
13. Removed gloves, washed hands, and documented results in patient's chart *(Work Product, Procedure 27-2)*.	10			
14. Completed the procedure within the appropriate time limit.	10			
Points Earned / Points Possible:	___ / 140			

Points possible reflect importance of step in meeting the task: Important = (5) Essential = (10).
Determine score by dividing points earned by total points possible, and multiplying results by 100.

Key Competencies		
ABHES	VI.A.1.a.4.j	Collect and Process Specimens
	VI.A.1.a.4.k	Perform CLIA Waived Tests (dipsticks)
	VI.A.1.a.4.q	Dispose of Biohazardous Materials
	VI.A.1.a.4.r	Practice Standard Precautions
	VI.A.1.a.4.y	Perform Urinalysis
CAAHEP	III.C.3.b.1.d	Dispose of Biohazardous Materials
	III.C.3.b.1.e	Practice Standard Precautions
	III.C.3.b.3.c.i	Perform Urinalysis

Student Name: _____   Date: _____   Score: _____

EVALUATION

Evaluator Signature: _____   Date: _____

Evaluator Comments:

DOCUMENTATION

Instructor Note: Retain work products with competency checklist.

Work Product, Procedure 27-2 (Progress Note)

Progress Note for Patient: Date:	**DOUGLASVILLE MEDICINE ASSOCIATES** **5076 BRAND BLVD** **DOUGLASVILLE, NY 01234** **(123) 456-7890**

Work Product, Procedure 27-2 (Urinalysis Report Form)

Patient's Name		**Date and Time of Collection**
Test Ordered	**Results**	**Reference Range**
Complete Urinalysis (UA):		
Physical UA:		
Color		Straw to Dark Yellow
Clarity/Transparency		Clear to Hazy
Abnormal Odor		None
Chemical UA/Reagent Strip:		
Specific Gravity		1.005-1.030
pH		5.0-8.0
Protein		Negative/trace
Glucose		Negative
Ketones		Negative
Blood		Negative
Bilirubin		Negative
Urobilinogen		0.1-1.0
Nitrite		Negative
Leukocytes		Negative

Work Product, Procedure 27-2 (In-House Urinalysis Dipstick Testing Log)

IN-HOUSE URINALYSIS DIPSTICK TESTING LOG																
Date	Patient Name/ ID	Ordering Provider	Manuf.	Exp. Date	Lot #	Gluc	Bili	Blood	Ketone	Specific Gravity	Pro	pH	Uro	Nitr	Leuk	MA Init

Key Competencies		
ABHES	VI.A.1.a.4.j	Collect and Process Specimens
	VI.A.1.a.4.k	Perform CLIA Waived Tests (dipsticks)
	VI.A.1.a.4.q	Dispose of Biohazardous Materials
	VI.A.1.a.4.r	Practice Standard Precautions
	VI.A.1.a.4.y	Perform Urinalysis
CAAHEP	III.C.3.b.1.d	Dispose of Biohazardous Materials
	III.C.3.b.1.e	Practice Standard Precautions
	III.C.3.b.3.c.i	Perform Urinalysis

Student Name: _____   Date: _____   Score: _____

Competency Checklist
PROCEDURE 28-1 Perform a Microhematocrit

Task: To perform a microhematocrit

Condition: Given the equipment and supplies as listed in the procedure, and a classmate to play the part of the patient, the student will demonstrate the proper steps for performing a microhematocrit, adhering to the steps listed below.

Standards: The student will have 15 minutes to complete the procedure and will need to score an 85% or above to pass the competency. Automatic failure results if any essential steps are omitted or performed incorrectly.

STEPS START TIME: END TIME:	Points Possible	First Attempt	Second Attempt	Third Attempt
1. Washed hands, applied PPE, and assembled equipment.	10			
2. Identified the patient using at least two identifiers, identified self, and explained the procedure.	10			
3. Performed a capillary puncture, wiped away the first drop of blood, and touched heparinized capillary tube to second drop of blood (not the skin).	10			
4. Applied gentle pressure by squeezing and releasing the fingertip until tube was three-fourths full. Sealed end with clay.	10			
5. Filled another hematocrit tube three-fourths full and sealed tube.				
6. Had patient apply pressure and applied an adhesive bandage to site.				
7. Placed tubes in microhematocrit centrifuge directly across from one another with sealed ends against gasket.	10			
8. Securely fastened both centrifuge lids, set timer for 5 minutes, and adjusted speed, if needed.	10			
9. Allowed centrifuge to stop completely before opening, removed both tubes, placed on reader, and determined results.	10			
10. Averaged the results of both tubes for final result.	10			
11. Properly disposed of used supplies and equipment, removed PPE, and washed hands.	10			
12. Documented procedure in patient's chart and on lab reporting form (*Work Product, Procedure 28-1*).	10			
13. Completed the procedure within the appropriate time limit.	10			
Points Earned / Points Possible:	___ / 110			

Points possible reflect importance of step in meeting the task: Important = (5) Essential = (10).
Determine score by dividing points earned by total points possible, and multiplying results by 100.

EVALUATION
Evaluator Signature: _____   Date: _____

Evaluator Comments:

Key Competencies		
ABHES	VI.A.1.a.4.q	Dispose of Biohazardous Materials
	VI.A.1.a.4.r	Practice Standard Precautions
	VI.A.1.a.4.z	Perform Hematology
CAAHEP	III.C.3.b.1.d	Dispose of Biohazardous Materials
	III.C.3.b.1.e	Practice Standard Precautions
	III.C.3.b.3.c.ii	Perform Hematology Testing

Student Name: _____   Date: _____   Score: _____

DOCUMENTATION

Instructor Note: Retain work products with competency checklist.

Work Product, Procedure 28-1 (Progress Note)

Progress Note for Patient: Date:	**DOUGLASVILLE MEDICINE ASSOCIATES** **5076 BRAND BLVD** **DOUGLASVILLE, NY 01234** **(123) 456-7890**

Work Product, Procedure 28-1 (Hematology Reporting Form)

HEMATOLOGY REPORTING FORM

Patient's Name:		Date and Time of Collection:
Test Ordered	**Results**	**Reference Range**
Complete Blood Count (CBC):		
White Blood Cell Count		4,500-11,000/cu mm
Red Blood Cell Count		M: 4.5-6.0 million/cu mm F: 4.0-5.5/ cu mm
Hemoglobin		M: 13-18 gm/dL F: 12-16 gm/dL
Hematocrit		M: 42-52% F: 36-45%
MCV		82-98 fL
MCH		26-34 pG
MCHC		32-36 g/dL
Platelet Count		150,000-400,000/ cu mm
Differential White Blood Cell Count:		
Neutrophilic Bands		0-2%
Neutrophils		40-65%
Eosinophils		1-3%
Basophils		0-1%
Lymphocytes		25-40%
Monocytes		3-9%
RBC Morphology:		
Doctor's Name:		Name of Person Conducting the Test:

Key Competencies		
ABHES	VI.A.1.a.4.q	Dispose of Biohazardous Materials
	VI.A.1.a.4.r	Practice Standard Precautions
	VI.A.1.a.4.z	Perform Hematology
CAAHEP	III.C.3.b.1.d	Dispose of Biohazardous Materials
	III.C.3.b.1.e	Practice Standard Precautions
	III.C.3.b.3.c.ii	Perform Hematology Testing

Student Name: _____   Date: _____   Score: _____

Competency Checklist
PROCEDURE 28-2 Prepare a Differential Blood Smear

Task: To prepare a differential blood smear

Condition: Given the equipment and supplies as listed in the procedure, and a classmate to play the part of the patient, the student will demonstrate the proper steps for preparing a differential blood smear, adhering to the steps listed below.

Standards: The student will have 10 minutes to complete the procedure and will need to score an 85% or above to pass the competency. Automatic failure results if any essential steps are omitted or performed incorrectly.

STEPS START TIME: END TIME:	Points Possible	First Attempt	Second Attempt	Third Attempt
1. Assembled equipment, labeled frosted end of slide (in pencil) with patient information, washed hands, and applied PPE.	10			
2. Filled a capillary tube with well-mixed EDTA blood and placed a drop of blood on a clean slide.	10			
3. Placed spreader slide in front of drop of blood at a 30- to 35-degree angle, pulled spreader slide back into drop of blood and allowed drop to spread approximately three-fourths of the width of the slide.	10			
4. Pushed the spreader slide forward with a quick, smooth motion.	10			
5. Repeated procedure until 2 acceptable smears were obtained, allowed smears to air dry. (Fixed slide with methanol if applicable.)	10			
6. Disposed of used slides in sharps container and other contaminated supplies in biohazard waste.	10			
7. Placed slides in protective covering for transport to lab.	10			
8. Removed PPE and washed hands.	10			
9. Completed the procedure within the appropriate time limit.	10			
Points Earned / Points Possible:	___ / 90			

Points possible reflect importance of step in meeting the task: Important = (5) Essential = (10).
Determine score by dividing points earned by total points possible, and multiplying results by 100.

EVALUATION
Evaluator Signature: _____   Date: _____

Evaluator Comments:

Key Competencies		
ABHES	VI.A.1.a.4.q	Dispose of Biohazardous Materials
	VI.A.1.a.4.r	Practice Standard Precautions
	VI.A.1.a.4.z	Perform Hematology
CAAHEP	III.C.3.b.1.d	Dispose of Biohazardous Materials
	III.C.3.b.1.e	Practice Standard Precautions
	III.C.3.b.3.c.ii	Perform Hematology Testing

Student Name: _____   Date: _____   Score: _____

Competency Checklist
PROCEDURE 28-3 Perform an Erythrocyte Sedimentation Rate

Task:　　　　To perform an erythrocyte sedimentation rate using the Sediplast® system

Condition:　 Given the equipment and supplies as listed in the procedure, the student will demonstrate the proper steps for preparing performing an ESR, adhering to the steps listed below.

Standards:　 The student will have 75 minutes to complete the procedure and will need to score an 85% or above to pass the competency. Automatic failure results if any essential steps are omitted or performed incorrectly.

STEPS START TIME:　　　　　END TIME:	Points Possible	First Attempt	Second Attempt	Third Attempt
1.　Washed hands, applied PPE, and assembled equipment.	10			
2.　Mixed blood well for 2 minutes, removed stopper of sedivial and filled with 0.8 mL of blood to the indicated mark, replaced stopper, and mixed blood well.	10			
3.　Placed sedivial in Sediplast rack on a level surface.	10			
4.　Inserted Sediplast tube through stopper using a twisting motion, pushed down until tube rested on bottom of vial and blood reached the zero line.	10			
5.　Set timer for 1 hour and read results immediately when timer sounded.	10			
6.　Cleaned work area and properly disposed of used Sediplast equipment in the biohazardous trash and the tube of blood in the sharps container.	10			
7.　Removed PPE and washed hands.	10			
8.　Recorded results in patient's chart and on lab log (*Work Product, Procedure 28-3*).	10			
9.　Completed the procedure within the appropriate time limit.	10			
Points Earned / Points Possible:	___ / 90			

Points possible reflect importance of step in meeting the task: Important = (5) Essential = (10).
Determine score by dividing points earned by total points possible, and multiplying results by 100.

EVALUATION
Evaluator Signature: _____   Date: _____

Evaluator Comments:

Key Competencies		
ABHES	VI.A.1.a.4.q	Dispose of Biohazardous Materials
	VI.A.1.a.4.r	Practice Standard Precautions
	VI.A.1.4.a.z	Perform Hematology
CAAHEP	III.C.3.b.1.d	Dispose of Biohazardous Materials
	III.C.3.b.1.e	Practice Standard Precautions
	III.C.3.b.3.c.ii	Perform Hematology Testing

Student Name: _____   Date: _____   Score: _____

DOCUMENTATION

Instructor Note: Retain work products with competency checklist.
Work Product, Procedure 28-3 (Progress Note)

Progress Note for	**DOUGLASVILLE MEDICINE ASSOCIATES**
	5076 BRAND BLVD
Patient:	**DOUGLASVILLE, NY 01234**
Date:	**(123) 456-7890**

Work Product, Procedure 28-3 (In-House Kit Testing Log)

IN-HOUSE KIT TESTING LOG

Date	Time	Patient Name/ID	Test Name	Ordering Provider	Manufacturer	Exp Date	Lot #	Results	Initials

Key Competencies			
ABHES	VI.A.1.a.4.q	Dispose of Biohazardous Materials	
	VI.A.1.a.4.r	Practice Standard Precautions	
	VI.A.1.4.a.z	Perform Hematology	
CAAHEP	III.C.3.b.1.d	Dispose of Biohazardous Materials	
	III.C.3.b.1.e	Practice Standard Precautions	
	III.C.3.b.3.c.ii	Perform Hematology Testing	

Student Name: _____ Date: _____ Score: _____

Competency Checklist
PROCEDURE 29-1 Prepare a Urine Specimen for Culture and Sensitivity Using a Urine Transport System

Task: To prepare a urine specimen for culture and sensitivity using a urine transport system

Condition: Given the equipment and supplies as listed in the procedure, and a urine sample to prepare for transport, the student will demonstrate the proper steps for preparing a urine specimen for culture and sensitivity, using a urine transport system, adhering to the steps listed below.

Standards: The student will have 5 minutes to complete the procedure and will need to score an 85% or above to pass the competency. Automatic failure results if any essential steps are omitted or performed incorrectly.

STEPS START TIME: END TIME:	Points Possible	First Attempt	Second Attempt	Third Attempt
1. Washed hands, applied PPE, and assembled equipment.	10			
2. Checked provider's order, completed lab requisition form and labeled tubes.	10			
3. Made sure urine specimen was properly labeled and checked expiration date on transport system before beginning transfer.	10			
4. Opened and assembled urine transport kit and inserted urine tube into holder without piercing stopper.	10			
5. Opened urine specimen (placed lid upside down on work surface). Inserted straw of transport system into the specimen and pushed vacuum tube onto sheathed needle inside the holder.	10			
6. Allowed tube to fill completely, removed tube from holder, and properly disposed of unit.	10			
7. Cleaned and disinfected work area and disposed of contaminated supplies following institutional guidelines.	10			
8. Removed PPE, washed hands, and correctly documented procedure on lab requisition form, in patient's chart, and on outside lab log.	10			
9. Completed the procedure within the appropriate time limit.	10			
Points Earned / Points Possible:	___ /90			

Points possible reflect importance of step in meeting the task: Important = (5) Essential = (10).
Determine score by dividing points earned by total points possible, and multiplying results by 100.

EVALUATION
Evaluator Signature: _____ Date: _____

Evaluator Comments:

Key Competencies		
ABHES	VI.A.1.a.4.j	Collect and Process Specimens
	VI.A.1.a.4.q	Dispose of Biohazardous Materials
	VI.A.1.a.4.r	Practice Standard Precautions
CAAHEP	III.C.3.b.1.d	Dispose of Biohazardous Materials
	III.C.3.b.1.e	Practice Standard Precautions
	III.C.3.b.2.c	Obtain Specimens for Microbiological Testing

Student Name: _____   Date: _____   Score: _____

DOCUMENTATION

Instructor Note: Retain work products with competency checklist.
Work Product, Procedure 29-1 (Progress Note)

Progress Note for Patient: Date:	**DOUGLASVILLE MEDICINE ASSOCIATES** **5076 BRAND BLVD** **DOUGLASVILLE, NY 01234** **(123) 456-7890**

Work Product, Procedure 29-1 (Outstanding Lab Results Tracking Report)

OUTSTANDING LAB RESULTS TRACKING REPORT

Date Sent	Patient Name/ ID	Ordering Provider	Tests Ordered	Number and Type of Specimens Sent to (include tube colors)	Prepared By	Laboratory	Date Results Received	Results Received By

Work Product, Procedure 29-1 (Lab Requisition Form)

Form located on following page.

Key Competencies			
ABHES	VI.A.1.a.4.j	Collect and Process Specimens	
	VI.A.1.a.4.q	Dispose of Biohazardous Materials	
	VI.A.1.a.4.r	Practice Standard Precautions	
CAAHEP	III.C.3.b.1.d	Dispose of Biohazardous Materials	
	III.C.3.b.1.e	Practice Standard Precautions	
	III.C.3.b.2.c	Obtain Specimens for Microbiological Testing	

LAB REQUISITION FORM

BILL	PLEASE LEAVE BLANK	C-3 REQUEST FORM	USA Biomedical Labs
☐ ACCOUNT	AREA _____	INSTRUCTIONS ① FOR PATIENT BILLING, COMPLETE BOX A.	957 Central Avenue
☐ PATIENT SEE ①	DEPT. _____	② FOR 3RD PARTY BILLING, COMPLETE BOX A	Heartland, NY 11112
☐ 3RD PARTY SEE ②	BILL CD _____	AND FILL IN DIAGNOSIS, THEN EITHER B, C, or D.	

N7708

PATIENT NAME (LAST)   (FIRST)   SPECIES   SEX   AGE YRS. MOS.   DATE COLLECTED MO. DAY YR.   TIME COLLECTED

PATIENT ADDRESS   STREET   MISC. INFORMATION   DR. I.D.   MEDICARE: #

CITY   STATE   ZIP   DIAGNOSIS

PHYSICIAN   WELFARE: #   CASE NAME:

PROGRAM: PATIENT 1ST NAME: DATE OF BIRTH MO. DAY YR. ALL CLAIMS

INSURANCE   I.D.   SERVICE CODE. GR. #

SUBSCRIBER NAME: RELATION: PHONE

STANDARD PROFILES

2987 ( ) Diagnostic (Multi-Chem) Profile	8350 ( ) Immunologic Evaluation*		
2804 ( ) Health Survey (SMA-12)	2814 ( ) Lipid Profile A		
2824 ( ) Executive Profile A	2817 ( ) Lipid Profile B		
2825 ( ) Executive Profile B	2003 ( ) Lipid Profile C		
2826 ( ) Executive Profile C	2805 ( ) Liver Profile A		
2858 ( ) Amenorrhea Profile	2867 ( ) Liver Profile B		
7330 ( ) Anticonvulsant Group	2868 ( ) MMR Immunity Panel		
2927 ( ) Autoimmune Profile	2869 ( ) Myocardial Infarction Profile		
2801 ( ) Calcium Metabolism Profile	2585 ( ) Parathyroid Panel A (Mid-Molecule)		
2859 ( ) Diabetes Management Profile	2586 ( ) Parathyroid Panel B (Dialysis)		
7701 ( ) Drug Abuse Screen	2587 ( ) Parathyroid Panel C (Adenoma)		
( ) Drug Analysis Comprehensive (S & U or G)	2818 ( ) Prenatal Profile A		
( ) Drug Analysis, Qual (U/G)	2819 ( ) Prenatal Profile B		
7340 ( ) Drug Analysis, Quant. (S)	2820 ( ) Prenatal Profile C		
2022 ( ) Electrolyte Profile	2877 ( ) Prenatal Profile D		
( ) Exanthem Group	( ) Respiratory Infection Profile A		
( ) Glucose/Insulin Response	( ) Respiratory Infection Profile B		
2871 ( ) Hepatitis Profile I	( ) Respiratory Infection Profile C		
2872 ( ) Hepatitis Profile II	( ) Respiratory Infection Profile D		
2873 ( ) Hepatitis Profile III	2821 ( ) Rheumatoid Profile A		
2874 ( ) Hepatitis Profile IV	2878 ( ) Rheumatoid Profile B		
2875 ( ) Hepatitis Profile V	2882 ( ) T & B Lymphocyte Differential Panel		
2876 ( ) Hepatitis Profile VI	2883 ( ) Testicular Function Profile		
2879 ( ) Hepatitis Profile VII	2832 ( ) Thyroid Panel A		
2864 ( ) Hirsutism Profile	2032 ( ) Thyroid Panel B		
2865 ( ) Hypertension Screen	2833 ( ) Thyroid Panel C		

SINGLE TESTS

5165 ( ) ABO and Rho (B) (S)	6526 ( ) Neonatal T$_4$ (S)
6555 ( ) Alpha-Fetoprotein RIA (S)	6525 ( ) Neonatal TSH (S)
3015 ( ) Alk. Phosphatase (S)	7941 ( ) Neonatal T$_4$ Blood Spot
3041 ( ) Amylase (S)	3019 ( ) Phosphorus (S)
5163 ( ) Antibody Screen ( ) If pos. ID & Titer (S) (B)	4132 ( ) Platelet Count (B) (S)
5166 ( ) Antibody ID (B&S)	3026 ( ) Potassium (S)
5164 ( ) Antibody Titer (B&S)	( ) Pregnancy Test, (S or U)
(Previous Pat. #_____)	5187 ( ) Premarital RPR (S)
5208 ( ) ANA. Fluorescent (S)	6505 ( ) Prostatic Acid Phosphatase (RIA) (S)*
5169 ( ) ASO Titer (B) (S)	2992 ( ) Protein Electrophoresis (S)
3147 ( ) Bilirubin, Direct (S)	IEP if Abnormal ( ) 9085
3010 ( ) BUN (S)	4149 ( ) Prothrombin Time (P)*
3018 ( ) Calcium (S)	4144 ( ) Reticulocyte Count (B)
6472 ( ) CEA (RIA) (Plasma Only)	5207 ( ) RA Latex Fixation (S)
2995 ( ) CBC with Automated Diff.	5194 ( ) RPR
(Abnormal Follow-Up Studies) (B) (SL)	5195 ( ) Rubella H.I. (S)
2996 ( ) CBC less Diff. (B)	3016 ( ) SGOT (S)
3022 ( ) Cholesterol (S)	3045 ( ) SGPT (S)
3042 ( ) CPK (S)	3031 ( ) T-3 Uptake (S)
6500 ( ) Digoxin (S)	3032 ( ) T-4 (S)
6501 ( ) Digitoxin (S)	2832 ( ) Thyroxine Index, Free (T$_7$) (S)
3606 ( ) GGT (S)	3036 ( ) Triglycerides (S)
3006 ( ) Glucose (S) Fasting	4111 ( ) Urinalysis (U)
3009 ( ) Glucose (P) Fasting	5277 ( ) Urogenital GC Assay
3023 ( ) Glucose P.P. (P)	UNLISTED TESTS OR PROFILES
Hrs. _____	
3650 ( ) HDL Cholesterol (S)	_____
5180 ( ) Heterophile Screen (Mono) (S)	_____
5179 ( ) Heterophile Absorption (S)	_____
3342 ( ) Hemoglobin A$_{1C}$ (B)	_____
6416 ( ) IgE (S)	_____
3078 ( ) Iron and T.I.B.C. (S)	_____

★ FROZEN   (B) BLOOD   (P) PLASMA   (U) URINE   (S) SERUM   (SL) SLIDES   (Rev. 1-84)

FOLD THIS FORM IN HALF SO TEST(S) ORDERED IS CLEARLY VISIBLE

Student Name: _____   Date: _____   Score: _____

Competency Checklist
PROCEDURE 29-2   Collect a Throat Specimen and Perform a Rapid Strep Test

Task: To collect a throat swab and perform a rapid strep test

Condition: Given the equipment and supplies as listed in the procedure, and a student to play the role of the patient, the student will collect a throat specimen and perform a rapid strep test, adhering to the steps listed below.

Standards: The student will have 15 minutes to complete the procedure and will need to score an 85% or above to pass the competency. Automatic failure results if any essential steps are omitted or performed incorrectly.

STEPS START TIME: END TIME:	Points Possible	First Attempt	Second Attempt	Third Attempt
1. Assembled equipment, washed hands, and applied PPE.	10			
2. Identified the patient using at least two identifiers, identified self, and explained procedure.	10			
3. Adjusted light source, instructed patient to stick out tongue and say "ahhhh." Depressed tongue with tongue depressor, and rolled sterile swab against the back of throat and tonsillar area.	10			
4. While still holding tongue down, removed swab from mouth without touching the sides of the mouth or tongue.	10			
5. If sending swab to lab for culture, swab was placed in appropriate transport media and accompanied by a lab requisition form.	10			
6. If performing a rapid strep test, ran a control and followed manufacturer's directions for performing testing.	10			
7. Properly disposed of contaminated equipment and supplies, removed PPE, washed hands, and documented procedure/results on reporting form, in patient's chart and lab log. If control was performed results of control were recorded in control log.	10			
8. Completed the procedure within the appropriate time limit.	10			
Points Earned / Points Possible:	___ / 80			

Points possible reflect importance of step in meeting the task: Important = (5) Essential = (10).
Determine score by dividing points earned by total points possible, and multiplying results by 100.

EVALUATION
Evaluator Signature: _____   Date: _____

Evaluator Comments:

Key Competencies		
ABHES	VI.A.1.a.4.q	Dispose of Biohazardous Materials
	VI.A.1.a.4. r	Practice Standard Precautions
	VI.A.1.a.4.k	Perform Selected CLIA-Waived Tests
	VI.A.1.a.4.i	Use Quality Control
	VI.B.1.a.4.u	Obtain Throat Specimen for Microbiological Testing
CAAHEP	III.C.3.b.1.d	Dispose of Biohazardous Materials
	III.C.3.b.1.e	Practice Standard Precautions
	III.C.3.b.2.c	Obtain Specimens for Microbiological Testing
	III.C.3.b.3.c.v	Perform Microbiology Testing
	III.C.3.c.4.d	Use Methods of Quality Control

Student Name: _____   Date: _____   Score: _____

DOCUMENTATION
Instructor Note: Retain work products with competency checklist.
Work Product, Procedure 29-2 (Progress Note)

Progress Note for Patient: Date:	**DOUGLASVILLE MEDICINE ASSOCIATES** **5076 BRAND BLVD** **DOUGLASVILLE, NY 01234** **(123) 456-7890**

Work Product, Procedure 29-2 (Miscellaneous Laboratory Test Report Form)

MISCELLANEOUS LABORATORY TEST REPORT FORM		
Patient's Name	**Date and Time of Collection**	
Test Ordered	**Results**	**Reference Range**
Pregnancy Test		
Rapid Strep Test		Negative
Mono Test		Negative
Influenza Test		Negative
H. Pylori		Negative

Work Product, Procedure 29-2 (In-House Testing Log)

IN-HOUSE TESTING LOG									
Date	**Time**	**Patient Name/ID**	**Test Name**	**Ordering Provider**	**Manufacturer**	**Exp. Date**	**Lot #**	**Results**	**Initials**

Work Product, Procedure 29-2 (Rapid Strep QC Log)

RAPID STREP QC LOG								
Date	**Test Name**	**Manufacturer's Name**	**Type of Control**	**Lot #**	**Expiration Date**	**Reference Range or Result**	**Result**	**Initials**

Key Competencies		
ABHES	VI.A.1.a.4.q	Dispose of Biohazardous Materials
	VI.A.1.a.4. r	Practice Standard Precautions
	VI.A.1.a.4.k	Perform Selected CLIA-Waived Tests
	VI.A.1.a.4.i	Use Quality Control
	VI.B.1.a.4.u	Obtain Throat Specimen for Microbiological Testing
CAAHEP	III.C.3.b.1.d	Dispose of Biohazardous Materials
	III.C.3.b.1.e	Practice Standard Precautions
	III.C.3.b.2.c	Obtain Specimens for Microbiological Testing
	III.C.3.b.3.c.v	Perform Microbiology Testing
	III.C.3.c.4.d	Use Methods of Quality Control

Student Name: _____   Date: _____   Score: _____

Competency Checklist
PROCEDURE 29-3 Collect a Wound Specimen

Task: To collect a wound specimen

Condition: Given the equipment and supplies as listed in the procedure, and a student to play the role of the patient, the student will collect a wound specimen using sterile technique, adhering to the steps listed below.

Standards: The student will have 15 minutes to complete the procedure and will need to score an 85% or above to pass the competency. Automatic failure results if any essential steps are omitted or performed incorrectly.

STEPS START TIME: END TIME:	Points Possible	First Attempt	Second Attempt	Third Attempt
1. Washed hands, applied PPE, and assembled equipment.	10			
2. Checked provider's order and completed lab requisition form.	10			
3. Identified the patient using at least two identifiers, identified self, and explained procedure.	10			
4. Set up sterile tray, draped patient, washed hands, and applied sterile gloves.	10			
5. *For Wound:* Cleaned any purulent matter from wound following office protocol. Rotated swab deep within the wound being careful not to touch the skin when withdrawing the swab. *For Abscess:* Applied an antiseptic before beginning procedure. Rotated swab over abscessed tissue being careful not to touch the surrounding skin when withdrawing the swab.	10			
6. Immediately placed swab in properly labeled transport media. Dressed wound according to physician's instructions.	10			
7. Properly disposed of contaminated materials.	10			
8. Removed PPE, washed hands, and documented in patient's chart and in lab log.	10			
9. Completed the procedure within the appropriate time limit.	10			
Points Earned / Points Possible:	___ / 90			

Points possible reflect importance of step in meeting the task: Important = (5) Essential = (10).
Determine score by dividing points earned by total points possible, and multiplying results by 100.

EVALUATION
Evaluator Signature: _____   Date: _____

Evaluator Comments:

Key Competencies		
ABHES	VI.A.1.a.4.q	Dispose of Biohazardous Materials
	VI.A.1.a.4.r	Practice Standard Precautions
	VI.A.1.a.4.v	Perform Wound Collection Procedure for Microbiological Testing
CAAHEP	III.C.3.b.1.d	Dispose of Biohazardous Materials
	III.C.3.b.1.e	Practice Standard Precautions
	III.C.3.b.2.c	Obtain Specimens for Microbiological Testing

Student Name: _____   Date: _____   Score: _____

DOCUMENTATION
Instructor Note: Retain work products with competency checklist.
Work Product, Procedure 29-3 (Progress Note)

Progress Note for Patient: Date:	**DOUGLASVILLE MEDICINE ASSOCIATES** **5076 BRAND BLVD** **DOUGLASVILLE, NY 01234** **(123) 456-7890**

Work Product, Procedure 29-3 (Outside Lab Tracking Log)

OUTSIDE LAB TRACKING LOG

Date Sent	Patient Name/ID	Ordering Provider	Tests Ordered	Number and Type of Specimens Sent to Laboratory (Include Tube Colors)	Prepared By	Laboratory	Date Results Received	Results Received By

Key Competencies			
ABHES	VI.A.1.a.4.q	Dispose of Biohazardous Materials	
	VI.A.1.a.4.r	Practice Standard Precautions	
	VI.A.1.a.4.v	Perform Wound Collection Procedure for Microbiological Testing	
CAAHEP	III.C.3.b.1.d	Dispose of Biohazardous Materials	
	III.C.3.b.1.e	Practice Standard Precautions	
	III.C.3.b.2.c	Obtain Specimens for Microbiological Testing	

Student Name: _____ Date: _____ Score: _____

Competency Checklist
PROCEDURE 29-4 Prepare a Wet Mount or Hanging Drop Slide

Task: To prepare a wet mount or hanging drop slide

Condition: Given the equipment and supplies as listed in the procedure, the student will prepare a wet mount or hanging drop slide, adhering to the steps listed below.

Standards: The student will have 15 minutes to complete the procedure and will need to score an 85% or above to pass the competency. Automatic failure results if any essential steps are omitted or performed incorrectly.

STEPS START TIME: END TIME:	Points Possible	First Attempt	Second Attempt	Third Attempt
1. Washed hands, applied PPE, and assembled equipment and supplies.	10			
Wet mount slide preparation:				
2. Deposited drop of bacterial suspension in middle of clean glass slide.	10			
3. Smeared petroleum jelly around edges of clean cover slip, placed cover slip over drop of suspension, and gently pressed cover slip to seal edges.	10			
Hanging drop slide preparation:				
4. Smeared petroleum jelly around edges of clean cover slip and deposited drop of bacterial suspension in middle of cover slip.	10			
5. Inverted slide and placed concave well slide over drop of bacterial suspension, gently pressed down on slide to seal edges of cover slip, and turned slide right side-up for microscopic examination by physician.	10			
6. Completed the procedure within the appropriate time limit.	10			
Points Earned / Points Possible:	___ / 60			

Points possible reflect importance of step in meeting the task: Important = (5) Essential = (10).
Determine score by dividing points earned by total points possible, and multiplying results by 100.

EVALUATION
Evaluator Signature: _____ Date: _____

Evaluator Comments:

Key Competencies			
ABHES	VI.A.1.a.4.q	Dispose of Biohazardous Materials	
	VI.A.1.a.4.r	Practice Standard Precautions	
	VI.A.1.a.4.j	Collect and Process Specimens	
CAAHEP	III.C.3.b.1.d	Dispose of Biohazardous Materials	
	III.C.3.b.1.e	Practice Standard Precautions	
	III.C.3.b.2.c	Obtain Specimens for Microbiological Testing	

Student Name: _____   Date: _____   Score: _____

Competency Checklist
PROCEDURE 29-5 Instruct a Patient on Fecal Specimen Collection
for Ova and Parasite Testing

Task: To instruct a patient on proper specimen handling technique when collecting a fecal specimen for ova and parasite testing

Condition: Given the equipment and supplies as listed in the procedure, the student will demonstrate the proper steps for instructing a patient on the proper method for collecting and handling a fecal specimen for ova and parasite testing, adhering to the steps listed below.

Standards: The student will have 5 minutes to complete the procedure and will need to score an 85% or above to pass the competency. Automatic failure results if any essential steps are omitted or performed incorrectly.

STEPS START TIME: END TIME:	Points Possible	First Attempt	Second Attempt	Third Attempt
1. Washed hands and assembled equipment.	10			
2. Identified the patient using at least two identifiers and identified self.	10			
3. Gave the patient the appropriate containers including a stool collection basin (Hat) as well as the O & P containers.	10			
4. Instructed the patient to:				
a. Collect the specimen in the wide-mouthed container being careful not to contaminate the specimen with urine.	10			
b. Follow the instructions on the vials for preparing each specimen.	10			
c. Collect a total of three specimens over three days per the provider's orders.	10			
d. Transfer each vial into a plastic sealable storage bag following collection. Store and return specimens according to instructions on lab form.	10			
5. Encouraged the patient to ask questions.	10			
6. Supplied patient with written instructions.	10			
7. Documented education in the patient's chart (*Work Product, Procedure 29-5*).	10			
8. Completed the procedure within the appropriate time limit.	10			
Points Earned / Points Possible:	___ /110			

Points possible reflect importance of step in meeting the task: Important = (5) Essential = (10).
Determine score by dividing points earned by total points possible, and multiplying results by 100.

EVALUATION
Evaluator Signature: _____   Date: _____

Evaluator Comments:

Key Competencies		
ABHES	VI.A.1.a.4.j	Collect and Process Specimens
CAAHEP	III.C.3.b.2.c	Obtain Specimens for Microbiological Testing

Student Name: _____   Date: _____   Score: _____

DOCUMENTATION

Instructor Note: Retain work products with competency checklist.
Work Product, Procedure 29-5 (Progress Note)

Progress Note for Patient: Date:	**DOUGLASVILLE MEDICINE ASSOCIATES** **5076 BRAND BLVD** **DOUGLASVILLE, NY 01234** **(123) 456-7890**

Key Competencies		
ABHES	VI.A.1.a.4.j	Collect and Process Specimens
CAAHEP	III.C.3.b.2.c	Obtain Specimens for Microbiological Testing

Student Name: _____   Date: _____   Score: _____

Competency Checklist
PROCEDURE 30-1 Measure Blood Glucose Using a Handheld Monitor

Task: To measure blood glucose using a hand-held monitor

Condition: Given the equipment and supplies as listed in the procedure, and a student to play the role of the patient, the student will perform a blood glucose, adhering to the steps listed below.

Standards: The student will have 15 minutes to complete the procedure and will need to score an 85% or above to pass the competency. Automatic failure results if any essential steps are omitted or performed incorrectly.

STEPS START TIME: END TIME:	Points Possible	First Attempt	Second Attempt	Third Attempt
1. Washed hands, applied PPE, and assembled equipment and supplies.	10			
2. Checked the expiration date on the glucose strips and controls.	10			
3. Performed a control, following manufacturer's instructions.	10			
4. Identified the patient using at least two identifiers, identified self, explained procedure, and verified compliance of fasting instructions.	10			
5. Instructed patient to wash and dry hands.	10			
6. Cleansed site with alcohol. (Allowed site to air dry.)				
7. Inserted strip into monitor and verified strip and unit code numbers matched.	10			
8. Performed capillary puncture using a safety lancet. (Disposed of lancet and wiped away first drop of blood.)	10			
9. When blood drop icon appeared or equivalent, touched edge of strip to drop of blood—allowing blood to be absorbed by strip.	10			
10. Instructed patient to apply pressure to puncture site and observed reading on monitor screen.	10			
11. Removed strip from monitor, checked puncture site, and applied adhesive bandage if needed.	10			
12. Disposed of contaminated materials in the biohazardous trash, and other supplies in the regular trash. Removed PPE, and washed hands.	10			
13. Documented in patient's chart, lab log, and control log and on lab reporting form.	10			
14. Completed the procedure within the appropriate time limit.	10			
Points Earned / Points Possible:	___ / 130			

Points possible reflect importance of step in meeting the task: Important = (5) Essential = (10).
Determine score by dividing points earned by total points possible, and multiplying results by 100.

EVALUATION
Evaluator Signature: _____   Date: _____

Evaluator Comments:

Key Competencies		
ABHES	VI.A.1.a.4.q	Dispose of Biohazardous Materials
	VI.A.1.a.4.r	Practice Standard Precautions
	VI.A.1.a.4.k	Perform Selected CLIA-Waived Tests
CAAHEP	III.C.3.b.1.d	Dispose of Biohazardous Materials
	III.C.3.b.1.e	Practice Standard Precautions
	III.C.3.b.3.c	CLIA-Waived Tests
	III.C.3.b.3.c.iii	Perform Chemistry Testing

Student Name: _____   Date: _____   Score: _____

DOCUMENTATION

Instructor Note: Retain work products with competency checklist.

Work Product, Procedure 30-1 (Progress Note)

Progress Note for Patient: Date:	**DOUGLASVILLE MEDICINE ASSOCIATES** **5076 BRAND BLVD** **DOUGLASVILLE, NY 01234** **(123) 456-7890**

Work Product, Procedure 30-1 (Miscellaneous Laboratory Test Report Form)

MISCELLANEOUS LABORATORY TEST REPORT FORM		
Patient's Name	**Date and Time of Collection**	
Test Ordered	**Results**	**Reference Range**
Pregnancy Test		
Rapid Strep Test		Negative
Glucose Test		70-110 mg/dL
Mono Test		Negative
Influenza Test		Negative
H. Pylori		Negative

Work Product, Procedure 30-1 (In-House Testing Log)

IN-HOUSE TESTING LOG									
Date	**Time**	**Patient Name/ID**	**Test Name**	**Ordering Provider**	**Manufacturer**	**Exp. Date**	**Lot #**	**Results**	**Initials**

Work Product, Procedure 30-1 (Glucose QC Log)

GLUCOSE QC LOG								
Date	**Test Name**	**Manufacturer's Name**	**Type of Control**	**Lot #**	**Expiration Date**	**Reference Range or Result**	**Result**	**Initials**

Key Competencies		
ABHES	VI.A.1.a.4.q	Dispose of Biohazardous Materials
	VI.A.1.a.4.r	Practice Standard Precautions
	VI.A.1.a.4.k	Perform Selected CLIA-Waived Tests
CAAHEP	III.C.3.b.1.d	Dispose of Biohazardous Materials
	III.C.3.b.1.e	Practice Standard Precautions
	III.C.3.b.3.c	CLIA-Waived Tests
	III.C.3.b.3.c.iii	Perform Chemistry Testing

Student Name: _____   Date: _____   Score: _____

Competency Checklist
PROCEDURE 30-2 Perform a Urine Pregnancy Test

Task: To perform a urine pregnancy test

Condition: Given the equipment and supplies as listed in the procedure, and a urine sample on which to perform the testing, the student will perform a urine pregnancy test, adhering to the steps listed below.

Standards: The student will have 15 minutes to complete the procedure and will need to score an 85% or above to pass the competency. Automatic failure results if any essential steps are omitted or performed incorrectly.

STEPS START TIME: END TIME:	Points Possible	First Attempt	Second Attempt	
1. Washed hands, applied PPE, assembled equipment and supplies, and read the kit's directions.	10			
2. Performed control.	10			
3. Opened test unit, added three drops of urine to well, and allowed test to develop for precisely 3 minutes or followed instructions on school's pregnancy test kit.	10			
4. Read test and control windows.	10			
5. Disposed of contaminated materials, removed PPE, and washed hands.	10			
6. Documented results on lab reporting form, in patient's chart, and lab log.	10			
7. Completed the procedure within the appropriate time limit.	10			
Points Earned / Points Possible:	___ / 70			

Points possible reflect importance of step in meeting the task: Important = (5) Essential = (10).
Determine score by dividing points earned by total points possible, and multiplying results by 100.

EVALUATION
Evaluator Signature: _____   Date: _____

Evaluator Comments:

Key Competencies		
ABHES	VI.B.1.a.4.i	Use Quality Control
	VI.B.1.a.4.k	Perform Selected CLIA-Waived Tests
	VI.B.1.a.4.q	Dispose of Biohazardous Materials
	VI.B.1.a.4.r	Practice Standard Precautions
CAAHEP	III.C.3.b.1.d	Dispose of Biohazardous Materials
	III.C.3.b.1.e	Practice Standard Precautions
	III.C.3.b.3.c	Perform CLIA-Waived Tests

Student Name: _____   Date: _____   Score: _____

DOCUMENTATION

Instructor Note: Retain work products with competency checklist.
Work Product, Procedure 30-2 (Progress Note)

Progress Note for	**DOUGLASVILLE MEDICINE ASSOCIATES**
Patient:	**5076 BRAND BLVD**
Date:	**DOUGLASVILLE, NY 01234**
	(123) 456-7890

Work Product, Procedure 30-2 (Miscellaneous Laboratory Test Report Form)

MISCELLANEOUS LABORATORY TEST REPORT FORM		
Patient's Name	**Date and Time of Collection**	
Test Ordered	**Results**	**Reference Range**
Pregnancy Test		
Rapid Strep Test		Negative
Glucose Test		70-110 mg/dL
Mono Test		Negative
Influenza Test		Negative
H. Pylori		Negative

Work Product, Procedure 30-2 (In-House Testing Log)

IN-HOUSE TESTING LOG									
Date	**Time**	**Patient Name/ID**	**Test Name**	**Ordering Provider**	**Manufacturer**	**Exp. Date**	**Lot #**	**Results**	**Initials**

Work Product, Procedure 30-2 (Pregnancy QC Log)

PREGNANCY QC LOG								
Date	**Test Name**	**Manufacturer's Name**	**Type of Control**	**Lot #**	**Expiration Date**	**Reference Range or Result**	**Result**	**Initials**

Key Competencies		
ABHES	VI.B.1.a.4.i	Use Quality Control
	VI.B.1.a.4.k	Perform Selected CLIA-Waived Tests
	VI.B.1.a.4.q	Dispose of Biohazardous Materials
	VI.B.1.a.4.r	Practice Standard Precautions
CAAHEP	III.C.3.b.1.d	Dispose of Biohazardous Materials
	III.C.3.b.1.e	Practice Standard Precautions
	III.C.3.b.3.c	Perform CLIA-Waived Tests

Student Name: _____   Date: _____   Score: _____

Competency Checklist
PROCEDURE 30-3 Perform a CLIA Waived Mono Test

Task:　　　　　To perform a CLIA waived mono test

Condition:　　Given the equipment and supplies as listed in the procedure, and a capillary specimen on which to perform the testing, the student will perform a CLIA waived mono test, adhering to the steps listed below.

Standards:　　The student will have 15 minutes to complete the procedure and will need to score an 85% or above to pass the competency. Automatic failure results if any essential steps are omitted or performed incorrectly.

STEPS START TIME:　　　　　　　END TIME:	Points Possible	First Attempt	Second Attempt	Third Attempt
1.　Washed hands, applied PPE, assembled equipment and patient's sample (usually comes from a capillary sample).	10			
2.　Performed control before testing patient sample.	10			
3.　Read the kit directions and performed test according to manufacturer's instructions.	10			
4.　Disposed of contaminated equipment and supplies, removed PPE, and washed hands.	10			
5.　Documented results in patient's chart, lab log, and quality control log.	10			
6.　Completed the procedure within the appropriate time limit.	10			
Points Earned / Points Possible:	___ / 60			

Points possible reflect importance of step in meeting the task: Important = (5) Essential = (10).
Determine score by dividing points earned by total points possible, and multiplying results by 100.

EVALUATION
Evaluator Signature: _____   Date: _____

Evaluator Comments:

Key Competencies			
ABHES	VI.A.1.a.4.i	Use Quality Control	
	VI.A.1.a.4.k	Perform Selected CLIA-Waived Tests	
	VI.A.1.a.4.q	Dispose of Biohazardous Materials	
	VI.A.1.a.4.r	Practice Standard Precautions	
CAAHEP	III.C.3.b.1.d	Dispose of Biohazardous Materials	
	III.C.3.b.1.e	Practice Standard Precautions	
	III.C.3.b.3.c. iv	CLIA-Waived Tests; Perform Immunology Testing	

Student Name: _____   Date: _____   Score: _____

DOCUMENTATION

Instructor Note: Retain work products with competency checklist.
Work Product, Procedure 30-3 (Progress Note)

Progress Note for Patient: Date:	**DOUGLASVILLE MEDICINE ASSOCIATES** **5076 BRAND BLVD** **DOUGLASVILLE, NY 01234** **(123) 456-7890**

Work Product, Procedure 30-3 (Miscellaneous Laboratory Test Report Form)

MISCELLANEOUS LABORATORY TEST REPORT FORM		
Patient's Name	**Date and Time of Collection**	
Test Ordered	**Results**	**Reference Range**
Pregnancy Test		
Rapid Strep Test		Negative
Glucose Test		70-110 mg/dL
Mono Test		Negative
Influenza Test		Negative
H. Pylori		Negative

Work Product, Procedure 30-3 (In-House Testing Log)

IN-HOUSE TESTING LOG									
Date	**Time**	**Patient Name/ID**	**Test Name**	**Ordering Provider**	**Manufacturer**	**Exp. Date**	**Lot #**	**Results**	**Initials**

Work Product, Procedure 30-3 (Mono QC Log)

MONO QC LOG								
Date	**Test Name**	**Manufacturer's Name**	**Type of Control**	**Lot #**	**Expiration Date**	**Reference Range or Result**	**Result**	**Initials**

Key Competencies		
ABHES	VI.A.1.a.4.i	Use Quality Control
	VI.A.1.a.4.k	Perform Selected CLIA-Waived Tests
	VI.A.1.a.4.q	Dispose of Biohazardous Materials
	VI.A.1.a.4.r	Practice Standard Precautions
CAAHEP	III.C.3.b.1.d	Dispose of Biohazardous Materials
	III.C.3.b.1.e	Practice Standard Precautions
	III.C.3.b.3.c. iv	CLIA-Waived Tests; Perform Immunology Testing

Student Name: _____   Date: _____   Score: _____

Competency Checklist
PROCEDURE 32-1 Maintain Medication and Immunization Records

Task: To maintain medication and immunization records

Condition: Given the equipment and supplies as listed in the procedure, the student will demonstrate the correct procedure for documenting medications and maintaining medication and immunization records, adhering to the steps listed below. Instructor will need to tell student what immunization was administered. Student will need to make up the administration information.

Standards: The student will have 10 minutes to complete the procedure and will need to score an 85% or above to pass the competency. Automatic failure results if any essential steps are omitted or performed incorrectly.

STEPS START TIME: END TIME:	Points Possible	First Attempt	Second Attempt	Third Attempt
1. Washed hands following medication administration and prior to charting.	10			
2. Assembled chart, medication label information, medication logs, and writing utensil.	10			
3. Recorded the medication procedure within the chart. Note included the following: date and time of administration, name of drug, form of drug, amount or dosage given, location (if applicable), route, ordering physician, and the medical assistant's signature. Post-injection observation should be documented as well. (Manufacturer's name, lot number, and expiration date may be necessary as well.)	10			
3. Filed Vaccination Informed Consent within the chart.	10			
4. Recorded required information in appropriate log within the chart if applicable.	10			
5. Recorded information in universal log if applicable.	10			
6. Placed chart and logs in their proper storage areas.	10			
7. Completed the procedure within the appropriate time limit.	10			
Points Earned / Points Possible:	___ / 70			

Points possible reflect importance of step in meeting the task: Important = (5) Essential = (10).
Determine score by dividing points earned by total points possible, and multiplying results by 100.

EVALUATION
Evaluator Signature: _____   Date: _____

Evaluator Comments:

Key Competencies		
ABHES	VI.A.1.a.4.n	Maintain medication and immunization records
CAAHEP	III.C.3.c.4.h	Maintain medication and immunization records

Student Name: _____   Date: _____   Score: _____

DOCUMENTATION

Instructor Note: Retain work products with competency checklist.
Work Product, Procedure 32-1 (Progress Note)

Progress Note for Patient: Date:	**DOUGLASVILLE MEDICINE ASSOCIATES** **5076 BRAND BLVD** **DOUGLASVILLE, NY 01234** **(123) 456-7890**

Work Product, Procedure 32-1 (Global Immunization Log)

GLOBAL IMMUNIZATION LOG

Today's Date	Patient's Name	Ordering Physician	Vaccine Name	Amt. Given	Manufacturer's Name	Lot Number	Exp. Date	MA

Work Product, Procedure 32-1 (Patient Vaccination Log)

PATIENT VACCINATION LOG

Patient's Name _____   DOB _____

Date	Time	Ordering Physician	Immunization Name	Number in Series (if applicable)	Amt. Given	Location	Route	Person who Administered Injection

Key Competencies		
ABHES	VI.A.1.a.4.n	Maintain medication and immunization records
CAAHEP	III.C.3.c.4.h	Maintain medication and immunization records

Student Name: _____   Date: _____   Score: _____

Competency Checklist
PROCEDURE 32-2 Write a Prescription

Task: To create a prescription

Condition: Given the equipment and supplies as listed in the procedure and a student to play the part of the physician, the student will demonstrate the correct procedure for creating a prescription, adhering to the steps listed below.

Standards: The student will have 10 minutes to complete the procedure and will need to score an 85% or above to pass the competency. Automatic failure results if any essential steps are omitted or performed incorrectly.

STEPS START TIME: END TIME:	Points Possible	First Attempt	Second Attempt	Third Attempt
1. Assembled chart, order for medication, and prescription pad.	10			
2. Read order and asked any questions necessary.	10			
3. Wrote in the patient's name, address, and DOB/age.	10			
4. If not on form already, wrote in the superscription or Rx symbol.	10			
5. Wrote the information included in the inscription (name, form and strength of the medication).	10			
6. Wrote in the information included in the subscription (dispense amount, numeric followed by written amount in parentheses).	10			
7. Wrote in the information included in the signature (instructions for taking).	10			
8. If applicable, checked the box that states: Dispense as Written/ Do Not Substitute.	10			
9. Circled the amount of refills.	10			
10. Inserted DEA number if applicable.	10			
11. Gave to physician to read and sign.	10			
12. Documented the order into the chart.	10			
13. Completed the procedure within the appropriate time limit.	10			
Points Earned / Points Possible:	___ / 130			

Points possible reflect importance of step in meeting the task: Important = (5) Essential = (10).
Determine score by dividing points earned by total points possible, and multiplying results by 100.

EVALUATION
Evaluator Signature: _____   Date: _____

Evaluator Comments:

Key Competencies		
ABHES	VI.A.1.a.4.m	Prepare and administer oral and parenteral medications as directed by physician
CAAHEP	III.C.3.c.4.g	Apply pharmacology principles to prepare and administer oral and parenteral (excluding IV) medications

Student Name: _____   Date: _____   Score: _____

DOCUMENTATION
Instructor Note: Retain work products with competency checklist.
Work Product, Procedure 32-2 (Prescription)

DOUGLASVILLE MEDICINE ASSOCIATES 5076 BRAND BLVD DOUGLASVILLE, NY 01234 (123) 456-7890

Patient's Name: _____   DOB: _____

Address: _____   Date: _____

Rx

Dispense as Written/Do Not Substitute   Signature:

Refills 1 2 3 4 5 6   DEA # _____

Key Competencies		
ABHES	VI.A.1.a.4.m	Prepare and administer oral and parenteral medications as directed by physician
CAAHEP	III.C.3.c.4.g	Apply pharmacology principles to prepare and administer oral and parenteral (excluding IV) medications

Student Name: _____   Date: _____   Score: _____

Competency Checklist
PROCEDURE 32-3 Administer an Oral Medication

Task: To administer oral medication

Condition: Given the equipment and supplies as listed in the procedure and a classmate to play the part of the patient, the student will demonstrate the correct procedure for administering an oral medication, adhering to the steps listed below.

Standards: The student will have 10 minutes to complete the procedure and will need to score an 85% or above to pass the competency. Automatic failure results if any essential steps are omitted or performed incorrectly.

STEPS START TIME: END TIME:	Points Possible	First Attempt	Second Attempt	Third Attempt
1. Verified the physician's order.	10			
2. Washed hands and gloved if necessary. Assembled medication and supplies. Checked label (Label Check # 1).	10			
3. Compared written drug order with drug label before preparing drug (Label Check # 2). Performed dosage calculation if necessary.	10			
4. Loosened cap and removed from bottle—placing lid on counter so that the inside of lid was pointing upward.	10			
5. *Solids:* Poured correct amount of pills into the cap of the medication and then into the medication cup. *Liquids:* Student poured medication into medication cup while palming the label. The cup was at eye level during the measurement. Student read the lowest point of the curve in the liquid—meniscus. (Did not contaminate the cap or medicine cup while preparing.)	10			
6. Replaced the cap to the medication and returned it to its proper storage area. Read label once more before returning to verify correct drug and dosage (Label Check # 3).	10			
7. Properly transported medication to the patient. Identified the patient using two identifiers.	10			
8. Identified self and explained procedure to the patient.	10			
9. Gave the patient the medication to swallow and observed the patient to make sure they experienced no difficulty in taking the medication. (Gave water for pill form, but not for liquid medication unless stated it was okay on package insert.)	10			
10. Properly disposed of the medication cup and other disposable equipment into the garbage and removed gloves and washed hands.	10			
11. Provided patient with educational materials and asked patient to repeat back any instructions to confirm the patient comprehended the information.	10			
12. Documented the procedure in the patient's chart and appropriate logs (if applicable).	10			
13. Completed the procedure within the appropriate time limit and instituted the "Seven Rights" of drug administration at the appropriate points in the procedure.	10			
Points Earned / Points Possible:	___ / 130			

Key Competencies		
ABHES	VI.A.1.a.4.m	Prepare and administer oral and parenteral medications as directed by physician
CAAHEP	III.C.3.c.4.g	Apply pharmacology principles to prepare and administer oral and parenteral (excluding IV) medications

Student Name: _____   Date: _____   Score: _____

Points possible reflect importance of step in meeting the task: Important = (5) Essential = (10).
Determine score by dividing points earned by total points possible, and multiplying results by 100.

EVALUATION

Evaluator Signature: _____   Date: _____

Evaluator Comments:

DOCUMENTATION

Instructor Note: Retain work products with competency checklist.
Work Product, Procedure 32-3 (Progress Note)

Progress Note for Patient: Date:	**DOUGLASVILLE MEDICINE ASSOCIATES** **5076 BRAND BLVD** **DOUGLASVILLE, NY 01234** **(123) 456-7890**

Work Product, Procedure 32-3 (Medication Log)

MEDICATION LOG

Date	Patient Name/ID	Ordering Provider	Name of Drug	Strength/ Amt. Given	Route	Manufacturer	Lot #	Exp. Date	Initials

Key Competencies		
ABHES	VI.A.1.a.4.m	Prepare and administer oral and parenteral medications as directed by physician
CAAHEP	III.C.3.c.4.g	Apply pharmacology principles to prepare and administer oral and parenteral (excluding IV) medications

Student Name: _____   Date: _____   Score: _____

Competency Checklist
PROCEDURE 32-4 Administer a Topical Medication

Task: To administer a topical medication

Condition: Given the equipment and supplies as listed in the procedure and a classmate to play the part of the patient, the student will demonstrate the correct procedure for administering a topical medication, adhering to the steps listed below.

Standards: The student will have 10 minutes to complete the procedure and will need to score an 85% or above to pass the competency. Automatic failure results if any essential steps are omitted or performed incorrectly.

STEPS START TIME: END TIME:	Points Possible	First Attempt	Second Attempt	Third Attempt
1. Verified the physician's order.	10			
2. Washed hands. Assembled medication and supplies. Checked label of medication when removing from cabinet (Label Check # 1).	10			
3. Compared written drug order with drug label before preparing drug. Checked the expiration date (Label Check # 2).	10			
4. Read the medication label again prior to placing the medication on the tray (Label Check # 3).	10			
5. Placed all other supplies on the tray (4x4s, cotton tip applicator, tongue blades).	5			
6. Properly transported medication to the patient.	5			
7. Identified the patient, identified self, and explained procedure to the patient.	10			
8. Asked patient to expose the affected area.	10			
9. Washed hands and applied gloves.	10			
10. Placed drape under the affected area.	10			
11. Loosened the lid and removed cap—placing cap so that the inside was facing up before placing on table.	10			
12. Carefully applied the medication directly over the affected area with a sterile cotton tip applicator, *working from the inside out.* (If applying an ointment to intact skin—did not have to use sterile technique but rather clean technique.)	10			
13. Inquired about patient's pain tolerance or comfort during the procedure.	10			
14. Covered area with clean/sterile dressing if necessary.	10			
15. Properly disposed of the used disposable supplies in the garbage and removed gloves and washed hands. (If body fluids were on any of the disposables, they should have been discarded in the biohazardous trash.)	10			
16. Provided patient with home care instructions and asked patient to repeat back any instructions to confirm the patient comprehended the information.	10			
17. Returned medication to its appropriate cabinet (outside of the container was clean before replacing back in storage).	10			
18. Documented the procedure in the patient's chart.	10			
19. Student instituted the "Seven Rights" of drug administration at the appropriate points during the procedure.				
20. Completed the procedure within the appropriate time limit.	10			
Points Earned / Points Possible:	___ / 180			

Key Competencies		
ABHES	VI.A.1.a.4.m	Prepare and administer oral and parenteral medications as directed by physician
CAAHEP	III.C.3.c.4.g	Apply pharmacology principles to prepare and administer oral and parenteral (excluding IV) medications

Student Name: _____   Date: _____   Score: _____

Points possible reflect importance of step in meeting the task: Important = (5) Essential = (10).
Determine score by dividing points earned by total points possible, and multiplying results by 100.

EVALUATION
Evaluator Signature: _____   Date: _____

Evaluator Comments:

DOCUMENTATION
Instructor Note: Retain work products with competency checklist.
Work Product, Procedure 32-4 (Progress Note)

Progress Note for Patient: Date:	**DOUGLASVILLE MEDICINE ASSOCIATES** **5076 BRAND BLVD** **DOUGLASVILLE, NY 01234** **(123) 456-7890**

Work Product, Procedure 32-4 (Medication Log)

				MEDICATION LOG					
Date	**Patient Name/ID**	**Ordering Provider**	**Name of Drug**	**Strength/ Amt. Given**	**Route**	**Manufacturer**	**Lot #**	**Exp. Date**	**Initials**

Key Competencies		
ABHES	VI.A.1.a.4.m	Prepare and administer oral and parenteral medications as directed by physician
CAAHEP	III.C.3.c.4.g	Apply pharmacology principles to prepare and administer oral and parenteral (excluding IV) medications

Student Name: _____   Date: _____   Score: _____

Competency Checklist
PROCEDURE 32-5 Administer a Transdermal Medication

Task: To administer a transdermal medication

Condition: Given the equipment and supplies as listed in the procedure and a classmate to play the part of the patient, the student will demonstrate the correct procedure for administering a transdermal medication, adhering to the steps listed below.

Standards: The student will have 10 minutes to complete the procedure and will need to score an 85% or above to pass the competency. Automatic failure results if any essential steps are omitted or performed incorrectly.

STEPS START TIME: END TIME:	Points Possible	First Attempt	Second Attempt	Third Attempt
1. Washed hands.	10			
2. Retrieved medication from drug cabinet—checking label before removing from shelf (Label Check # 1). (Checked name and strength of drug.)	10			
3. Removed unopened transdermal patch from the box.	10			
4. Compared written drug order with drug label before preparing drug. Checked the expiration date (Label Check # 2).	10			
5. Read package insert prior to returning other patches to shelf to find out proper application directions. Read label before returning to cabinet once again to verify correct dose and drug (Label Check # 3).	10			
6. Properly transported the medication to the patient.	10			
7. Correctly identified the patient using two identifiers, identified self, and explained the procedure.	10			
8. Washed hands and applied gloves.	10			
9. Asked patient to expose the area in which the medication is to be applied. Selected area that was free from hair growth, lesions, wounds, moles or rashes. (If area was soiled or oily, cleaned skin with alcohol. Allowed to completely dry before applying patch.)	10			
10. Peeled protective plastic backing off dermal patch. Ensured patch was not accidentally torn or crushed during the opening process.	10			
11. Gently placed sticky side of the patch over correct area of skin. Applied gentle pressure to the patch to ensure patch adhered to patient's skin properly.	10			
12. Observed patient for appropriate time period for any signs of allergic reaction.	10			
13. Properly disposed of the medication package and other disposable supplies into the garbage.	10			
14. Removed gloves and washed hands.	10			
15. Provided patient with verbal instructions and educational brochures and asked patient to repeat back instructions.	10			
16. Had patient wait appropriate time period (20–30 minutes following application to check for any local or system reaction).				
17. Dismissed the patient and documented the procedure in the patient's chart and appropriate log.	10			
18. Student instituted the "Seven Rights" of proper drug administration at the appropriate times throughout the procedure.				
19. Completed the procedure within the appropriate time limit.	10			
Points Earned / Points Possible:	___ / 170			

Key Competencies		
ABHES	VI.B.1.a.4.m	Prepare and administer oral and parenteral medications as directed by physician
CAAHEP	III.C.3.c.4.g	Apply pharmacology principles to prepare and administer oral and parenteral (excluding IV) medications

Student Name: _____   Date: _____   Score: _____

Points possible reflect importance of step in meeting the task: Important = (5) Essential = (10).
Determine score by dividing points earned by total points possible, and multiplying results by 100.

EVALUATION
Evaluator Signature: _____   Date: _____

Evaluator Comments:

DOCUMENTATION
Instructor Note: Retain work products with competency checklist. Retain this section along with EKG tracing for Work Product documentation.
Work Product, Procedure 32-5 (Progress Note)

Progress Note for Patient: Date:	**DOUGLASVILLE MEDICINE ASSOCIATES** **5076 BRAND BLVD** **DOUGLASVILLE, NY 01234** **(123) 456-7890**

Work Product, Procedure 32-5 (Medication Log)

MEDICATION LOG

Date	Patient Name/ID	Ordering Provider	Name of Drug	Strength/ Amt. Given	Route	Manufacturer	Lot #	Exp. Date	Initials

Key Competencies		
ABHES	VI.B.1.a.4.m	Prepare and administer oral and parenteral medications as directed by physician
CAAHEP	III.C.3.c.4.g	Apply pharmacology principles to prepare and administer oral and parenteral (excluding IV) medications

Student Name: _____   Date: _____   Score: _____

Competency Checklist
PROCEDURE 32-6 Administer a Rectal Suppository

Task: To administer a rectal suppository to a patient

Condition: Given the equipment and supplies as listed in the procedure and a classmate to play the part of the patient, the student will demonstrate the correct procedure for administering a rectal suppository, adhering to the steps listed below.

Standards: The student will have 10 minutes to complete the procedure and will need to score an 85% or above to pass the competency. Automatic failure results if any essential steps are omitted or performed incorrectly.

STEPS START TIME: END TIME:	Points Possible	First Attempt	Second Attempt	Third Attempt
1. Washed hands.	10			
2. Retrieved medication from refrigerator checking to make certain of right medication (Label Check # 1).	10			
3. Compared written drug order with drug label before preparing drug; checked the name, strength, expiration date (Label Check # 2).	10			
4. Removed the suppository from the box and returned other suppositories back to the refrigerator checking label one more time (Label Check # 3).	10			
5. Placed the unopened suppository on tray with 4x4s and lubricant; properly transported the medication to the patient.	10			
6. Correctly identified the patient using two identifiers, identified self, and explained procedure.	10			
7. Gave patient drape and gown and instructed how to disrobe.				
8. Washed hands and applied gloves.	10			
9. Placed disposable underpad on the table for the patient to lie on.	10			
10. Carefully opened the foil pack and removed suppository, being careful not to mash it.	10			
11. Instructed patient to lie in Sims' position on the exam table.	10			
12. Applied lubricant to the suppository tip. Instructed patient to take in a deep breath and to blow it out while the suppository is being inserted.	10			
13. Gently spread the cheeks of the buttocks with one hand while inserting the suppository with index or middle finger of the other hand, guiding it past the internal anal sphincter along the side of the rectal wall	10			
14. Asked patient to remain in Sims' position for allotted time listed in instructions.	10			
15. Removed gloves and washed hands. Observed patient for appropriate reaction to the medication.	10			
16. Assisted the patient into seated position when proper length of time had been reached for adequate medication absorption. Checked patient for any reactions at that time.	10			
17. Dismissed the patient and documented the procedure in the patient's chart and appropriate log (*Work Product, Procedure 32-6*).	10			
18. Student instituted the "Seven Rights" of proper drug administration at the appropriate times throughout the procedure.	10			
19. Completed the procedure within the appropriate time limit.	10			
Points Earned / Points Possible:	___ / 180			

Key Competencies		
ABHES	VI.A.1.a.4.m	Prepare and administer oral and parenteral medications as directed by physician
CAAHEP	III.C.3.c.4.g	Apply pharmacology principles to prepare and administer oral and parenteral (excluding IV) medications

Student Name: _____   Date: _____   Score: _____

Points possible reflect importance of step in meeting the task: Important = (5) Essential = (10).
Determine score by dividing points earned by total points possible, and multiplying results by 100.

EVALUATION
Evaluator Signature: _____   Date: _____

Evaluator Comments:

DOCUMENTATION
Instructor Note: Retain work products with competency checklist.
Work Product, Procedure 32-6 (Progress Note)

Progress Note for Patient: Date:	**DOUGLASVILLE MEDICINE ASSOCIATES** **5076 BRAND BLVD** **DOUGLASVILLE, NY 01234** **(123) 456-7890**

Work Product, Procedure 32-6 (Medication Log)

MEDICATION LOG

Date	Patient Name/ID	Ordering Provider	Name of Drug	Strength/ Amt. Given	Route	Manufacturer	Lot #	Exp. Date	Initials

Key Competencies		
ABHES	VI.A.1.a.4.m	Prepare and administer oral and parenteral medications as directed by physician
CAAHEP	III.C.3.c.4.g	Apply pharmacology principles to prepare and administer oral and parenteral (excluding IV) medications

Student Name: _____   Date: _____   Score: _____

Competency Checklist
PROCEDURE 34-1 Withdraw Medication from a Vial

Task: To withdraw medication from a vial

Condition: Given the equipment and supplies as listed in the procedure, the student will demonstrate the correct procedure for withdrawing medication from a vial, adhering to the steps listed below.

Standards: The student will have 7 minutes to complete the procedure and will need to score an 85% or above to pass the competency. Automatic failure results if any essential steps are omitted or performed incorrectly

STEPS START TIME: END TIME:	Points Possible	First Attempt	Second Attempt	Third Attempt
1. Washed hands and applied gloves.	10			
2. Assembled equipment and supplies.	10			
3. Selected correct medication by checking the medication label (Label Check # 1).	10			
4. Checked expiration date on drug label; compared medication label to physician's order; calculated correct dose if needed (Label Check # 2).	10			
5. Opened syringe and needle (assembled if necessary).	10			
6. Cleaned the vial with antiseptic wipe.	10			
7. Holding syringe at eye level, pulled back on plunger of syringe—to draw the amount of air into the syringe—equal to amount of medication to be withdrawn.	10			
8. Checked to make certain needle was firmly attached to syringe and removed needle cap; inserted needle through rubber stopper until it reached the empty space between the stopper and the medication fluid.	10			
9. Pushed forward on plunger to inject air into the vial; inverted vial without contaminating the needle or hub of syringe.	10			
10. Withdrew the proper amount of medication; removed air bubbles by flicking the side of syringe where bubbles were located.	10			
11. Removed any remaining air in the tip of the syringe; made necessary adjustments to ascertain correct medication amount. Removed the needle from the rubber stopper; replaced the needle cap following institutional policy or replaced needle with a new needle/cap setup.	10			
12. Read medication label (Label Check # 3) and replaced the medication vial to the correct storage cabinet.	10			
13. Placed syringe on a clean tray for administration with necessary supplies to administer injection.	10			
14. Completed the procedure within the appropriate time limit.	10			
Points Earned / Points Possible:	___ / 140			

Points possible reflect importance of step in meeting the task: Important = (5) Essential = (10).
Determine score by dividing points earned by total points possible, and multiplying results by 100.

EVALUATION
Evaluator Signature: _____   Date: _____

Evaluator Comments:

Key Competencies		
ABHES	VI.A.1.a.4.m	Prepare and administer oral and parenteral medications as directed by the physician
CAAHEP	III.C.3.b.4.g	Apply pharmacology principles to prepare and administer oral and parenteral (excluding IV) medications

Student Name: _____   Date: _____   Score: _____

Competency Checklist
PROCEDURE 34-2 Withdraw Medication from an Ampule

Task: To withdraw medication from an ampule

Condition: Given the equipment and supplies as listed in the procedure, the student will demonstrate the correct procedure for withdrawing medication from an ampule, adhering to the steps listed below.

Standards: The student will have 7 minutes to complete the procedure and will need to score an 85% or above to pass the competency. Automatic failure results if any essential steps are omitted or performed incorrectly.

STEPS START TIME: END TIME:	Points Possible	First Attempt	Second Attempt	Third Attempt
1. Washed hands and applied gloves.	10			
2. Assembled equipment and supplies.	10			
3. Selected correct medication by checking the medication label (Label check # 1).	10			
4. Checked expiration date on drug label; compared medication label to physician's order; calculated the correct dose if needed (Label Check # 2).	10			
5. Opened and assembled syringe and filter needle.	10			
6. Tapped the stem of ampule lightly to remove medication in the neck of the ampule.	10			
7. Cleaned the ampule with antiseptic wipe and allowed to completely dry.	10			
8. Placed a piece of gauze around neck of ampule; quickly and firmly broke off stem of ampule—breaking it away from the body.	10			
9. Discarded stem of ampule into sharps container.	10			
10. Removed needle cap from a prepared filter needle while checking to make certain the needle was firmly attached to syringe.	10			
11. Inserted the needle into the ampule below the fluid level. Held ampule at slight angle while drawing up entire contents of ampule.	10			
12. Removed needle from ampule without touching the edges of ampule; Disposed of ampule into sharps container checking the medication label one last time (Label Check # 3).	10			
13. Removed air bubbles in the syringe.	10			
14. Slightly pulled back on plunger of syringe to withdraw any residual medication left in filter needle. Engaged safety device and removed filter needle from syringe—disposing of needle in sharp's container. Opened new needle and firmly attached to syringe.	10			
15. Pushed slightly forward on plunger to remove air in the tip of the syringe and shaft of new needle. Replaced needle cap.	10			
16. Placed syringe on a clean tray for administration along with necessary items to administer injection to the patient.	10			
17. Completed the procedure within the appropriate time limit.	10			
Points Earned / Points Possible:	___ / 170			

Points possible reflect importance of step in meeting the task: Important = (5) Essential = (10).
Determine score by dividing points earned by total points possible, and multiplying results by 100.

Key Competencies		
ABHES	VI.A.1.a.4.m	Prepare and administer oral and parenteral medications as directed by the physician
CAAHEP	III.C.3.b.4.g	Apply pharmacology principles to prepare and administer oral and parenteral (excluding IV) medications

Student Name: _____   Date: _____   Score: _____

EVALUATION
Evaluator Signature: _____   Date: _____

Evaluator Comments:

Key Competencies		
ABHES	VI.A.1.a.4.m	Prepare and administer oral and parenteral medications as directed by the physician
CAAHEP	III.C.3.b.4.g	Apply pharmacology principles to prepare and administer oral and parenteral (excluding IV) medications

Student Name: _____   Date: _____   Score: _____

Competency Checklist
PROCEDURE 34-3 Reconstitute a Powdered-Base Medication with a Diluent

Task: To reconstitute a powdered-base medication

Condition: Given the equipment and supplies as listed in the procedure, the student will demonstrate the correct procedure for reconstituting a powdered-base medication, adhering to the steps listed below.

Standards: The student will have 7 minutes to complete the procedure and will need to score an 85% or above to pass the competency. Automatic failure results if any essential steps are omitted or performed incorrectly

STEPS START TIME: END TIME:	Points Possible	First Attempt	Second Attempt	Third Attempt
1. Washed hands and applied gloves.	10			
2. Assembled equipment and supplies.	10			
3. Selected correct medication and diluent by carefully checking both labels while removing from cabinet (Label Check # 1).	10			
4. Checked expiration dates on both drug labels; compared medication label to physician's order; calculated correct dose if needed (Label Check # 2).	10			
5. Opened the syringe and needle and assembled if necessary.				
6. Cleaned rubber stoppers of both vials with alcohol wipes.	10			
7. Pulled back on the plunger to fill the syringe with the amount of air equal to the amount of diluting liquid required for reconstitution from the vial containing the diluent.	10			
8. Checked to make certain that needle was firmly attached to syringe and removed needle cap.	10			
9. Inserted needle into the diluent vial; pushed in plunger forcing air into the vial of diluent.	10			
10. Inverted vial; withdrew desired amount of solution; checked for air bubbles.	10			
11. Removed needle from vial; inserted needle into vial containing powered medication.	10			
12. Added the appropriate amount of reconstituting liquid to powdered drug; slowly rotated vial while injecting fluid into vial.	10			
13. Replaced needle cap; rolled vial between hands to mix the medication.	10			
14. Recorded the new date of expiration on the label of the medication vial.	10			
15. Rechecked medication label and diluent vials before returning vial to proper storage area.	10			
16. Prepared to administer medication to the patient. Placed necessary items on tray to administer injection to the patient.	10			
17. Completed the procedure within the appropriate time limit.	10			
Points Earned / Points Possible:	___ / 160			

Points possible reflect importance of step in meeting the task: Important = (5) Essential = (10).
Determine score by dividing points earned by total points possible, and multiplying results by 100.

Key Competencies		
ABHES	VI.A.1.a.4.m	Prepare and administer oral and parenteral medications as directed by the physician
CAAHEP	III.C.3.b.4.g	Apply pharmacology principles to prepare and administer oral and parenteral (excluding IV) medications

Student Name: _____   Date: _____   Score: _____

EVALUATION
Evaluator Signature: _____   Date: _____

Evaluator Comments:

Key Competencies		
ABHES	VI.A.1.a.4.m	Prepare and administer oral and parenteral medications as directed by the physician
CAAHEP	III.C.3.b.4.g	Apply pharmacology principles to prepare and administer oral and parenteral (excluding IV) medications

Student Name: _____   Date: _____   Score: _____

Competency Checklist
PROCEDURE 34-4 Mix Two Medications into One Syringe

Task: To mix two medications into one syringe

Condition: Given the equipment and supplies as listed in the procedure, the student will demonstrate the correct procedure for mixing two medications into one syringe, adhering to the steps listed below.

Standards: The student will have 7 minutes to complete the procedure and will need to score an 85% or above to pass the competency. Automatic failure results if any essential steps are omitted or performed incorrectly.

STEPS START TIME: END TIME:	Points Possible	First Attempt	Second Attempt	Third Attempt
1. Washed hands and applied gloves.	10			
2. Assembled equipment and supplies.	10			
3. Removed medications from drug cabinet while checking their labels (Label check # 1).	10			
4. Checked expiration dates on both drug labels; compared medications to physician's instructions; calculated correct doses if needed (Label check # 2).	10			
5. Opened syringe and needle; firmly attached needle to syringe.	10			
6. Cleaned rubber stoppers of both vials with alcohol wipes.	10			
7. Determined which medication was primary; drew up air into syringe equal to amount of medication required to be withdrawn from *second vial*.	10			
8. Checked to make certain needle was firmly attached to syringe and removed cap to needle.	10			
Move to the second vial:				
9. Inserted needle into second vial and pushed air from syringe into the vial to replace the medication to be aspirated later. *Did not allow needle touch the liquid.*	10			
10. Carefully removed needle; drew up amount of air into syringe equal to the amount of medication required to be removed from the *primary vial*.	10			
Move back to first vial:				
11. Inserted needle into primary vial; pushed forward on the plunger forcing air from syringe into vial without touching the medication.	10			
12. Inverted vial; kept needle immersed in medication solution while drawing the proper amount of medication into the barrel of the syringe; checked for air bubbles.	10			
13. Removed any excess air in the tip of the syringe. If medication is lacking in syringe, pulled back on the plunger to the correct amount of medication.	10			
14. Removed needle from first stopper of first vial, engaged safety device and discarded into sharps container.	10			
Moved back to first vial:				
15. Replaced syringe with new needle and inserted into secondary vial.	10			
16. Inverted vial and slowly withdrew medication to correct calibration mark on the syringe. Removed needle from vial.	10			

Key Competencies		
ABHES	VI.A.1.a.4.m	Prepare and administer oral and parenteral medications as directed by the physician
CAAHEP	III.C.3.b.4.g	Apply pharmacology principles to prepare and administer oral and parenteral (excluding IV) medications

Student Name: _____   Date: _____   Score: _____

17. Checked for air bubbles and replaced needle cap following institutional policy or replaced entire needle unit. Checked that the total amount of medication in the syringe was correct and returned vials to proper storage area. Checked labels on medication vials again to ascertain they were the correct medications (Label check # 3).	10			
18. Placed medication and necessary items on tray for patient administration of injection.	10			
19. Completed the procedure within the appropriate time limit.	10			
Points Earned / Points Possible:	___ / 190			

Points possible reflect importance of step in meeting the task: Important = (5) Essential = (10).
Determine score by dividing points earned by total points possible, and multiplying results by 100.

EVALUATION
Evaluator Signature: _____   Date: _____

Evaluator Comments:

Key Competencies		
ABHES	VI.A.1.a.4.m	Prepare and administer oral and parenteral medications as directed by the physician
CAAHEP	III.C.3.b.4.g	Apply pharmacology principles to prepare and administer oral and parenteral (excluding IV) medications

Student Name: _____   Date: _____   Score: _____

Competency Checklist
PROCEDURE 34-5 Load a Cartridge or Injector Device

Task: To load a cartridge or injector device

Condition: Given the equipment and supplies as listed in the procedure, the student will demonstrate the correct procedure for loading a cartridge or injector device, adhering to the steps listed below.

Standards: The student will have 7 minutes to perform the procedure and will need to score an 85% or above to pass the competency. Automatic failure results if any essential steps are omitted or performed incorrectly.

STEPS START TIME: END TIME:	Points Possible	First Attempt	Second Attempt	Third Attempt
1. Washed hands and applied gloves.	10			
2. Assembled equipment and supplies.	10			
3. Removed cartridge from storage location—while carefully checking the drug label (Label Check # 1).	10			
4. Checked expiration date; compared medication with doctor's order; calculated the correct dose if necessary (Label Check # 2).	10			
5. Picked up cartridge unit holder (injector).	10			
6. Turned ribbed collar toward the "Open" arrow until it stopped.	10			
7. Held injector with the open end up and fully inserted sterile cartridge into the injector.	10			
8. Tightened ribbed collar of the injector by turning ribbed collar toward the "Close" arrow. (Held cartridge to prevent unit from swiveling inside the holder.)	10			
9. Threaded plunger rod tightly onto cartridge unit until resistance was felt.	10			
10. Prepared the medication tray.	10			
11. After use, did not recap needle. Disengaged the plunger rod from the injector while holding needle down and away from fingers or hands.	10			
12. Loosened the ribbed collar of the injector.	10			
13. Held needle over biohazard sharps container allowing the needle and cartridge to drop into the sharps container.	10			
14. Cleaned cartridge holder with an antiseptic cleanser and returned to storage area.	10			
15. Cleaned work area, removed gloves, and washed hands.	10			
16. Completed the procedure within the appropriate time limit.	10			
Points Earned / Points Possible:	___ / 160			

Points possible reflect importance of step in meeting the task: Important = (5) Essential = (10).
Determine score by dividing points earned by total points possible, and multiplying results by 100.

EVALUATION
Evaluator Signature: _____   Date: _____

Evaluator Comments:

Key Competencies		
ABHES	VI.A.1.a.4.m	Prepare and administer oral and parenteral medications as directed by the physician
CAAHEP	III.C.3.b.4.g	Apply pharmacology principles to prepare and administer oral and parenteral (excluding IV) medications

Student Name: _____   Date: _____   Score: _____

Competency Checklist
PROCEDURE 34-6 Administer an Intradermal Injection

Task: To administer an intradermal injection

Condition: Given the equipment and supplies as listed in the procedure, and a classmate or injection pad to perform the injection on, the student will demonstrate the correct procedure for administering an intradermal injection, adhering to the steps listed below.

Standards: The student will have 10 minutes to complete the procedure (not including the post-injection observation) and will need to score an 85% or above to pass the competency. Automatic failure results if any essential steps are omitted or performed incorrectly.

STEPS START TIME: END TIME:	Points Possible	First Attempt	Second Attempt	Third Attempt
1. Washed hands.	10			
2. Assembled equipment and supplies.	10			
3. Identified the patient using at least two identifiers, identified self, and explained the procedure.	10			
4. Asked patient about any drug or latex allergies.	10			
5. Properly located and selected injection site.	10			
6. Cleaned the injection site in circular manner and allowed site to air dry.	10			
7. Prepared equipment and applied gloves.	10			
8. Removed needle guard without contaminating it.	10			
9. Selected the location; stretched the skin; Inserted needle at a 10- to 15-degree angle with the bevel up.	10			
10. Injected medication slowly—while allowing a wheal to form. Removed needle at same angle of insertion.	10			
11. Gently placed cotton ball over injection site; did not press on cotton or massage the site.	10			
12. Engaged safety device and placed needle/syringe unit into sharps container.	10			
13. Gave patient home care and waiting instructions and performed a post-injection observation on patient 20–30 minutes following injection. (If applicable, instructed patient when to return to the office to have site evaluated—48–72 hours.)	10			
14. Correctly documented procedure on progress note and in appropriate logs.	10			
15. Completed the procedure within the appropriate time limit and instituted the "Seven Rights" of proper drug administration at the appropriate times throughout the procedure.	10			
Points Earned / Points Possible:	___ / 150			

Points possible reflect importance of step in meeting the task: Important = (5) Essential = (10).
Determine score by dividing points earned by total points possible, and multiplying results by 100.

Key Competencies		
ABHES	VI.A.1.a.4.m	Prepare and administer oral and parenteral medications as directed by the physician
	VI.A.1.a.4.n	Maintain medication and immunization records
CAAHEP	III.C.3.b.4.g	Apply pharmacology principles to prepare and administer oral and parenteral (excluding IV) medications
	III.C.3.b.4.h	Maintain medication and immunization records

Student Name: _____   Date: _____   Score: _____

EVALUATION
Evaluator Signature: _____   Date: _____

Evaluator Comments:

DOCUMENTATION
Instructor Note: Retain work products with competency checklist. Retain this section along with EKG tracing for Work Product documentation.
Work Product, Procedure 34-6 (Progress Note)

Progress Note for Patient: Date:	**DOUGLASVILLE MEDICINE ASSOCIATES** **5076 BRAND BLVD** **DOUGLASVILLE, NY 01234** **(123) 456-7890**

Work Product, Procedure 28-3 (Medication Log)

MEDICATION LOG

Date	Patient Name/ID	Ordering Provider	Name of Drug	Strength/ Amt. Given	Route	Manufacturer	Lot #	Exp. Date	Initials

Key Competencies		
ABHES	VI.A.1.a.4.m	Prepare and administer oral and parenteral medications as directed by the physician
	VI.A.1.a.4.n	Maintain medication and immunization records
CAAHEP	III.C.3.b.4.g	Apply pharmacology principles to prepare and administer oral and parenteral (excluding IV) medications
	III.C.3.b.4.h	Maintain medication and immunization records

Student Name: _____   Date: _____   Score: _____

Competency Checklist
PROCEDURE 34-7 Administer a Subcutaneous Injection

Task: To administer a subcutaneous injection

Condition: Given the equipment and supplies as listed in the procedure, and a classmate or injection pad to perform the injection on, the student will demonstrate the correct procedure for administering a subcutaneous injection, adhering to the steps listed below.

Standards: The student will have 10 minutes to complete the procedure (not including the post-injection observation) and will need to score an 85% or above to pass the competency. Automatic failure results if any essential steps are omitted or performed incorrectly.

STEPS START TIME: END TIME:	Points Possible	First Attempt	Second Attempt	Third Attempt
1. Washed hands.	10			
2. Assembled equipment and supplies. Instituted the "Seven Rights" of drug administration.	10			
3. Identified the patient using at least two identifiers, identified self, and explained the procedure.	10			
4. Asked patient about possible drug, latex, or adhesive allergies.	10			
5. Selected proper injection site.	10			
6. Cleaned the injection site in circular motion working outward and allowed site to air dry.	10			
7. Prepared equipment and applied gloves.	10			
8. Removed needle guard without contaminating.	10			
9. Pinched/grasped the skin with one hand while inserting needle using a 45-degree angle with the other hand.	10			
10. Aspirated to ascertain not in a blood vessel and injected medication slowly and steadily.	10			
11. Removed needle at same angle of insertion.				
12. Placed cotton ball over injection site and gently massaged area.	10			
13. Engaged needle's safety device. Placed needle and syringe unit into sharps container.	10			
14. Applied adhesive bandage and had patient wait in a designated area for 20–30 minutes.	10			
15. Cleaned area, removed gloves, and washed hands.	10			
16. Performed post-injection observation of the injection site and patient at the proper time and gave patient home care instructions.	10			
17. Correctly documented procedure and post-injection observation on progress note and in appropriate logs.	10			
18. Completed the procedure within the appropriate time limit and instituted the "Seven Rights" of proper drug administration at the appropriate times throughout the procedure.	10			
Points Earned / Points Possible:	___ / 180			

Points possible reflect importance of step in meeting the task: Important = (5) Essential = (10).
Determine score by dividing points earned by total points possible, and multiplying results by 100.

Key Competencies		
ABHES	VI.A.1.a.4.m	Prepare and administer oral and parenteral medications as directed by the physician
	VI.A.1.a.4.n	Maintain medication and immunization records
CAAHEP	III.C.3.b.4.g	Apply pharmacology principles to prepare and administer oral and parenteral (excluding IV) medications
	III.C.3.b.4.h	Maintain medication and immunization records

Student Name: _____   Date: _____   Score: _____

EVALUATION
Evaluator Signature: _____   Date: _____

Evaluator Comments:

DOCUMENTATION
Instructor Note: Retain work products with competency checklist.
Work Product, Procedure 34-7 (Progress Note)

Progress Note for Patient: Date:	**DOUGLASVILLE MEDICINE ASSOCIATES** **5076 BRAND BLVD** **DOUGLASVILLE, NY 01234** **(123) 456-7890**

Work Product, Procedure 34-7 (Medication Log)

MEDICATION LOG

Date	Patient Name/ID	Ordering Provider	Name of Drug	Strength/ Amt. Given	Route	Manufacturer	Lot #	Exp. Date	Initials

Key Competencies		
ABHES	VI.A.1.a.4.m	Prepare and administer oral and parenteral medications as directed by the physician
	VI.A.1.a.4.n	Maintain medication and immunization records
CAAHEP	III.C.3.b.4.g	Apply pharmacology principles to prepare and administer oral and parenteral (excluding IV) medications
	III.C.3.b.4.h	Maintain medication and immunization records

Student Name: _____   Date: _____   Score: _____

Competency Checklist
PROCEDURE 34-8 Administer an Intramuscular Injection

Task: To administer an intramuscular injection

Condition: Given the equipment and supplies as listed in the procedure, and a classmate or injection pad to perform the injection on, the student will demonstrate the correct procedure for administering an intramuscular injection, adhering to the steps listed below.

Standards: The student will have 10 minutes to complete the procedure (not including the post-injection observation) and will need to score an 85% or above to pass the competency. Automatic failure results if any essential steps are omitted or performed incorrectly.

STEPS START TIME: END TIME:	Points Possible	First Attempt	Second Attempt	Third Attempt
1. Washed hands.	10			
2. Assembled equipment and supplies.	10			
3. Identified the patient using at least two identifiers, identified self, and explained the procedure.	10			
4. Asked the patient about drug, latex and adhesive allergies.	10			
5. Located proper injection site.	10			
6. Cleaned the injection site in circular motion working outward and allowed site to air dry.	10			
7. Prepared equipment and applied gloves.	10			
8. Removed needle guard without contaminating needle or sticking self.	10			
9. Held the skin taut with one hand while inserting the needle smoothly and swiftly using a 90-degree angle with the other hand.	10			
10. Aspirated to ascertain not in a blood vessel; if blood was in syringe, started all over again. Stabilized needle within the tissue.	10			
11. Injected medication slowly and steadily into the tissue—removed needle at same angle of insertion.	10			
12. Placed cotton ball over injection site and gently massaged area (if not contraindicated).	10			
13. Engaged safety device; placed needle/syringe unit into sharps container.	10			
14. Observed patient for a reaction; removed gloves and washed hands.	10			
15. Applied adhesive bandage and gave patient both home care and waiting instructions.	10			
16. Performed post-injection observation of patient and site 20–30 minutes following the injection.	10			
17. Correctly documented procedure and post-injection observation on progress note and in appropriate logs.	10			
18. Completed the procedure within the appropriate time limit and instituted the "Seven Rights" of proper drug administration at the appropriate times throughout the procedure.	10			
Points Earned / Points Possible:	___ / 180			

Points possible reflect importance of step in meeting the task: Important = (5) Essential = (10).
Determine score by dividing points earned by total points possible, and multiplying results by 100.

Key Competencies		
ABHES	VI.A.1.a.4.m	Prepare and administer oral and parenteral medications as directed by the physician
	VI.A.1.a.4.n	Maintain medication and immunization records
CAAHEP	III.C.3.b.4.g	Apply pharmacology principles to prepare and administer oral and parenteral (excluding IV) medications
	III.C.3.b.4.h	Maintain medication and immunization records

Student Name: _____   Date: _____   Score: _____

EVALUATION
Evaluator Signature: _____   Date: _____

Evaluator Comments:

DOCUMENTATION
Instructor Note: Retain work products with competency checklist.
Work Product, Procedure 34-8 (Progress Note)

Progress Note for Patient: Date:	**DOUGLASVILLE MEDICINE ASSOCIATES** **5076 BRAND BLVD** **DOUGLASVILLE, NY 01234** **(123) 456-7890**

Work Product, Procedure 34-8 (Medication Log)

MEDICATION LOG

Date	Patient Name/ID	Ordering Provider	Name of Drug	Strength/ Amt. Given	Route	Manufacturer	Lot #	Exp. Date	Initials

Key Competencies			
ABHES	VI.A.1.a.4.m	Prepare and administer oral and parenteral medications as directed by the physician	
	VI.A.1.a.4.n	Maintain medication and immunization records	
CAAHEP	III.C.3.b.4.g	Apply pharmacology principles to prepare and administer oral and parenteral (excluding IV) medications	
	III.C.3.b.4.h	Maintain medication and immunization records	

Student Name: _____   Date: _____   Score: _____

Competency Checklist
PROCEDURE 34-9 Administer a Z-Track Medication

Task: To administer a Z-Track Medication

Condition: Given the equipment and supplies as listed in the procedure, and a classmate or injection pad to perform the injection on, the student will demonstrate the correct procedure for administering a Z-track medication, adhering to the steps listed below.

Standards: The student will have 10 minutes to complete the procedure (not including the post-injection observation) and will need to score an 85% or above to pass the competency. Automatic failure results if any essential steps are omitted or performed incorrectly.

STEPS START TIME: END TIME:	Points Possible	First Attempt	Second Attempt	Third Attempt
1. Washed hands.	10			
2. Assembled equipment and supplies.	10			
3. Identified the patient using at least two identifiers, identified self, and explained the procedure.	10			
4. Asked patient about drug, latex, and adhesive allergies.	10			
5. Selected and located the proper injection site (dorsogluteal or dorsoventral).	10			
6. Cleaned the injection site using a circular motion working outward and allowed site to air dry.	10			
7. Prepared equipment and applied gloves.	10			
8. Removed needle guard without contaminating the needle or sticking self.	10			
9. Using one hand, pulled the tissue laterally 1–2 inches away from injection site.	10			
10. With the other hand inserted needle swiftly and smoothly using a 90-degree angle; aspirated using the one hand technique.	10			
11. Injected medication slowly and steadily and waited 10 seconds before removing needle at the same angle of insertion.	10			
12. Released tissue *after* removing needle from the site. Placed cotton ball over injection site. *Did not massage site.*	10			
13. Engaged safety device; placed needle and syringe into sharps container.	10			
14. Applied adhesive bandage over injection site and gave patient home care instructions. Had patient wait for the proper amount of time following the injection.	10			
15. Performed post-injection observation 20–30 minutes following the injection. Observed patient for a reaction; removed gloves and washed hands.	10			
16. Correctly documented procedure and post-injection observation on progress note and in appropriate logs.	10			
17. Completed the procedure within the appropriate time limit and instituted all "Seven Rights" of drug administration at the appropriate times throughout the procedure.	10			
Points Earned / Points Possible:	___ /170			

Points possible reflect importance of step in meeting the task: Important = (5) Essential = (10).
Determine score by dividing points earned by total points possible, and multiplying results by 100.

Key Competencies		
ABHES	VI.A.1.a.4.m	Prepare and administer oral and parenteral medications as directed by the physician
	VI.A.1.a.4.n	Maintain medication and immunization records
CAAHEP	III.C.3.b.4.g	Apply pharmacology principles to prepare and administer oral and parenteral (excluding IV) medications
	III.C.3.b.4.h	Maintain medication and immunization records

Student Name: _____   Date: _____   Score: _____

EVALUATION
Evaluator Signature: _____   Date: _____

Evaluator Comments:

DOCUMENTATION
Instructor Note: Retain work products with competency checklist.
Work Product, Procedure 34-9 (Progress Note)

Progress Note for Patient: Date:	**DOUGLASVILLE MEDICINE ASSOCIATES** **5076 BRAND BLVD** **DOUGLASVILLE, NY 01234** **(123) 456-7890**

Work Product, Procedure 34-9 (Medication Log)

MEDICATION LOG

Date	Patient Name/ID	Ordering Provider	Name of Drug	Strength/ Amt. Given	Route	Manufacturer	Lot #	Exp. Date	Initials

Key Competencies		
ABHES	VI.A.1.a.4.m	Prepare and administer oral and parenteral medications as directed by the physician
	VI.A.1.a.4.n	Maintain medication and immunization records
CAAHEP	III.C.3.b.4.g	Apply pharmacology principles to prepare and administer oral and parenteral (excluding IV) medications
	III.C.3.b.4.h	Maintain medication and immunization records

Student Name: _____   Date: _____   Score: _____

Competency Checklist
PROCEDURE 35-1 Apply First Responder Principles during an Emergency to an Adult

Task: To apply first responder principles during an emergency to an adult

Condition: Given the equipment and supplies as listed in the procedure, and a few classmates to play the parts of victim and other staff members, the student will demonstrate the correct procedure for administering first responder principles to an adult during an emergency, adhering to the steps listed below.

Standards: The student will have 15 minutes to complete the procedure and will need to score an 85% or above to pass the competency. Automatic failure results if any essential steps are omitted or performed incorrectly.

Student comes upon the scene of _____.

STEPS START TIME: END TIME:	Points Possible	First Attempt	Second Attempt	Third Attempt
1. Determined scene safety (traffic, live wires, gassy odors).	10			
2. Applied PPE.	10			
3. Established unresponsiveness of the victim and rated victim's consciousness using AVPU scale. Checked for MedicAlert product.	10			
4. Alerted medical staff and physician *stat*. Instructed staff members to call 911.	10			
5. "A": Opened the airway (head tilt-chin lift). If head or neck injury used jaw thrust procedure to open airway.	10			
6. "B": Assessed breathing and gave two breaths if applicable.	10			
7. "C": Checked carotid pulse and for other signs of circulation. If no pulse administered five sets of 30 compressions to two ventilations over a 2-minute period. Continued until victim's heartbeat was restored, or until an AED arrived, or until the EMS arrived.	10			
8. "D": If there was no pulse, and an AED was available, applied AED and followed directions from unit for proving shocks and continuous CPR.	10			
9. "D": Checked for disabilities (head to toe evaluation of victim using the DOTS mnemonic: Deformities, Open injuries, Tenderness, or Swelling).	10			
10. "R": Appropriately responded to victim's condition or injuries (controlled bleeding, immobilized joints by splinting, etc.).	10			
11. Assessed victim's vital signs.	10			
12. Continued to observe victim until physician or EMS arrived. Reported findings to emergency personnel or physician.	10			
13. Disposed of biohazardous wastes.	10			
14. Washed hands.	10			
15. Correctly documented procedure on progress note.	10			
16. Completed the procedure within the appropriate time limit.	10			
Points Earned / Points Possible:	___ / 160			

Points possible reflect importance of step in meeting the task: Important = (5) Essential = (10).
Determine score by dividing points earned by total points possible, and multiplying results by 100.

Key Competencies		
ABHES	VI.A.1.a.4.e	Recognize emergencies
	VI.A.1.a.4.f	Perform first aid and CPR

Student Name: _____   Date: _____   Score: _____

EVALUATION

Evaluator Signature: _____   Date: _____

Evaluator Comments:

DOCUMENTATION

Instructor Note: Retain work products with competency checklist.

Work Product, Procedure 35-1 (Progress Note)

Progress Note for Patient: Date:	**DOUGLASVILLE MEDICINE ASSOCIATES** **5076 BRAND BLVD** **DOUGLASVILLE, NY 01234** **(123) 456-7890**

Key Competencies		
ABHES	VI.A.1.a.4.e	Recognize emergencies
	VI.A.1.a.4.f	Perform first aid and CPR

Student Name: _____ Date: _____ Score: _____

Competency Checklist
PROCEDURE 35-2 Control Bleeding in the Medical Office

Task: To control bleeding in the medical office

Condition: Given the equipment and supplies as listed in the procedure, and a few classmates to play the parts of the victim and physician, the student will demonstrate the correct steps for controlling bleeding on a patient that is profusely bleeding in the office, adhering to the steps listed below.

Standards: The student will have 15 minutes to complete the procedure and will need to score an 85% or above to pass the competency. Automatic failure results if any essential steps are omitted or performed incorrectly.

STEPS START TIME: END TIME:	Points Possible	First Attempt	Second Attempt	Third Attempt
1. Washed hands and applied PPE.	10			
2. Assembled equipment and supplies.	10			
3. Identified the patient, identified self, and determined extent of bleeding emergency.	10			
4. If area was bandaged and bleeding was coming through the bandage, applied 4x4s over top of existing bandage. If no bandage was present, applied sterile 4x4s over bleeding wound and applied direct pressure to the site.	10			
5. Elevated patient's limb above the level of patient's heart.	10			
6. Applied direct pressure to the artery between the point of attachment and the site of the injury (brachial artery for upper limbs and femoral artery for lower limbs).	10			
7. If bleeding was still not controlled, alerted physician so that he or she could apply tourniquet above the affected area (attached note indicating time tourniquet was applied).	10			
8. Treated patient for shock and helped patient to remain calm while waiting for EMS.	10			
9. Monitored patient for breathing and heart function.	10			
10. Correctly documented incident on progress note.	10			
11. Completed the procedure within the appropriate time limit.	10			
Points Earned / Points Possible:	___ / 110			

Points possible reflect importance of step in meeting the task: Important = (5) Essential = (10).
Determine score by dividing points earned by total points possible, and multiplying results by 100.

EVALUATION
Evaluator Signature: _____ Date: _____

Evaluator Comments:

Key Competencies			
ABHES	VI.A.1.a.4.e	Recognize emergencies	
	VI.A.1.a.4.f	Perform first aid and CPR	

Student Name: _____   Date: _____   Score: _____

DOCUMENTATION
Instructor Note: Retain work products with competency checklist
Work Product, Procedure 35-2 (Progress Note)

Progress Note for Patient: Date:	**DOUGLASVILLE MEDICINE ASSOCIATES** **5076 BRAND BLVD** **DOUGLASVILLE, NY 01234** **(123) 456-7890**

Key Competencies			
ABHES	VI.A.1.a.4.e	Recognize emergencies	
	VI.A.1.a.4.f	Perform first aid and CPR	

Student Name: _____   Date: _____   Score: _____

Competency Checklist
PROCEDURE 35-3 Splint an Arm

Task: To splint an arm

Condition: Given the equipment and supplies as listed in the procedure, and a classmate to play the part of the patient (victim), the student will demonstrate the correct steps for applying a splint to the arm, adhering to the steps listed below.

Standards: The student will have 15 minutes to complete the procedure and will need to score an 85% or above to pass the competency. Automatic failure results if any essential steps are omitted or performed incorrectly.

STEPS START TIME: END TIME:	Points Possible	First Attempt	Second Attempt	Third Attempt
1. Washed hands.	10			
2. Assembled equipment and supplies.	10			
3. Identified the patient using at least two identifiers, identified self, and explained the procedure.	10			
4. Followed steps on commercial splint for preparing splint.	10			
5. Positioned arm in the position in which it was to be splinted, stabilizing joint above and below the injury.	10			
6. Checked pulse point *distal* to the injury, checking the strength of the pulse, and for sensation and movement of fingers while arm was in the splinted position.	10			
7. Applied splint according to manufacturer's directions. Applied sling if applicable.	10			
8. Checked *distal* pulse point for pulse strength and checked fingers for sensation and movement after applying splint.	10			
9. Applied ice to reduce swelling.	10			
10. Washed hands.	10			
11. Correctly documented procedure on progress note.	10			
12. Completed the procedure within the appropriate time limit.	10			
Points Earned / Points Possible:	___ / 120			

Points possible reflect importance of step in meeting the task: Important = (5) Essential = (10).
Determine score by dividing points earned by total points possible, and multiplying results by 100.

EVALUATION
Evaluator Signature: _____   Date: _____

Evaluator Comments:

Key Competencies		
ABHES	VI.A.1.a.4.e	Recognize emergencies
CAAHEP	VI.A.1.a.4.f	Perform first aid and CPR

Student Name: _____   Date: _____   Score: _____

DOCUMENTATION
Instructor Note: Retain work products with competency checklist.
Work Product, Procedure 35-3 (Progress Note)

Progress Note for Patient: Date:	**DOUGLASVILLE MEDICINE ASSOCIATES** **5076 BRAND BLVD** **DOUGLASVILLE, NY 01234** **(123) 456-7890**

Key Competencies		
ABHES	VI.A.1.a.4.e	Recognize emergencies
CAAHEP	VI.A.1.a.4.f	Perform first aid and CPR

Student Name: _____   Date: _____   Score: _____

Competency Checklist
PROCEDURE 35-4 Treat the Patient for Shock

Task: To treat a patient for shock

Condition: Given the equipment and supplies as listed in the procedure, and a classmate to play the part of the patient (victim), the student will demonstrate the correct steps for treating a patient in shock, adhering to the steps listed below.

Standards: The student will have 15 minutes to complete the procedure and will need to score an 85% or above to pass the competency. Automatic failure results if any essential steps are omitted or performed incorrectly.

STEPS START TIME: END TIME:	Points Possible	First Attempt	Second Attempt	Third Attempt
1. Washed hands.	10			
2. Recognized the patient may be going into shock and took the patient's vital signs.	10			
3. Alerted physician *stat* and/or alerted EMS.	10			
4. Elevated patient's legs (used pillows or blankets if table does not allow for trendelenburg position).	10			
5. Placed a blanket or sheet over patient to keep warm.	10			
6. Monitored patient's airway, breathing and circulation.	10			
7. Kept the patient calm and reassured patient that help was on the way.	10			
8. Correctly documented procedure on progress note.	10			
9. Completed the procedure within the appropriate time limit.	10			
Points Earned / Points Possible:	___ / 90			

Points possible reflect importance of step in meeting the task: Important = (5) Essential = (10).
Determine score by dividing points earned by total points possible, and multiplying results by 100.

EVALUATION
Evaluator Signature: _____   Date: _____

Evaluator Comments:

Key Competencies		
ABHES	VI.A.1.a.4.e	Recognize emergencies
	VI.A.1.a.4.f	Perform first aid and CPR

Student Name: _____   Date: _____   Score: _____

DOCUMENTATION
Instructor Note: Retain work products with competency checklist.
Work Product, Procedure 35-4 (Progress Note)

Progress Note for Patient: Date:	**DOUGLASVILLE MEDICINE ASSOCIATES** **5076 BRAND BLVD** **DOUGLASVILLE, NY 01234** **(123) 456-7890**

Key Competencies		
ABHES	VI.A.1.a.4.e	Recognize emergencies
	VI.A.1.a.4.f	Perform first aid and CPR

System Requirements for SynapseEHR 1.1

- Microsoft Windows 2000, Windows XP (Service Pack 3), or Vista (Service Pack 1), MS Office 2003, MS Office 2007
- Pentium or Celeron PC with 300 MHz or higher processor recommended; 233 MHz minimum required
- 128 megabytes of RAM or higher recommended
- 1.5 gigabytes of available hard disk space (if using a USB Flash Drive, must have at least 50 MB of free space available)
- Super VGA (800 x 600) or higher-resolution video adapter and monitor
- CD-ROM or DVD drive; USB port if using a USB Flash Drive
- Keyboard and mouse or compatible pointing device

Installation Instructions for SynapseEHR 1.1

1. Insert the CD in your computer's CD drive. It should automatically begin the setup process. If not, continue to step 3.
2. Follow the installation prompts on the screen. Continue to steps 7–10 if you would like to use Synapse with a USB Flash Drive. If you are not using a USB Flash Drive, the installation is complete.
3. Double click "My Computer."
4. Double click the Control Panel icon.
5. Double click Add/Remove Programs.
6. Click the Install button and follow the on-screen prompts from there. Follow steps 7–10 if you would like to use Synapse with a USB Flash Drive. If you are not using a USB Flash Drive, the installation is complete.

Note: Only follow steps 7–10 if you are using Synapse with a USB Flash Drive.

7. Insert a USB Flash Drive into your computer USB port. Your USB Flash Drive must have at least 50 MB of free space available.
8. Copy the SynapseEHR database, SynapseEHR.mdb, from C:\Program Files\SynapseEHR to your USB Flash Drive:
   - Open "My Computer."
   - Double click on C: (Drive).
   - Double click on Program Files.
   - Double click on the SynapseEHR folder.
   - Click one time on SynapseEHR.mdb to highlight the file.
   - Right click and select Copy.
   - Next, open "My Computer" again.
   - Double click to open your Flash Drive (if not already open).
   - Right click and select Paste.
   - SynapseEHR.mdb should now appear on your Flash Drive.
   - Close all open windows.
9. To open Synapse, select your Flash Drive and double click on SynapseEHR.mdb.
10. You can now begin working in the Synapse program. If you have questions regarding steps 7–10, please contact Delmar's Technical Support at 800-648-7450, Monday–Friday, 8:30 a.m. to 5:30 p.m. EST.

Signing into SynapseEHR 1.1

The default log-on is already populated (Student1, Student1), and the first-time user will only need to click "enter." Once in the program, the user may change the user name and/or password.

IMPORTANT! READ CAREFULLY: This End User License Agreement ("Agreement") sets forth the conditions by which Cengage Learning will make electronic access to the Cengage Learning-owned licensed content and associated media, software, documentation, printed materials, and electronic documentation contained in this package and/or made available to you via this product (the "Licensed Content"), available to you (the "End User"). BY CLICKING THE "I ACCEPT" BUTTON AND/OR OPENING THIS PACKAGE, YOU ACKNOWLEDGE THAT YOU HAVE READ ALL OF THE TERMS AND CONDITIONS, AND THAT YOU AGREE TO BE BOUND BY ITS TERMS, CONDITIONS, AND ALL APPLICABLE LAWS AND REGULATIONS GOVERNING THE USE OF THE LICENSED CONTENT.

1.0 SCOPE OF LICENSE

1.1 Licensed Content. The Licensed Content may contain portions of modifiable content ("Modifiable Content") and content which may not be modified or otherwise altered by the End User ("Non-Modifiable Content"). For purposes of this Agreement, Modifiable Content and Non-Modifiable Content may be collectively referred to herein as the "Licensed Content." All Licensed Content shall be considered Non-Modifiable Content, unless such Licensed Content is presented to the End User in a modifiable format and it is clearly indicated that modification of the Licensed Content is permitted.

1.2 Subject to the End User's compliance with the terms and conditions of this Agreement, Cengage Learning hereby grants the End User, a nontransferable, nonexclusive, limited right to access and view a single copy of the Licensed Content on a single personal computer system for noncommercial, internal, personal use only. The End User shall not (i) reproduce, copy, modify (except in the case of Modifiable Content), distribute, display, transfer, sublicense, prepare derivative work(s) based on, sell, exchange, barter or transfer, rent, lease, loan, resell, or in any other manner exploit the Licensed Content; (ii) remove, obscure, or alter any notice of Cengage Learning's intellectual property rights present on or in the Licensed Content, including, but not limited to, copyright, trademark, and/or patent notices; or (iii) disassemble, decompile, translate, reverse engineer, or otherwise reduce the Licensed Content.

2.0 TERMINATION

2.1 Cengage Learning may at any time (without prejudice to its other rights or remedies) immediately terminate this Agreement and/or suspend access to some or all of the Licensed Content, in the event that the End User does not comply with any of the terms and conditions of this Agreement. In the event of such termination by Cengage Learning, the End User shall immediately return any and all copies of the Licensed Content to Cengage Learning.

3.0 PROPRIETARY RIGHTS

3.1 The End User acknowledges that Cengage Learning owns all rights, title and interest, including, but not limited to all copyright rights therein, in and to the Licensed Content, and that the End User shall not take any action inconsistent with such ownership. The Licensed Content is protected by U.S., Canadian and other applicable copyright laws and by international treaties, including the Berne Convention and the Universal Copyright Convention. Nothing contained in this Agreement shall be construed as granting the End User any ownership rights in or to the Licensed Content.

3.2 Cengage Learning reserves the right at any time to withdraw from the Licensed Content any item or part of an item for which it no longer retains the right to publish, or which it has reasonable grounds to believe infringes copyright or is defamatory, unlawful, or otherwise objectionable.

4.0 PROTECTION AND SECURITY

4.1 The End User shall use its best efforts and take all reasonable steps to safeguard its copy of the Licensed Content to ensure that no unauthorized reproduction, publication, disclosure, modification, or distribution of the Licensed Content, in whole or in part, is made. To the extent that the End User becomes aware of any such unauthorized use of the Licensed Content, the End User shall immediately notify Cengage Learning. Notification of such violations may be made by sending an e-mail to infringement@cengage.com.

5.0 MISUSE OF THE LICENSED PRODUCT

5.1 In the event that the End User uses the Licensed Content in violation of this Agreement, Cengage Learning shall have the option of electing liquidated damages, which shall include all profits generated by the End User's use of the Licensed Content plus interest computed at the maximum rate permitted by law and all legal fees and other expenses incurred by Cengage Learning in enforcing its rights, plus penalties.

6.0 FEDERAL GOVERNMENT CLIENTS

6.1 Except as expressly authorized by Cengage Learning, Federal Government clients obtain only the rights specified in this Agreement and no other rights. The Government acknowledges that (i) all software and related documentation incorporated in the Licensed Content is existing commercial computer software within the meaning of FAR 27.405(b)(2); and (2) all other data delivered in whatever form, is limited rights data within the meaning of FAR 27.401. The restrictions in this section are acceptable as consistent with the Government's need for software and other data under this Agreement.

7.0 DISCLAIMER OF WARRANTIES AND LIABILITIES

7.1 Although Cengage Learning believes the Licensed Content to be reliable, Cengage Learning does not guarantee or warrant (i) any information or materials contained in or produced by the Licensed Content, (ii) the accuracy, completeness or reliability of the Licensed Content, or (iii) that the Licensed Content is free from errors or other material defects. THE LICENSED PRODUCT IS PROVIDED "AS IS," WITHOUT ANY WARRANTY OF ANY KIND AND CENGAGE LEARNING DISCLAIMS ANY AND ALL WARRANTIES, EXPRESSED OR IMPLIED, INCLUDING, WITHOUT LIMITATION, WARRANTIES OF MERCHANTABILITY OR FITNESS FOR A PARTICULAR PURPOSE. IN NO EVENT SHALL CENGAGE LEARNING BE LIABLE FOR: INDIRECT, SPECIAL, PUNITIVE OR CONSEQUENTIAL DAMAGES INCLUDING FOR LOST PROFITS, LOST DATA, OR OTHERWISE. IN NO EVENT SHALL CENGAGE LEARNING'S AGGREGATE LIABILITY HEREUNDER, WHETHER ARISING IN CONTRACT, TORT, STRICT LIABILITY OR OTHERWISE, EXCEED THE AMOUNT OF FEES PAID BY THE END USER HEREUNDER FOR THE LICENSE OF THE LICENSED CONTENT.

8.0 GENERAL

8.1 Entire Agreement. This Agreement shall constitute the entire Agreement between the Parties and supercedes all prior Agreements and understandings oral or written relating to the subject matter hereof.

8.2 Enhancements/Modifications of Licensed Content. From time to time, and in Cengage Learning's sole discretion, Cengage Learning may advise the End User of updates, upgrades, enhancements and/or improvements to the Licensed Content, and may permit the End User to access and use, subject to the terms and conditions of this Agreement, such modifications, upon payment of prices as may be established by Cengage Learning.

8.3 No Export. The End User shall use the Licensed Content solely in the United States and shall not transfer or export, directly or indirectly, the Licensed Content outside the United States.

8.4 Severability. If any provision of this Agreement is invalid, illegal, or unenforceable under any applicable statute or rule of law, the provision shall be deemed omitted to the extent that it is invalid, illegal, or unenforceable. In such a case, the remainder of the Agreement shall be construed in a manner as to give greatest effect to the original intention of the parties hereto.

8.5 Waiver. The waiver of any right or failure of either party to exercise in any respect any right provided in this Agreement in any instance shall not be deemed to be a waiver of such right in the future or a waiver of any other right under this Agreement.

8.6 Choice of Law/Venue. This Agreement shall be interpreted, construed, and governed by and in accordance with the laws of the State of New York, applicable to contracts executed and to be wholly performed therein, without regard to its principles governing conflicts of law. Each party agrees that any proceeding arising out of or relating to this Agreement or the breach or threatened breach of this Agreement may be commenced and prosecuted in a court in the State and County of New York. Each party consents and submits to the nonexclusive personal jurisdiction of any court in the State and County of New York in respect of any such proceeding.

8.7 Acknowledgment. By opening this package and/or by accessing the Licensed Content on this Web site, THE END USER ACKNOWLEDGES THAT IT HAS READ THIS AGREEMENT, UNDERSTANDS IT, AND AGREES TO BE BOUND BY ITS TERMS AND CONDITIONS. IF YOU DO NOT ACCEPT THESE TERMS AND CONDITIONS, YOU MUST NOT ACCESS THE LICENSED CONTENT AND RETURN THE LICENSED PRODUCT TO CENGAGE LEARNING (WITHIN 30 CALENDAR DAYS OF THE END USER'S PURCHASE) WITH PROOF OF PAYMENT ACCEPTABLE TO CENGAGE LEARNING, FOR A CREDIT OR A REFUND. Should the End User have any questions/comments regarding this Agreement, please contact Cengage Learning at delmar.help@cengage.com.